DISABILITY IN INDUSTRIAL BRITAIN

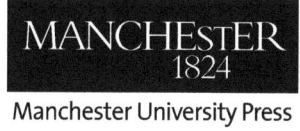

Manchester University Press

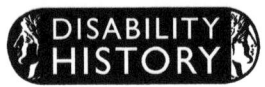

Series editors
Dr Julie Anderson, Professor Walton O. Schalick, III

This series published by Manchester University Press responds to the growing interest in disability as a discipline worthy of historical research. The series has a broad international historical remit, encompassing issues that include class, race, gender, age, war, medical treatment, professionalisation, environments, work, institutions and cultural and social aspects of disablement including representations of disabled people in literature, film, art and the media.

Already published
Deafness, community and culture in Britain: leisure and cohesion, 1945–1995
Martin Atherton
Rethinking modern prostheses in Anglo-American commodity cultures, 1820–1939
Claire L. Jones (ed.)
Destigmatising mental illness? Professional politics and public education in Britain, 1870–1970
Vicky Long
Intellectual disability: a conceptual history, 1200–1900
Patrick McDonagh, C. F. Goodey and Tim Stainton (eds)
Fools and idiots? Intellectual disability in the Middle Ages
Irina Metzler
Framing the moron: the social construction of feeble-mindedness in the American eugenics era
Gerald V. O'Brien
Recycling the disabled: army, medicine, and modernity in WWI Germany
Heather R. Perry
Disability in the Industrial Revolution: physical impairment in British coalmining, 1780–1880
David M. Turner and Daniel Blackie
Worth saving: disabled children during the Second World War
Sue Wheatcroft

DISABILITY IN INDUSTRIAL BRITAIN

A CULTURAL AND LITERARY HISTORY OF IMPAIRMENT IN THE COAL INDUSTRY, 1880–1948

Kirsti Bohata, Alexandra Jones, Mike Mantin and Steven Thompson

Manchester University Press

Copyright © Kirsti Bohata, Alexandra Jones, Mike Mantin and Steven Thompson 2020

The rights of Kirsti Bohata, Alexandra Jones, Mike Mantin and Steven Thompson to be identified as the authors of this work have been asserted by them in accordance with the Copyright, Designs and Patents Act 1988.

An electronic version of this book is also available under a Creative Commons (CC-BY-NC-ND) licence, thanks to the support of the Wellcome Trust, which permits non-commercial use, distribution and reproduction provided the authors and Manchester University Press are fully cited and no modifications or adaptations are made. Details of the licence can be viewed at https://creativecommons.org/licenses/by-nc-nd/4.0/.

Published by Manchester University Press
Altrincham Street, Manchester M1 7JA
www.manchesteruniversitypress.co.uk

British Library Cataloguing-in-Publication Data
A catalogue record for this book is available from the British Library

ISBN   978 1 5261 2431 9   hardback

ISBN   978 1 5261 2432 6   open access

First published 2020

The publisher has no responsibility for the persistence or accuracy of URLs for any external or third-party internet websites referred to in this book, and does not guarantee that any content on such websites is, or will remain, accurate or appropriate.

Typeset
by Toppan Best-set Premedia Limited

Contents

List of figures	page vi
Series editors' foreword	vii
Acknowledgements	viii
List of abbreviations	ix
Introduction	1
1 Work, economy and disability in the British coalfields	18
2 Medicalising miners? Medicine, care and rehabilitation	64
3 Systems of financial support for impaired miners and their families	105
4 The social relations of disability	140
5 The politics and politicisation of disability	178
6 Sites of struggle: disability in working-class coalfields literature	211
Conclusion	249
Select bibliography	256
Index	269

Figures

1	A miner is tested for nystagmus using 'the head test'. From the First Report of the Miners' Nystagmus Committee, 1922. National Archives.	page 84
2	Miners partaking in exercises and handicraft at a rehabilitation centre, 1940s. National Archives.	91
3	Miners practise archery at Uddingston Rehabilitation Centre, near Glasgow. Courtesy of the National Mining Museum Scotland Trust.	92
4	Disabled miner George Preece, c.1909. National Museum of Wales.	151
5	Crochet panel depicting a naval gunship made by George Preece during his re-habilitation after a mining accident at Abercynon Colliery in 1909. National Museum of Wales.	152
6	Pneumoconiosis banner in NUM march, 1952.	230
7	'The Toll of Industry': a plate from *The Labour Leader*, 1911. British Library.	231

Series editors' foreword

You know a subject has achieved maturity when a book series is dedicated to it. In the case of disability, while it has co-existed with human beings for centuries the study of disability's history is still quite young.

In setting up this series, we chose to encourage multi-methodologic history rather than a purely traditional historical approach, as researchers in disability history come from a wide variety of disciplinary backgrounds. Equally 'disability' history is a diverse topic which benefits from a variety of approaches in order to appreciate its multi-dimensional characteristics.

A test for the team of authors and editors who bring you this series is typical of most series, but disability also brings other consequential challenges. At this time disability is highly contested as a social category in both developing and developed contexts. Inclusion, philosophy, money, education, visibility, sexuality, identity and exclusion are but a handful of the social categories in play. With this degree of politicisation, language is necessarily a cardinal focus.

In an effort to support the plurality of historical voices, the editors have elected to give fair rein to language. Language is historically contingent, and can appear offensive to our contemporary sensitivities. The authors and editors believe that the use of terminology that accurately reflects the historical period of any book in the series will assist readers in their understanding of the history of disability in time and place.

Finally, disability offers the cultural, social and intellectual historian a new 'take' on the world we know. We see disability history as one of a few nascent fields with the potential to reposition our understanding of the flow of cultures, society, institutions, ideas and lived experience. Conceptualisations of 'society' since the early modern period have heavily stressed principles of autonomy, rationality and the subjectivity of the individual agent. Consequently we are frequently oblivious to the historical contingency of the present with respect to those elements. Disability disturbs those foundational features of 'the modern.' Studying disability history helps us resituate our policies, our beliefs and our experiences.

Julie Anderson
Walton O. Schalick, III

Acknowledgements

This book has been written as part of the Wellcome Trust Programme Award in Medical History, 'Disability and Industrial Society: A Comparative Cultural History of British Coalfields, 1780–1948' [grant number 095948/Z/11/Z]. It draws on the work of the research team: Professor Anne Borsay, Professor David Turner, Professor Kirsti Bohata, Dr Mike Mantin and Dr Alexandra Jones (Swansea University); Dr Daniel Blackie (University of Oulu); Dr Steven Thompson (Aberystwyth University); Dr Ben Curtis (University of Wolverhampton); Dr Vicky Long (Newcastle University) and Dr Victoria Brown (Glasgow Caledonian University); and Professor Arthur McIvor and Dr Angela Turner (Strathclyde University).

We are grateful to the Wellcome Trust for the generous support that made the research project and this publication possible, and to the various members of the research team and the Advisory Board who helped make involvement in it so enjoyable and intellectually stimulating. We are grateful too to our respective institutions, Swansea and Aberystwyth universities, for the support and assistance that we have received over a number of years. Many archivists and librarians have been so very helpful and knowledgeable when gathering resources for this book and we acknowledge our considerable debt to them. We have also benefited from comments and suggestions of the many scholars who attended the academic papers and public lectures we gave at various workshops and conferences over recent years. Lastly, we have been particularly fortunate to benefit from the comments, suggestions and criticisms of Alun Burge, Hywel Francis, Angela V. John, Huw Walters and Daniel G. Williams.

We are grateful to the following for permission to reproduce images: Richard Burton Archives, Swansea University (cover image), the National Archives (figures 1 & 2), National Museum of Wales (figures 3 & 4), British Library (figure 7). Figure 3 is reproduced courtesy of the National Mining Museum Scotland. We have been unsuccessful in identifying the copyright holder of figure 6; the image is held by National Museum of Wales.

The research project from which this book derives was planned and initially led by Professor Anne Borsay. Our debts to Anne, both intellectual and personal, are incalculable and it is difficult to conceive of this project having been started without her wisdom, guidance and expertise. Anne was intended as the lead author for this volume but, tragically, passed away before work could be started. We dedicate this book to Anne's memory and hope that she would be pleased with the way in which we have attempted to realise her ambitions for the project.

Abbreviations

DCRO	Durham County Record Office
GA	Glamorgan Archives
ILP	International Labour Party
MFGB	Miners' Federation of Great Britain
ML	Mitchell Library, Glasgow City Archives
MP	Member of Parliament
NA	Northumberland Archives
NAS	National Archives of Scotland
NCB	National Coal Board
NEEMARC	North East Mining Archive and Research Centre
NHS	National Health Service
NLS	National Library of Scotland
NUM	National Union of Mineworkers
SOHC	Scottish Oral History Centre
SWCC	South Wales Coalfield Collection
SWML	South Wales Miners' Library
TNA	The National Archives, Kew
TUC	Trades Union Congress
TWAS	Tyne and Wear Archives Service
WGAS	West Glamorgan Archives Service

Introduction

On 5 September 1908, Frank Eaves, a collier from Tonypandy in the Rhondda Fawr valley, south Wales, stood before Judge Bryn Roberts at Pontypridd County Court. Eaves had met with an accident while working underground in Blaenclydach Colliery in 1906, when a stone of half a hundredweight had fallen on his foot. He had not worked since that time and had been in receipt of compensation from the insurance company that covered the liabilities of the Blaenclydach Colliery Company. The company had exerted pressure on Eaves to accept a lump-sum payment for some time and had now brought a case before Judge Bryn Roberts to terminate the compensation payments on the grounds that he was sufficiently recovered to resume work. The insurance company drew upon the expert medical testimony of four doctors who all testified that Eaves now suffered 'neurasthenia', an ill-defined condition of the nerves, and one often associated with malingering, rather than the effects of the accident in 1906. For their part, the South Wales Miners' Federation, who supported Eaves in his case, instructed medical opinion and three doctors testified that Eaves was suffering from a 'functional disorder', loss of sensation in his leg, and that he was unable to use his foot and to continue work underground.

In the event, the judge found in favour of the insurance company and ordered the termination of the compensation payments. He stated that he believed that Eaves' present condition was due to his 'long abstention from physical labour'. He did not accuse him of malingering, he said, but he did think that Eaves would be much better if he had gone back to work. Expressing his concern at the larger number of neurasthenic cases coming before the courts, Judge Bryn Roberts stated that 'he was convinced that the man would have recovered if he had only made a determined effort … he thought it was absolutely in the man's own interests to go back to work, otherwise he would become an incurable invalid'.[1]

Miners' leaders in the Rhondda valley reacted with fury to the decision. Dai Watts Morgan, the Agent for the Rhondda No. 1 District of the Miners' Federation, opined at a meeting of lodge delegates of the District that Eaves was a man of 'unblemished character', who had led 'as clean a life as anyone of them' present, but the moment he met with an accident, 'he became a vagabond and a dishonest person'.[2] Watts Morgan's reaction in this case was also coloured by the numerous compensation cases that had been decided against miners by Judge Bryn Roberts in these years. Again and again, it was noted, Roberts had found against injured miners and had dismissed cases or else terminated payments at the request of coal companies and their insurance companies.³ The feeling was such that delegates at that Rhondda No. 1 District meeting discussed the possibility of strike action to protest Roberts' judgement. Another trade union leader, the fiery Charles Butt Stanton, was even more critical of Judge Bryn Roberts and referred to him scathingly as 'boss union smasher' who tried to ruin the miners' union by bleeding the Federation's resources through his numerous decisions against its members in compensation cases.⁴

The legal case would have had profound consequences for Eaves. His ability to access compensation payments was crucially important to his standard of living and to the well-being of his family, while the experience of standing in court to hear a judge tell him that he needed to try harder to overcome his impairment – thus constructing his disability as a personal challenge to be overcome if only he were sufficiently determined – would have been damaging to his self-esteem and his sense of himself as a respectable workman. Some comfort might have been derived from the sympathy, moral support and practical help provided by his trade union comrades, but the benefits of this would have extended only so far. On another level, however, Eaves' case is rather mundane. These kinds of accidents and injuries were daily occurrences in the British coal industry, while the contestation of compensation cases in the courts was similarly an everyday reality in mining communities. The everyday and mundane nature of the case, however, is precisely the point, and it illustrates many of the major themes of this study of disability in industrial Britain.

In the first place, Eaves' case highlights the centrality of the compensation system to the understandings and experiences of disability in coalfield society in the twentieth century. It shows the ways in which medical diagnosis defined a person's status and determined their access to resources. The case also hints at the possibility of, indeed the requirement for, continued employment in order to make ends meet, regardless of bodily ability to carry out any such work. But the case also demonstrates that medical definitions of impairment were contested and politicised in a struggle between capital and labour. The case offers an excellent example of the centrality of impairment and disability to industrial relations in the coal industry, and the extent to which such issues both mobilised activism and could be used in a rhetorical fashion to mobilise workers in class struggle. The words of Judge Bryn Roberts are also a striking articulation of the widespread narrative which saw disability as a personal tragedy in which 'accommodation to the impairment is squarely [the disabled person's] own responsibility or that of their families' while demanding a 'strenuous effort toward improvement'.⁵ The individual is enjoined to overcome (or adjust to) their disability by, in the words of Judge Bryn Roberts, 'determined effort'.

Significantly, Eaves passes out of history after this brief moment of attention and his case communicates a fundamental truth about the experiences of disabled people in the past. Eaves' case was reported in the local and regional newspapers and was minuted in the trade union district meetings, and these sources allow us to put together the basic outline of his circumstances, but Eaves' voice is never heard at any point and we have little idea of any aspect of his life not connected to his injury and his claim for compensation. As with so many disabled people in the past, we are unable to get a real sense of his feelings or emotions, his sense of self and his experience of disability in an ableist society. In his disappearance from historical view, Eaves suffered the fate of so many disabled people in the past. This book cannot restore the voices of disabled people in industrial society, but it does trace the material circumstances, political interventions and social and cultural contexts of disabled people's lives in order to understand both the lived experience and the rhetoric of disability. It explores the ways in which disabled people and a politicised discourse of disability influenced the nature of coalfields society along material, political and cultural axes. Indeed, disability can be seen at the pivotal centre, as a site of struggle, in industrial society.[6] In this interdisciplinary study, we trace the way in which disability was central to campaigns for reform to employment law, welfare, medicine, political agitation and the imaginative literature which sought to reflect, in a highly mediated way, the daily and structural conditions of coalfield society.

The coal industry provides an excellent case study for any such attempt to locate disability in industrial society, since the extent of impairment was considerable. Frank Eaves would have been very aware that he was not the only miner to experience impairment or to suffer injustice. He could pick up his local newspaper on any day of the week and see numerous reports of men similar to himself injured in accidents in any one of the numerous collieries in the Rhondda valley. When he attended the doctor's surgery for medical assessment, he would have joined a long queue of men with injuries and ailments that required treatment or certification. If he attended any of the regular meetings of his colliery trade union lodge, he would have heard accounts of numerous cases very similar to his own in which liability was denied by the coal company and the trade union was forced to decide how to assist their stricken member. In the cultural sphere, he would hear of disabling accidents in ballads and, though it would be a few more years before his fellow colliers began to fictionalise his experience, soon he would be able to see his experiences reflected in a burgeoning working-class literature. If it has become a truism that disability is ubiquitous, that, in the words of Douglas C. Baynton, 'Disability is everywhere in history, once you begin looking for it, but conspicuously absent in the histories we write', then it is in coalmining communities that this assertion is most apposite.[7]

Whether it is in the dry and statistical approach to accidents and disasters in parliamentary papers, the sensationalist and melodramatic portrayals of popular journalism, the rhetorical and self-righteous indignation of trade union campaign materials, the potent disability metaphors and stories in coalfields literature, or the heroic self-portrayals of miners in oral history reminiscences and working-class autobiographies, the dangers to life and limb in the coal industry loom large. Phrases such as 'blood on the coal' and 'the toll of the mine', or 'traul y pwll' in Welsh, have become well-worn tropes intended to convey danger and to elicit sympathy or even anger. Whatever the rhetorical or melodramatic aspects of such portrayals, they do nevertheless communicate an essential truth, for the coal industry was undeniably dangerous. Work underground was an inherently dangerous business and there were innumerable ways in which miners suffered accidents, experienced injuries and became impaired. Impacts from heavy machinery or tools, the fall of the roof or sides of underground passages, collisions with fast-moving and heavy trams of coal, the misfiring of explosive 'shots', flooding, explosions, fires, electrocution and a great many other perils all posed a threat to a miner's well-being. In the period between 1868 and 1919, for example, 'a miner was killed every six hours, seriously injured every two hours and injured badly ... every two or three minutes'.[8] Relative to other industries, this was a significant toll of injury: in the few years just before the First World War, 16.5 per cent of coalminers were injured every year compared with 8.3 per cent of metal smelters, 5.3 per cent of railway workers, and 2 per cent of workers in the cotton industry.[9] Added to these threats, occupational diseases were a major cause of chronic illness and impairment. Miners' nystagmus, a condition that involved the oscillation of the eyeball, dizziness and other symptoms, caused many miners to give up their employment in the industry or else shift to surface work, while pneumoconiosis ('miners' lung' or 'black lung') incapacitated increasingly large numbers of miners by the mid-twentieth century.[10] As if these risks to miners' bodily well-being were not enough, miners also suffered impairment as a result of rheumatism and arthritis, a range of inflammation ailments, such as 'beat knee', 'beat hand' and 'beat elbow', and hernias and other strain injuries.[11] The high accident and occupational disease rates in the coal industry, and the large absolute numbers of individuals affected, are compelling reasons to choose coal as a case study in the analysis of disability and industrial society.

Of all the industries found in modern Britain, it is perhaps coal that has attracted most attention from labour historians, and a well-established historiography, both of the industry as a whole and of specific coalfields, has developed.[12]

Much of this work has its roots in the flowering of labour history from the 1960s and 1970s onwards and tends to be institutional in approach, focused on trade unions and the broader labour movements of which they were a part, and grounded in a class-struggle narrative that prioritises conflictual industrial relations and industrial disputes.[13] More recent historical work has broadened the field of vision somewhat and had added new perspectives on community, culture, women, gender, the body and sexuality, but attention to older themes such as solidarity, militancy and union organisation continues to be important.[14] Studies of the literary and cultural histories of coal follow a similar pattern, with an emphasis on class[15] broadening to include studies influenced by scholars working on gender and sexuality, race and ethnicity, dialect and nation, affect and humour.[16]

Despite the growth in disability studies, disability has been conspicuously absent from studies of industrial history and literature. Aside from David M. Turner and Daniel Blackie's book, *Disability in the Industrial Revolution*,[17] which emerged from the same research project as the present volume, disability is notable by its absence from the historiography of the coal industry despite the attention to related issues such as safety, accidents and occupational health.[18] Yet disability history, particularly an interdisciplinary approach that embraces cultural representations of disability in literature written from inside the communities themselves, has much to say that is new, innovative and fundamentally important about coalfield societies and about disability in industrial society. Disability, as already noted, was a very common experience in mining communities and, as such, became an important organising principle as trade unions and the broader labour movement fashioned industrial relations campaigns and political strategies to deal with the issues that arose. Similarly, in the working-class literature of the twentieth century, class, industrial politics and disability are represented as intimately related. Histories of coalfield societies have tended to focus on political and industrial radicalism, but, arguably, a more radical historiography can derive from work that looks at the confluence of forces and discourses that converge around disability and which also considers the experiences of disabled people and ideas about impairment, disability and normalcy in this particular context.

Like many works on disability history, our perspective borrows heavily from disability studies and the social model of disability, where a distinction is made between impairment and disability.[19] Impairment is based purely on physical difference, while disability is a social issue: the former does not simply 'cause' the latter, social barriers do, such as restricted access to medical activities, educational institutions and welfare provision. A medical model which sees disability solely as an individual, personal tragedy in need of cure has been categorically rejected. Industrialisation has long had an important role in key works of disability theory, and prominent scholars advanced the theory that the industrial revolution witnessed and, more importantly, brought about the exclusion of disabled people from the workplace and their economic and social isolation, often in institutions. One of the starkest portrayals of this came from Victor Finkelstein, who argued that while disabled people were oppressed in the pre-industrial period, they were nevertheless integrated into work placements.[20] This changed with industrialisation, however, which created a society based on 'large scale industry with production-lines geared to able-bodied norms', and with it the creation of institutions designed to separate those who did not conform to these norms.[21] The work of theorists such as Finkelstein was crucial in questioning narratives of industrialisation as a time of positive economic progress for disabled people. Yet the broad categorisation applied by Finkelstein has been seen as unsatisfactory. Other scholars have since constructed more detailed models of the structural disability caused by industrial modes of production.[22] Anne Borsay argues that the impact of the Industrial Revolution has been overemphasised, and the social exclusion of disabled people in spaces such as education, philanthropy and leisure had developed long before industrialisation.[23] The onset of industrialisation undoubtedly affected disabled people through some measure of exclusion from work, but the record of the British coal industry demonstrates there were still large numbers of disabled people within the industry with a number of different experiences which changed over time, and disabled people sometimes had the opportunity to take their own decisions regarding their welfare, social relations and place in the industrial economy. A case study of the coal industry presents an opportunity to examine in detail the relationship between physical disability, work and industrialisation, challenging existing assumptions about the place of disabled people in the industrial workplace.

This study of coalfield disability is not confined to male workers alone, however, and we have endeavoured to integrate disabled women into the study at all points. Coalfield history has focused predominantly, sometimes exclusively, on men. Historians such as Angela V. John, Griselda Carr, Sue Bruley and Valerie Gordon Hall challenged this male-dominated landscape with pioneering studies on women in the coalfields during the nineteenth and twentieth centuries.[24] Studies of *disabled* women in the coalfield are almost non-existent, given the tacit assumption that coalfield disability was an occupational issue, and women were legally banned from working in the pits from 1842. Yet the category of 'work' in the coalfields needs to be expanded to include the unpaid but no less arduous work generally done by women in the home, as well as the labour of care. Women's labour was equally dangerous and exhausting, and disabling injuries were common among miners' wives. Relatedly, congenital impairment has largely been ignored in coalfield communities and such disabilities, whether experienced by men or by women, would likely have most affected women care givers, at least in the early years. In expanding the category of work and considering disability in relation to work, this study builds on a special issue of *Disability Studies Quarterly* on 'Disability, Work and Representation: New Perspectives'.[25]

If women's experiences have been ignored, so too has the ethnic diversity of the coalfields been overlooked. The coalfields were far from ethnically homogeneous. Immigration from Ireland, Poland and the British empire was widespread as work in the coalfields became readily available, and in particular south Wales saw high levels of immigration from England.[26] As such, in researching disability we have aimed to avoid the assumption of a male, ethnically homogeneous coalfield workforce. This is not without its practical challenges. The lives of disabled women are – if historians wish to find them – visible in autobiographies, literature and oral testimony, as well as hidden in coalfield records. Not only were there many disabled women in the workforce, but women also had a huge role in the political battle over disability compensation and disabled people's rights in the coalfields. Ethnicity, however, has proved much more difficult to explore with our limited source base – that is, records which record both disability and minority ethnicities are scarce – though we have included ethnicity as a concern where possible and do, of course, foreground the sometimes signficiant ethnic (particularly linguistic and religious) differences between Wales, Scotland and England in our comparative study. Furthermore, while there is undoubtedly room for a transnational study which compares different countries' attitudes to disability and looks at the movement of labour and empire from a disability history perspective, our British focus limits us from tackling this subject in depth.

This study of disabled men and disabled women in coalfield communities adopts a comparative approach that utilises three coalfields as case studies. It is organised around a thematic approach to work and the economy, welfare, medicine, social relations and politics in the south Wales, north-east of England and Scottish coalfields. Relative to its companion volume, by Turner and Blackie, this study has an additional chapter on the place of disability in the unique body of industrial writing to emerge from the coalfields during our period, 1880–1948, and we draw on this literature throughout in a deliberately interdisciplinary methodology. Each coalfield had its own distinctive geographical, economic, political, cultural and literary features, and these could vary considerably from pit village to pit village, let alone from region to region. The three coalfields have been chosen for their importance within the British coalmining economy as well as the significant features that set them apart from each other. The smaller, more geographically diffuse Scottish coalfields, for instance, differ greatly from the more concentrated coal measures in the north-east of England and south Wales. Similarly, the Welsh and Scottish coalfields had reputations for industrial militancy and political radicalism that were not matched to the same degree in the north-east of England. In addition, each coalfield experienced a different chronology of development: the north-east of England was a well-established and mature coalfield society by 1880, while south Wales and parts of the Scottish coalfields underwent rapid industrialisation from this point onwards. This comparative approach to coalfields disability history complements the significant body of work that exists in relation to coalfield societies.[27] Other major coalfields, such as Lancashire, Yorkshire, north Wales and Staffordshire, and smaller areas in Bristol, Leicestershire, north Warwickshire, Cumberland and Kent, have their own rich disability histories and warrant study in their own right.

In its approach to cultural history, this book attempts where possible to foreground the perspectives and lived experiences of working-class disabled people in history. The challenge is to find such traces in the archives. As the author Gwyn Thomas once wrote: 'the family records of the proletariat do not stretch back so far, except in shadow form in the account books of the coal owners.'[28] As we have noted above, there are even fewer traces of the voices of disabled people in the archives, though some of the miner-writers we discuss were themselves temporarily or permanently disabled. A number of sources help to get closer to the lived experience of disability. Newspapers offer innumerable insights into the major issues in coalfield societies in addition to the micro-level experiences of individual miners and women; autobiographies of coalminers highlight the everyday occurence of injury and disease and the consequences for daily lives; existing collections of oral testimony offer first-hand perspectives of the emotional aspects of impairment; and contemporary coalfield literature included disabilty both as a trait of characters and as a metaphor for the industry. However, the vast majority of primary sources offer a top-down perspective, concerned with disability but where disabled voices are silent and disabled lives are accessible only in 'shadow form'. For this historically marginalised group, this is an issue that all disability historians are confronted with, but methodologies borrowed from 'history from below', in which sources are read 'against the grain' in order to extract some sort of meaning about the objects of these sources, can help turn such sources to our advantage, while recognising the limitations of reconstructing experience, particularly for oppressed groups with shifting identities.[29] Furthermore, compensation documents, registers of disabled employees, mutual aid records and medical records all help to piece together the institutional framework within which disabled people lived their lives.

Perhaps one of the most innovative dimensions of this book is its deliberately interdisciplinary approach, and this reflects our debt to the foundations of disability studies, which draw on a wide range of disciplines. It not only draws on literature as a rich source for the cultural historian attempting to foreground the perspectives and lived experiences of working-class disabled people in history; it goes further in exploring the cultural representations of disability in coalfields literature using methodologies taken from literary criticism. For the purposes of this book, 'coalfields literature' encompasses a range of genres and forms of literature which have as their primary focus the coalmining industry and people of coalfields communities. For much of the nineteenth century, ballads, autobiography (much of it unpublished),[30] and 'pit poetry' by 'miner-poets' such as Joseph Skipsey[31] were the most important forms.[32] Ballads and poems (often composed using a dialect of English such as 'pitmatic', or another language such as Scots or Welsh) record major accidents and disabilities. By the 1880s, a tradition of coalfields novels began to emerge, largely in the form of romance mainly by middle-class writers, including a number of female authors.[33] While sympathetic to the hardships of the workers, the narrative perspective was usually positioned outside the community depicted and suspicious of substantial challenge of the status quo. Victorian romances of the late nineteenth century were slowly replaced by increasingly ethnographic forms, which – though still at one remove – attempted to describe the everyday quality of life in mining districts.

By 1918 the vast majority of writers were working-class men[34] refining a broadly realist genre (with some notable modernist exceptions) that allowed them to write about work and life – and disability – in coalfields society. Our approach to this literature has been informed by the interdisciplinary work of disability scholars, including Rosemarie Garland Thompson, Lennard Davis and Tobin Siebers. A broadly historicist literary methodology draws on well-established literary critical praxis in which critics draw on a range of imaginative and non-literary texts in the study of cultural and historical manifestations of power, ideology and the linguistic underpinning of these. The significance of literature in understanding contemporary discourses has been acknowledged by some historians. In his ground-breaking volume *Slumming: Sexual and Social Politics in Victorian London*, Seth Koven adopts a mixed methodology which draws on journalism, Victorian photography and archival sources as well as literary fiction. He argues not only that novels provide valuable knowledge where traditional historical sources may be thin, but that an appreciation of literature offers a different kind of insight into cultural attitudes, assumptions and taboos:

> Novels register not just what can be said, but also what cannot be said, and sometimes, what cannot be fully understood by contemporaries. Novels can give us access to cultural attitudes – and fantasies ... [–] which may allow us to reread and put greater pressure on our traditional historical sources.[35]

In disability studies, which has tended to adopt interdisciplinary approaches from the outset, literary scholars such as David Mitchell and Sharon Snyder contend that since texts 'inevitably filter disability through the reigning ideologies of their day', a study of literature is an important element of disability history:

> the analysis of imaginative works allow scholars in the humanities to record a history of people with disabilities that comes closer to recapturing the 'popular' values of everyday lives. If disability is the product of an interaction between individual differences and social environments (architectural, legislative, familial, attitudinal, etc.), then the contrast between discourses of disability situates art and literature as necessary to reconstructing the dynamics of this historical interaction.[36]

Literature can provide a source for understanding the lives of disabled people in the past, but also more broadly a way of exploring attitudes to embodiment and structures of social relationships.

While this study confirms that literature is a crucial source for the cultural historian and a means whereby the historicist literary critic can engage with contemporary ideological values, our approach to literature is also attentive to disability theorists such as David T. Mitchell, Sharon L. Snyder and Ato Quayson, who foreground literary aesthetics – that is, the particular formal and creative ways in which literature constructs and conveys meaning. In order to understand how coalfields literature 'adds another tier of interpretation [of disability] that is comprehensible within the terms set by the literary aesthetic domain',[37] we need to understand the genesis, forms and exemplary tropes of this body of writing. Literary scholars would remind us that we cannot simply assume that there is a 'direct and mimetic relationship between literature and social attitudes towards disability'.[38] Rather, literature is a rich and complex art form which both informs and is influenced by social understandings and embodied experiences of disability. Thus, the final chapter of this book focuses on the literary history and a literary critique of disability in coalfields writing.

Language is central to the way we think about ourselves and others. In this volume, in referring to people with impairments we have used the term 'disabled people' rather than 'people with disabilities'. As Gleeson points out, the notion that 'people with disabilities' is a humanising improvement on the term 'disabled people' (the same may be said for the singular form) is problematic. He follows Abberley in declaring 'this to be a retrograde terminological change which effectively depoliticises the social discrimination that disabled people are subjected to'.[39] As Ato Quayson, a literary and cultural theorist, notes, 'In practice, it is almost impossible to keep the two [terms] separate, since "impairment" is "automatically" placed within a social discourse that interprets it and "disability" is produced by the interaction of impairment and a spectrum of social discourses on normality that serve to stipulate what counts as disability in the first place.'[40] Thus 'disability' itself is a shifting and historically contingent term; very few coalminers with impairments, injuries or diseases whom we would today label 'disabled' would have identified as 'disabled'. In the coalfields, disability is a concept closely bound to work, and many miners with impairments continued to work.

It is also worth noting the position of the authors of the present volume themselves, some of whom are non-disabled or non-physically disabled. Our role as historians and critics requires an awareness of positionality and our relationship to the historical subjects and discourses. In her essay 'Getting Personal', Kim V. L. England implores researchers of minority groups to consider their place in the social landscape, applying 'reflexivity' as 'self-critical sympathetic introspection and the self-conscious analytical scrutiny of the self as researcher'.[41] Although England is here talking mostly about field work (in particular, her project about a lesbian community), her points about the study of experience are crucial for disability historians and already embedded within literary and cultural studies:

> In our rush to be more inclusive and conceptualize difference and diversity, might we be guilty of appropriating the voices of 'others'? How do we deal with this when planning and conducting our research? And can we incorporate the voices of 'others' without colonizing them in a manner that reinforces patterns of domination?[42]

The position of the historian and critic, particularly a non-disabled scholar, with the research subject of impaired and disabled people is essential to consider and theorise, avoiding applying perspectives and opinions that may not have existed.

The scope and potential of disability history in the British coalfields is enormous, and this book is structured thematically to cover as much ground as possible. The chapters cover work and economy, medicine, welfare, social relations, politics and literature. This thematic structure facilitates the exploration of issues relating to disability in the coalfields, but it also creates limitations. Firstly, there is no linear chronological structure, though much of each chapter is structured around change over time and key events for disabled people such as the 1880 and 1897 Compensation Acts, and more general milestones such as the 1926 miners' lockout and the nationalisation of the industry after the Second World War. Secondly, there is inevitable overlap between these themes: disabled miners likely did not use these categories at all to describe their lives, and the boundaries that we draw here would have been crossed constantly. Welfare and socialising, for instance, could happen at the same time at the meeting of a friendly society in a public house. We flag these overlaps and connections between chapters where possible and certainly the flexibility of these categories allows us room to discuss the complexity of disability in the coalfields.

Chapter 1 outlines the world of work in the colliery districts. We consider the factors that led to impairment in mining districts and outline the character and variety of those impairments. The assessment of the working conditions of women in the home and the impairments they experienced in these highly segregated communities is an integral part of the discussion, reinserting the domestic sphere into industrial and disability history. The chapter also considers the ways disabled workers could find employment in the coal industry and how their opportunities for doing so changed over time. The second chapter outlines the medical and rehabilitation services accessed by impaired miners and the extent to which the miner's body was medicalised during the half century or so up to the founding of the National Health Service. Attention here comes to focus increasingly on the 1940s as orthopaedic medicine, the government and the trade unions came to prioritise the size, fitness and productivity of the mining workforce. We find that medicalisation was complex and varied, with impetus coming from miners and disabled people just as much, perhaps, as from the medical profession. Chapter 3 assesses the various sources of welfare available to miners and their families in their attempts to ameliorate the financial and economic consequences of impairment. The entry of statutory systems of relief into the mixed economy of social welfare care for disabled people and their families is a major theme here, as is the inadequacy of that statutory provision.

Chapter 4 adopts a spatial approach to the social relations of disability and considers the 'private', 'public', interstitial and liminal spaces of disability. Significant differences between men and women are outlined in this chapter and we assess the extent to which social isolation could be experienced in mining communities. The subsequent chapter assesses the considerable political activity undertaken in relation to disability. It claims that disability was central to the industrial relations strategies and political campaigns of miners' trade unions and the broader labour movement of which they were a part. The final chapter is an analysis of the cultural representations of disability in coalfields writing and the ways in which disability imagery is put to rhetorical use in working-class coalfields literature. While it picks up some of the literary threads running through the preceding chapters, it marks a change in approach – deliberately adopting a literary critical methodology which foregrounds form and aesthetic alongside historicist readings. We find that disability is pivotal in representations of economic, political, social and working lives depicted in coalfields literature.

Notes

1 *Evening Express*, 7 September 1908, p. 2.
2 South Wales Coalfield Collection, Swansea University, SWCC/MNA/NUM/3/8/10a, South Wales Miners' Federation, Rhondda No. 1 District, Monthly reports, 7 September 1908.
3 For further cases in which Roberts found against injured miners, see J. Eaton, '"Union Smasher of the Boss Class"? The Judgeship of John Bryn Roberts in Glamorgan, 1906–18', *Welsh History Review*, 13:1 (1986), pp. 58–61; for further details on Eaves' case, see Ben Curtis, 'Adding Insult to Injury: The Case of Frank Eaves, a Disabled Miner', *Llafur*, 11:2 (2013), pp. 148–53.
4 Eaton, '"Union Smasher of the Boss Class"?', p. 62.
5 Ato Quayson, *Disability Aesthetics: Disability and the Crisis of Representation* (New York: Columbia University Press, 2007), p. 2.
6 David T. Mitchell and Sharon L. Snyder refer to disability as an ideological and rhetorical, as well as a material, site of struggle in *Narrative Prosthesis: Disability and the Dependencies of Discourse* (Ann Arbor: University of Michigan Press, 2000), p. 24.
7 Douglas C. Baynton, 'Disability and the Justification of Inequality in American History', in Paul K. Longmore and Lauri Umansky (eds), *The New Disability History: American Perspectives* (New York: New York University Press, 2001), p. 52.
8 John Benson, *British Coalminers in the Nineteenth Century: A Social History* (Dublin: Gill and Macmillan, 1980), p. 43.
9 Arthur McIvor, *A History of Work in Britain, 1880–1950* (Basingstoke: Macmillan, 2001), p. 120.
10 On miners' chest diseases, see Arthur McIvor and Ronald Johnston, *Miners' Lung: A History of Dust Disease in British Coal Mining* (Aldershot: Ashgate, 2007).
11 McIvor and Johnston, *Miners' Lung*, p. 51; more generally, see Edgar L. Collis, *The Coal Miner: His Health, Diseases and General Welfare* (Glasgow: Industrial Health Education Society, 1920).
12 For examples of particularly notable works, see Roy A. Church, *The History of the British Coal Industry Volume 3: 1830–1913: Victorian Pre-Eminence* (Oxford: Clarendon

Press, 1986); Barry Supple, *The History of the British Coal Industry, Volume 4. 1913–1946: The Political Economy of Decline* (Oxford: Clarendon, 1987). For regional works, see Alan Campbell, *The Scottish Miners, 1874–1939* (Aldershot: Ashgate Publishing Limited, 2000); Hywel Francis and David Smith, *The Fed: A History of the South Wales Miners in the Twentieth Century* (London: Lawrence and Wishart, 1980); W. R. Garside, *The Durham Miners, 1919–1960* (London: Allen & Unwin, 1971). See also the introductory and other essays in John Benson (ed.), *Coal in Victorian Britain* (London: Pickering & Chatto, 2012), six volumes.

13 For an excellent overview of the historiography of trades unionism in the coal industry, see Keith Gildart, 'Introduction', in Keith Gildart (ed.), *Coal in Victorian Britain, Part II: Coal in Victorian Society, Volume 6, Industrial Relations and Trade Unionism* (London: Pickering & Chatto, 2012), pp. xi–xli.

14 On recent developments, see Gildart, 'Introduction'; also, Sue Bruley, *The Women and Men of 1926: A Gender and Social History of the General Strike and Miners' Lockout in South Wales* (Cardiff: University of Wales Press, 2010). See also Sue Bruley, 'The General Strike and Miners' Lockout of 1926 in South Wales: Oral Testimony and Public Representations', *Welsh History Review*, 26:2 (2012), pp. 271–96; Jaclyn J. Gier-Viskovatoff and Abigail Porter, 'Women of the British Coalfields on Strike in 1926 and 1984: Documenting Lives Using Oral History and Photography', *Frontiers: A Journal of Women Studies*, 19 (1998), pp. 199–230; Angela V. John, *By the Sweat of Their Brow: Women Workers at Victorian Coal Mines* (London: Croom Helm, 1980); Angela V. John, 'Scratching the Surface. Women, Work and Coalmining History in England and Wales', *Oral History*, 10 (1982), pp. 13–26.

15 See, for instance, Martha Vicinus, *The Industrial Muse: A Study of Nineteenth Century British Working-Class Literature* (London: Croom Helm, 1974); H. Gustav Klaus (ed.), *The Socialist Novel in Britain: Towards the Recovery of a Tradition* (Brighton: The Harvester Press, 1982); Dai Smith, 'A Novel History', in Tony Curtis (ed.), *Wales: The Imagined Nation, Essays in Cultural and National Identity* (Bridgend: Poetry Wales Press, 1986), pp. 129–58; H. Gustav Klaus and Stephen Knight (eds), *British Industrial Fictions* (Cardiff: University of Wales Press, 2000); Chris Hopkins, *English Fiction in the 1930s* (London: Continuum, 2006).

16 See for instance Pamela Fox, *Class Fictions: Shame and Resistance in the British Working-Class Novel, 1890–1945* (Durham, NC and London: Duke University Press, 1994); Katie Gramich, 'The Masquerade of Gender in the stories of Rhys Davies', in Meic Stevens (ed.), *Rhys Davies: Decoding the Hare* (Cardiff: University of Wales Press, 2001), pp. 205–15; Stephen Knight *A Hundred Years of Fiction: Writing Wales in English* (Cardiff: University of Wales Press, 2004); Daniel Williams, *Black Skin, Blue Books: African Americans and Wales, 1845–1945* (Cardiff: University of Wales Press, 2012); Nicola Wilson, *Home in British Working-Class Fiction* (Farnham: Ashgate 2015); Lisa Sheppard and Aidan Byrne, 'A Critical Minefield: The Haunting of the Welsh Working Class Novel', in John Goodridge and Bridget Keenan (eds), *A History of British Working Class Literature* (Cambridge: Cambridge University Press, 2017),

pp. 367–84; Laura Wainwright, *New Territories in Modernism: Anglophone Welsh Writing, 1930–1949* (Cardiff: University of Wales Press, 2018).
17 David M. Turner and Daniel Blackie, *Disability in the Industrial Revolution: Physical Impairment in British Coalmining, 1780–1880* (Manchester: Manchester University Press, 2018).
18 For an overview of some recent work, see John Benson, 'Introduction', in John Benson (ed.), *Coal in Victorian Britain, Part II: Coal in Victorian Society, Volume 5, Health and Accidents* (London: Pickering & Chatto, 2012), pp. xvi–xviii. The one exception to this neglect of disability by historians of the coal industry is McIvor and Johnston, *Miners' Lung*.
19 Union of the Physically Impaired Against Segregation, 'Fundamental Principles of Disability' (1965), www.disability-studies.leeds.ac.uk/wp-content/uploads/sites/40/library/UPIAS-fundamental-principles.pdf, accessed 13 September 2018. See, for example, Catherine J. Kudlick, 'Disability History: Why We Need Another "Other"', *The American Historical Review*, 108:3 (2003), pp. 763–93; Paul K. Longmore and Lauri Umansky, 'Disability History: From the Margins to the Mainstream', in Longmore and Umansky, *The New Disability History: American Perspectives* (New York: New York University Press), pp. 1–32; Elizabeth Bredberg, 'Writing Disability History: Problems, Perspectives and Sources', *Disability & Society*, 14:2 (1999), pp. 189–201.
20 Victor Finkelstein, *Attitudes and Disabled People: Issues for Discussion* (New York: International Exchange of Information in Rehabilitation, 1980), p. 6.
21 Finkelstein, *Attitudes and Disabled People*, p. 8.
22 For an early example, see Michael Oliver, *The Politics of Disability: A Sociological Approach* (Basingstoke: Palgrave Macmillan, 1990); more recently, see Sarah F. Rose, *No Right to be Idle: The Invention of Disability, 1840s–1930s* (Chapel Hill: University of North Carolina Press, 2017).
23 Anne Borsay, *Disability and Social Policy in Britain since 1750: A History of Exclusion* (Basingstoke: Palgrave Macmillan, 2005), p. 14.
24 Angela V. John, *By the Sweat of Their Brow: Women Workers at Victorian Coal Mines* (London: Croom Helm, 1979); Griselda Carr, *Pit Women: Coal Communities in Northern England in the Early Twentieth Century* (London: Merlin Press, 2001); Valerie G. Hall, *Women at Work, 1860–1939: How Different Industries Shaped Women's Experiences* (Woodbridge: Boydell Press, 2013); Bruley, *The Women and Men of 1926*.
25 David M. Turner, Kirsti Bohata and Steven Thompson (eds), 'Disability, Work and Representation: New Perspectives', Special Issue of *Disability Studies Quarterly*, 37:4 (2017).
26 Kenneth Lunn, 'Reactions to Lithuanian and Polish Immigrants in the Lanarkshire Coalfield 1880–1914', in Kenneth Lunn (ed.), *Hosts, Immigrants and Minorities: Historical Responses to Newcomers in British Society, 1870–1914* (Folkestone: Dawson, 1980), pp. 308–42; Paul O'Leary, *Immigration and Integration: The Irish in Wales, 1798–1922* (Cardiff: University of Wales Press, 2002); John Foster, Muir Houston

and Chris Madigan, 'Irish Immigrants in Scotland's Shipyards and Coalfields: Employment Relations, Sectarianism and Class Formation', *Historical Research*, 84:226 (2011), pp. 657–92.

27 Stefan Berger, Andy Croll and Norman LaPorte (eds), *Towards a Comparative History of Coalfield Societies* (Ashgate: Aldershot, 2005); John McIlroy, Alan Campbell and Keith Gildart (eds), *Industrial Politics and the 1926 Mining Lockout: The Struggle for Dignity* (Cardiff: University of Wales Press, 2004); Stefan Berger, 'Working-Class Culture and the Labour Movement in the South Wales and Ruhr Coalfields, 1850–2000: A Comparison', *Llafur*, 8:2 (2001), pp. 5–40; David Gilbert, *Class, Community, and Collective Action: Social Change in Two British Coalfields, 1850–1926* (Oxford: Clarendon Press, 1992); Roger Fagge, *Power, Culture and Conflict in the Coalfields: West Virginia and South Wales, 1900–1922* (Manchester: Manchester University Press, 1996); Leighton S. James, *The Politics of Identity and Civil Society in Britain and Germany: Miners in the Ruhr and South Wales 1890–1926* (Manchester: Manchester University Press, 2008).

28 Gwyn Thomas, *Sorrow for Thy Sons* (London: Lawrence & Wishart, 1986), pp. 16–17.

29 See Joan W. Scott, 'The Evidence of Experience', *Critical Inquiry*, 17:4 (1991), p. 795.

30 On miners' autobiographies, see William S. Howard, 'Miners' Autobiographies, 1790–1945: A Study of Life Accounts by English Miners and Their Families' (unpublished doctoral thesis, Sunderland: Sunderland Polytechnic, 1991); Emma Griffin: *A People's History of the Industrial Revolution* (New Haven and London: Yale University Press, 2013); Keith Gildart, 'Mining Memories: Reading Coalfield Autobiographies', *Labor History*, 50:2 (2009) pp. 139–61. See also Nan Hackett, *British Working-Class Autobiographies: An Annotated Bibliography* (New York: AMS Press, 1985).

31 According to Gustav Klaus, Joseph Skipsey was 'the first of a number of miner writers who resist[ed] the label "pit-poet", as they cherish[ed] greater ambitions and move[d] increasingly beyond the range of subjects provided by the mining milieu'. See Gustav H. Klaus, *The Literature of Labour: Two Hundred Years of Working-Class Writing* (Brighton: The Harvester Press, 1985), p. 76.

32 Aside from the well-known example of George Eliot's *Felix Holt, the Radical* (London, 1866), which is only tangentially concerned with mining, pre-1880 examples of fiction set in British coalfields include: Robert Douglas, 'The Miners: A Story of the Old Combination Laws', *The New Monthly Magazine and Humorist*, 3 (1844), pp. 25–52; G. Wharton Simpson, 'Colliers and Coal Mining', *The Working Man's Friend, and Family Instructor*, 6:71 (May, 1851); Anon. [Sarah Jane Mayne], *Jan Rutherford; or, The Miners' Strike* (London: Clarke, Beeton & Company, 1854); John Saunders, *Israel Mort, Overman: A Story of the Mine* (London: H. S. King, 1873); Frances Hodgson Burnett, *That Lass o Lowrie's: A Lancashire Story* (London: Ward, Locke & Co., 1878).

33 See Kirsti Bohata and Alexandra Jones, 'Welsh Women's Industrial Fiction, 1880–1910', *Women's Writing* 24:4 (2017), pp. 499–516.
34 The predominance of men reflects the lack of time, resources and access to education and libraries which was a feature of working-class women's lives. Middle-class women writers were a significant presence up to the First World War.
35 Seth Koven, *Slumming: Sexual and Social Politics in Victorian London* (Princeton: Princeton University Press, 2004), pp. 204–5.
36 Mitchell and Snyder, *Narrative Prosthesis*, p. 43.
37 Ato Quayson, *Aesthetic Nervousness: Disability and the Crisis of Representation* (New York: Columbia University Press, 2007), p. 14.
38 Alice Hall, *Literature and Disability* (London: Routledge, 2016), p. 62.
39 B. J. Gleeson, 'Disability Studies: A Historical Materialist View', *Disability & Society*, 12:2 (1997), p. 182.
40 Quayson, *Aesthetic Nervousness*, p. 3.
41 Kim V. L. England, 'Getting Personal: Reflexivity, Positionality, and Feminist Research', *The Professional Geographer*, 46:1 (1994), p. 82.
42 England, 'Getting Personal', p. 81.

I

WORK, ECONOMY AND DISABILITY IN THE BRITISH COALFIELDS

The period from 1880 to 1948 witnessed considerable economic, industrial and political change, and the coal industry was situated right at heart of the various transformations that took place. At the start of this period, the economy had experienced a number of decades of growth and Britain's worldwide economic and imperial pre-eminence was undoubted. By the end of the period, in contrast, Britain had experienced two periods of total war and a prolonged period of economic depression, and had fallen behind a number of its international competitors. Nothing encapsulated this transformation more than the coal industry, which itself had endured the loss of markets, severe dislocation and profound difficulties. War, international economic turbulence and structural problems in the industry had caused a period of sharp decline in the decades after the First World War and, while nationalisation in 1946 was greeted by miners and their supporters as a new beginning, the coal industry was nevertheless a much smaller industry by that time, as compared to its Edwardian heyday.

The lives and experiences of disabled people were affected in profound ways by these various developments in the coal industry and, indeed, were central to those changes. Numerous pieces of legislation were passed, intended to improve working conditions and safety standards, though with varying degrees of success, while technical innovations such as mechanical coal-cutting and electrification served to introduce new risks into the industry. Injury and disease continued to imperil life and limb, and impairment was the experience of a large number of the inhabitants of mining districts. These impairments had an impact on the ability of workers to earn an income – some miners were permanently excluded from the coalmining economy, their working lives permanently altered – but others continued to work in the industry, albeit in other capacities and with a resultant drop in income. In fact, this is an important theme in this chapter and the study as a whole. Impaired workers have been almost invisible in coalmining historiography, and this chapter argues for an economic history of British coal that recognises the centrality of disability. This theme also addresses a central contention within disability studies over many decades, that industrialisation was the major cause of the exclusion of disabled people from the economy in the modern period.[1]

The coal industry, 1880–1948

The history and nature of the coal industry in the period from 1880 to 1948 is the crucial context in which miners and their wives were impaired, individuals were disabled and understandings of disability were constructed. This context needs to be understood before the experiences of disabled people can be properly contextualised. The years from 1880 to the outbreak of the First World War found the coal industry enjoying what N. K. Buxton has called a 'comfortable superiority' at the head of British industry.[2] Its road to domination was a long-standing process equally informed by national industrial development and established regional economic and geological patterns. Coal production increased from ten million tons of fuel produced in 1800, to thirty million in 1840, 150 million in 1880 and finally 287 million by the eve of World War One.[3] This increase was matched by a corresponding rise in the labour force, and a little over a million men and boys, roughly a tenth of the entire occupied male population, were directly employed in the industry by that peak year of production in 1913.[4] Yet these figures belie the enormous regional variations, as individual coalfields developed at varied rates as a result of the different coals found in each coalfield, the various markets for such coals and the particular activities of local industrialists.

The 'Great Northern Coalfield', in Durham and Northumberland, attained a superior position in the late eighteenth century in terms of production, manpower and cultural and political significance, and retained this primacy up until the Edwardian period. Early development had taken place in the Tyne Valley and along the coast, but new collieries came to be opened in other parts of the two counties as the century progressed.[5] Such was the development that the north-east of England produced almost a quarter of Britain's coal by 1880 and employed a fifth of the industry's labour force, almost 100,000 individuals in total.[6] The north-east of England was finally surpassed, in terms of output and manpower, by south Wales just prior to the First World War. The deeper pits sunk in the central part of the coalfield to exploit the deeper coal reserves situated under the Cynon, Rhondda and Rhymney valleys from the 1870s onwards meant that south Wales had overtaken the north-east of England. By 1913 it was employing one fifth of British miners, almost a quarter of a million men and boys, and producing one fifth of coal in Britain, 56 million tons in total.[7] The region particularly benefited from an increase in demand for British coal from abroad, as exports rose from a total proportion of less than one tenth of British coal production in 1869 to a third in 1913.[8]

While the north-east of England and south Wales differed in terms of the chronologies of their development, they were nevertheless the two largest coalfields in Britain by 1880. Scotland differed from these two regions in that there were a number of distinct and separate fields, spread across a larger area than was the case with the more compact fields in the other two regions. Historians refer to two distinct regions of Scottish mining. Both regions were situated in a broad swathe of the country through the central lowlands but can be distinguished according to the East of Scotland coalfield, which included Clackmannanshire, Stirlingshire, Fifeshire and the Lothians, while the larger, West of Scotland coalfield included Dunbartonshire, Renfrewshire, Ayrshire and Lanarkshire.[9]

Following the peak year of production in 1913, the British coal industry faced a period of uncertainty and economic depression. While the First World War increased the economic and political importance of the industry, it also sowed the seeds of the industry's difficulties in the interwar decades. This was particularly the case for exporting regions, such as Scotland, the north-east of England and south Wales, as international customers were lost during the war and those countries found new suppliers or else developed their own coal industries to compensate for the loss of imports from Britain.[10]

The immediate post-war years seemed to herald a period of optimism and buoyancy, with the coal industry still enjoying the benefits of the large orders and full employment brought about by the war, but industrial strife and economic downturn brought such optimism to an end and heralded the start of a long period of mass unemployment. Many collieries closed in that first jolt of recession in 1921, while others succumbed to the worsening economic conditions from 1926 onwards and the worldwide economic recession from 1929. By 1929 a quarter of all coalminers were unemployed and the coalfields of south Wales, the north-east of England and the Scottish coalfields were among the worst-hit regions of Britain, with unemployment rates approaching 40 per cent, twice as great as the level in Britain as a whole.[11] The performance of the industry improved somewhat from the mid-1930s onwards, while rearmament and then the outbreak of war in 1939 served to increase demand for coal and helped to lessen unemployment. Indeed, the 1940s saw a shortage of labour in the mining industry as demand rose and many miners were drawn into the armed forces.[12]

Economic considerations were also crucial to the cultural production and thematic content of coalfields literature.[13] In the late Victorian and Edwardian period working-class writing on the coalfields primarily took the form of poetry, ballads and some autobiographical works. Poetry and ballads were often sold by the sheet, raising a supplementary income for the miner, with some of the more successful writers being published in collected editions later in life, or posthumously.[14] In regard to the coalfields novel, most authors in this period were middle class and often interested in religious subjects, particularly exploring Methodist topics in the industrial, working-class community.[15] These novels, as well as early examples of coalfields (auto-)biographies,[16] were largely published with the support of Christian publishing companies and by sponsorship from individual Methodist ministers.[17] In the period following the First World War, coalfields literature flourished as a genre, supported by an increasing number of politically left-leaning publishers,[18] as well as by developments in education, that afforded opportunities to be published that were not previously available to working-class writers.

Economic considerations were both key to the opportunity to write and a central theme in working-class literature of the interwar period interested in poverty, economic depression and unemployment. The majority of these 'miner-writers' were not employed as miners at the time of writing, and most took up writing following the prolonged industrial action of 1926. This includes miner-writers such as Idris Davies, Jack Jones, Lewis Jones, Joe Corrie and Harold Heslop, all of whom explored the interaction between the economic depression and industrial unrest. Jack Jones gives detailed descriptions of the money he earned from writing and lecturing in his autobiography, *Unfinished Journey*, but notes he was 'still destitute and entitled to Public Assistance'[19] under the definitions of the means-test investigator. Jones received £25 for his first novel, *Rhondda Roundabout*, but he describes how most of that money disappeared quickly when £5 had already been spent to pay a typist (initially he could not afford a typewriter) and the rest went to repay part of his debt to his son Glynne, the back-rent and half-year's rates. When a piece of writing, titled *Behold They Live*, was rejected for being 'too gloomy', Jones raved:

> How could it be other than gloomy? A hundred and fifty thousand unemployed for the best part of ten years – many of 'em longer than that. Hanging on to life by the skin of their teeth in narrow valleys where there's damn-all to look at but a couple of derelict pits and the man-made mountain of pit-refuse into which the men and boys of the 'dead' townships burrow for brassy coal to keep the home-fires burning. Gloom, yes, and gloom the world should be aware of.[20]

Jones was not alone in articulating a desire to make the world aware of the situation of the unemployed miners; this was a common statement from contemporary working-class coalfields writers. In this way, the economic depression had a significant impact on the underlying theme of much of the coalfields literature, as well as creating the unemployment that encouraged many of these former miners to take up their pens.

Work

While coalmining was not characterised by the same occupational diversity or variety of grades as other industries, still the types and character of work done by workers in the industry varied. Underground workers constituted roughly 80 per cent of the mining workforce but, here too, there were differences in the types of tasks carried out by different individuals each working day.[21] Of these, it was the 'hewer' or 'collier', in his work cutting coal at the face, who occupied the top position in the hierarchy of grades in the mining workforce.[22] Hewers were the largest group of underground workmen and, by 1905, constituted roughly 48 per cent of the total in the north-east of England, 56 per cent of those in south Wales and 59 per cent in Scotland.[23] Men tended to become hewers in their early twenties, after having worked at various different tasks previously, when their strength was at its greatest. Their work was the most onerous, but it was also the best paid and carried the highest status. To some degree, the precise character of the work of hewers varied from coalfield to coalfield: hewers in the north-east of England carried out less 'deadwork' than their counterparts elsewhere, since they did not, for example, cut, load, remove or set the props that held up the roof underground, whereas the Scottish hewers and the south Welsh colliers generally did most of their own deadwork. This was partly due to geological conditions underground – the more vulnerable roofs in south Wales and Scotland required immediate attention from colliers; it also meant that colliers in south Wales were better paid, but that their cousins in the north-east held a higher status in a more hierarchical labour force, since their work was a little more differentiated.[24]

Elsewhere underground, many of the other grades of workmen were engaged in haulage: 'putters' and 'drawers' pushed trams of coal, while 'hauliers' or 'drivers' handled the ponies or, later, engines that became the main means of transporting drams of coal underground from the late nineteenth century onwards. 'Hitchers' and 'onsetters' transferred the drams to the pit cages for ascent to the surface, while a variety of labourers ensured that the roadways and other areas were kept in working order: 'roadsmen' maintained the roofs and sides of passages underground, while 'bottomers' were responsible for keeping good order at the pit bottom. Changes in working methods also necessitated the employment of new types of workers underground: masons and bricklayers were required, for example, as the longwall method of mining coal was adopted and necessitated the erection of walls to channel the flow of air, while mechanisation created a demand for fitters and electricians to service the haulage and coal-cutting machines.[25] All of this work underground was overseen by colliery officials such as overmen, viewers, deputies and firemen.

Work on the surface tended to be of a lower status than underground work and was less well paid. It was also more heterogeneous than work underground, and a variety of tasks were completed by different types of worker. 'Enginemen' controlled the engine that raised and lowered the cage, while 'furnacemen' shovelled the coal that drove those engines. 'Banksmen' or 'pit-headmen' unloaded full drams from the cage and sent empty cages back down, while 'putters', 'drawers' and 'drivers' moved those drams from the pit-bank to the screens or tippers. The screens were themselves staffed by boys, old men and, in some coalfields, women who picked pieces of stone and muck out of the coal. Other surface workers included blacksmiths, who were needed to shoe pit ponies and also to make and mend the large number of metal objects that were utilised on a daily basis in a colliery, pick sharpeners, horsemen, saddlers, carpenters, waggon fillers and men in the lamp room who filled, distributed and collected the lamps each day.

The one type of surface workman who possessed as high a status as the underground hewer was the checkweighman, who ensured that the coal raised by each hewer was weighed and recorded fairly; checkweighmen were often also prominent trade union activists, since, chosen by the men, they could not be victimised by employers as easily. Therefore, the mining workforce, while not as heterogeneous as those in other industries, was nevertheless varied, and workers found themselves engaged in different tasks each day and faced by a variety of risks and perils in their daily work.

One of the characteristics of the realist coalfields literature was the detailed portrayal of the experience of work at the colliery, including the interactions between different roles. Here the hewer is similarly portrayed as the most prestigious role, even when there are job roles with more seniority, such as the 'firemen' who make decisions about safety. Indeed, 'firemen' are often portrayed as complicit with the management in hiding issues of poor safety from the records, such as not reporting high levels of gas or weak roofs. Tom Hanlin's novel *Yesterday Will Return* (1946), for example, shows a manager convince a fireman not to report gas, and bribe a young miner who was burned not to say anything, because 'Even if the fireman had not reported the gas, the boy might have claimed compensation for being burned by gas, and that would have meant an inquiry and a very expensive business for the Company.'[26] In this way certain roles in the pit were believed to be more aligned with the sympathies of the management, against the interests of the working men. The opposite, of course, was true for a role such as checkweighman, a man appointed by the miners to ensure fairness in the weighing of the coal and their payments. The less prestigious roles were often those performed by boys first starting out in work, by older men no longer able to keep up with the hard pace of hewing or, as we shall see, by miners who had been impaired in the course of their work and could not return to their original underground position.

The daily tasks of workmen clearly varied, and each was impacted differently by the process of mechanisation. Mechanisation was a crucially important aspect of working practices in the latter decades of the nineteenth century and the first half of the twentieth century, and had far-reaching consequences for the risks faced by miners in their daily work. Electric coal-cutting was developed from the end of the nineteenth century, but still only 8 per cent of British coal was machine-cut by 1914, compared to a fifth in the United States.[27] The spread of mechanised coal-cutting progressed according to geology and the policies of local companies. In Scotland, for example, difficult physical conditions, which included a largely depleted Lanarkshire coalfield, created a more pressing economic need to modernise, and so spurred efforts to mechanise, while the longwall method of mining utilised in the coalfield also lent itself to mechanisation.[28] In south Wales, on the other hand, coal was easier to cut by hand and so there was not the same motivation for companies to introduce mechanised forms of coal-cutting, despite the use of longwall methods there too.[29] Despite this, south Wales developed mechanical conveying at a comparatively faster rate than other coalfields, showing that mechanisation took many forms.[30] Nevertheless, 75 per cent of all coal was cut by mechanised methods by the late 1930s.[31]

The introduction of mechanisation, where it was achieved, changed the nature of work for miners and, in a variety of ways, created new risks for miners and increased certain dangers. The 1925 Royal Commission on the Coal Industry, for example, reported on the 'striking decrease in deaths from explosions and from shaft accidents' in previous years, but noted the increase in industrial diseases.[32] More significantly, the increased use of mechanised coal-cutting technology and haulage methods served to increase the amounts of dust in the atmosphere and thereby the risks posed by lung disease. In a series of investigative articles on the perils posed by dust, the *News Chronicle* attributed an increase in silicosis in the mining industry to mechanisation. An article entitled 'When Men Grow Old Too Soon' maintained that 'The alarming increase in silicosis is largely due to the mechanisation of boring.'[33] Mechanisation, therefore, had its role in creating injury as well as in preventing it.

Coalfields literature often picked up on mechanisation as a threat to men's health because of the new dangers it introduced. A new coal-cutting machine reduced the hard digging work, recalls Bert Coombes in *These Poor Hands* (1939), but added danger because the noise drowned out the subtle sounds of a weak roof about to collapse, while the timbers had to be set further apart to allow room for the machine. Coombes was trained to work one of these machines and describes his initial reluctance because 'the work was reputed to be very dangerous, even among men who had spent a lifetime in danger.'[34] He details both minor and major risks of being near the machine: 'the falling coal and clod, the tearing chain, the bursting cable, and the danger of that amount of electric current made every day's work full of risk.'[35] Following a particularly bad roof fall onto the cutter, it is assumed Coombes must have been buried and one colleague runs straight past him on his way to get help because he 'was so frightened that he did not recognise me.'[36] Coombes comments on how these accidents linger in the mind: 'these near escapes make us nervous for awhile [sic], especially if we think what might have happened. For some time we see a danger in every stone, then become hardened again.'[37] In one particularly disturbing narrative, in which he describes becoming trapped between the cutter and the roof, the traumatic nature of these incidences is clear:

> Already I could feel the pressure on my feet increasing, and I knew that even at that slow speed I would be under that lower part in two minutes, and all my body would have to go through a space that was only four inches in height. I screamed again and again, and struggled, but failed to get loose. [...] I was frantic with fear, for I could almost sense my bones being crushed under the top.[38]

Fortunately, his struggles knocked a sledge-hammer into the cutter chain, causing the machine's electrics to cut out. Coombes remarks how this incident stayed with him, that he never again attempted to crawl over the top of the machine and that he 'kept that sledge-head for some years after; it had the marks of the picks driven into it.'[39] Bert Coombes was by no means the only writer to focus on the hazards of the new machine. Lewis Jones includes a story of a young man losing his arm to a conveyor in his novel *Cwmardy* (1937) and Sid Chaplin describes a man's horrendous injuries after falling into the path of a cutter in *The Thin Seam* (1950).[40] A recurrent theme is the danger posed by the pressure to speed up and cut corners, particularly in the vulnerable conditions, following the 1926 lockout, in which men 'slaved their navels to their backbones with those damned conveyors grinding at their heels.'[41] One man pushing himself to the new, faster pace goes 'giddy' and falls into the machine, losing his arm as a consequence. In a less dramatic but more insidious example Durham miner and writer Sid Chaplin suggests that the need to feed the machine outweighs consideration for the worker's body. The worker, Daniel, is in perfect synchronisation, like a machine himself: 'Dig in, draw out, shoot forth, back, dig in, draw out – the big beautiful machine perfectly serving the other big beautiful machine'.[42] But the vulnerability of the human body is clear, since Daniel is working on, despite a partially broken shovel that promises a *'beat* hand' (a condition discussed below[43]):

> Daniel was living up to the canons of the pit: *dinna be soft*. Now, if it had been me I'd have thrown that shovel with its broken crutch into the goaf, and gone in search of another. That would have meant holding the cutter up for ten minutes or a quarter of an hour. But my hand means more to me that a ten minutes' delay. Or does it?[44]

As with the other literary examples, the introduction of machinery is seen as a benefit for the company, but to the detriment of men's safety.

Different methods of working the coal, whether longwall or versions of 'pillar and stall', by mechanised means or by hand, had important consequences for the organisation of labour underground, industrial relations and levels of union militancy, as Martin Daunton has shown.[45] In addition, they determined how workers in the industry were paid. Those men who worked at the face and cut the coal, whether described as 'hewers' or 'colliers', were paid piece rates, and thus their weekly wage was determined by the amount of coal they raised. This was crucially important to their experience of work and to the possibility of disability, though the consequences of this method of payment for injury, disease and impairment were complex. On the one hand, piece rates could work to encourage a faster pace of work that increased the risks of injury and impairment to the individual miner. Certainly some socialists and trade union activists laid a great deal of blame for increased risk at the door of the piece-rate system. One socialist newspaper in south Wales referred to the 'infernal bustle of the piece-rate system' in the period just before the First World War which, it claimed, was responsible for 'the tendency towards increased periods and possibilities of bad health and of shortening the length of life of the average miner underground'.[46] Labour MP John Swan wrote against both the piece-rate system and cavilling in his novel *The Mad Miner* (1933), claiming:

> Some day an enlightened public conscience will abolish this iniquitous piece-system in mines and give a measure of justice, by a reasonable daily wage, to the miner whose labour is so arduous whose risks are so great and labour so valuable.

Piece work and cavils[47] in mines are vices exploiting virtue. It is an alluring gamble which lends colour to its wickedness. It is an ingenious device and artifice to exploit the innocent helpless miners. It oscillates not only with the good and bad place, but brings the inevitable reaction of risks, accidents and premature age. The strong yesterday are weak to-day and cast aside.[48]

Using the well-worn image of the 'big hewer', Swan shows that even a very strong man would be unable to earn enough wages when working in a very poor, wet and hazardous section of the pit. In comparison to the 'big hewer', less fit men would be even more disadvantaged by drawing a bad lot. Enjoying the benefit of drawing a good lot is therefore cast as a bribe, an 'alluring gamble', to undercut the fight for a fairer minimum wage that goes against the wider interests of the miners and solidarity in the community. By the interwar period, such analysis of the effects of piece work underpinned union critiques of various aspects of the work process and resolutions were passed in favour of its abolition.[49]

On the other hand, and acting against this tendency towards an increased work pace, faceworkers did not work rigidly observed hours, or else missed days when the need or the desire arose precisely because they were paid by piece rates rather than by the hour. John Benson makes the point that while miners in the nineteenth century tended to work regular hours, needed to work hard to earn a decent living and were tied to set periods for ascending and descending the shaft, they nevertheless were more free to vary their working hours than other grades of workmen, who were paid by the hour and who worked set hours.[50] In his evidence to the Royal Commission on Labour in 1892, for example, the Ayrshire miners' leader Keir Hardie noted that 'The miners, with the exception of one very large colliery, are free to leave the pits when they please … They are free to go when they please, irrespective of what they have accomplished.'[51] In addition, as a result of the piece-rate system, miners tended to increase their output before holidays or in readiness for some period of greater need, but also lessened their productivity through less intense activity or even days off work when conditions were good. This presented a potential degree of flexibility for disabled workers who could not maintain regular, high productivity – issues of reduced productivity would not have affected their chances of employment because they would have been paid based only on what they had produced, but they would have come up against the commercial imperatives of colliery companies to maximise productivity in order to boost profits.

Voluntary absenteeism was common and, at times, faceworkers opted for greater leisure time rather than larger incomes when a certain standard had been achieved.⁵² This tendency, however, was probably more true of the period up to 1914, when buoyancy in the trade was more marked, than was the case during the years of the two wars or the interwar economic depression, when various pressures served to limit the amount of autonomy that workers were able to exercise in this context. At the same time, and crucial to the social history of disability in the coal industry, it is evident that voluntary absenteeism came to form a strategy for impaired workers in their attempts to manage their failing strength and the effects of occupational disease. The miner-writer Bert Coombes looked to defend his comrades from accusations that their absenteeism imperilled the war effort in the 1940s and asserted that many miners missed a shift or two each week as they felt their chests tightening as a result of pneumoconiosis: they 'hope to stave off the disease by losing time frequently and so clearing the lungs'.⁵³ In such instances, well-being and physical capacity were prioritised over additional income in the piece rate-system.

Not only did the organisation of work in a colliery have consequences for the form of payment made to coal workers, but it also determined the shift patterns and working hours in the different coalfields, which themselves were crucial to the work experience and the likelihood of disability. Until the Mines Regulation Act of 1908, hewers in the north-east of England worked one of two short shifts each day, either between 4am and about 11am or else from 10am to about 4pm. Their 'bank-to-bank' time (the time from pithead to pithead) was roughly six-and-a-half hours, while their time at the coalface was about five-and-a-half hours, giving them relatively short working hours in comparison with other types of workers and to other miners.⁵⁴ In contrast, and due to the longwall system utilised there, colliers in south Wales worked one long shift during the day. Efforts had been made during the nineteenth century to persuade workers to adopt the two-shift system, but, careful of their family lives and domestic arrangements, and keen not to share their stall with another miner, they had refused. The result was that by the early twentieth century south Wales colliers spent almost ten hours bank-to-bank and roughly eight hours at the coalface. Daunton has calculated that when short days are also taken into account the disparity between the north-east of England and south Wales was even more marked and that miners in parts of south Wales worked 48 per cent longer than their counterparts in the north-east.⁵⁵ Colliers in south Wales continued to work longer hours than miners in other coalfields by the time of the First World War, despite the 1908 legislation that supposedly brought the working day down to eight hours.⁵⁶

The differences in working hours between different coalfields explain the varied responses to the campaign to bring about statutory working hours in the coal industry. Through much of the latter part of the nineteenth century, coalminers' leaders, similar to union leaders in other industries, had campaigned for the introduction of an eight-hour day in the industry. Many Scottish miners, notably those in Fife, had gained an eight-hour day in the 1870s, and so any such change meant less to them than it did to miners in coalfields such as south Wales, where the introduction of such a measure would have made a material difference to their daily working lives.[57] In Durham and Northumberland, by contrast, an eight-hour day would have meant an increase in hours for many miners. In 1906, 74 per cent of miners in the north-east of England were already working fewer than eight hours a day, while in south Wales the number was 0.4 per cent.[58]

In the debates over the appropriate numbers of hours that miners should work, it is interesting to note that safety, injury and impairment played a role.[59] In discussions over an eight-hour day in the 1890s, for example, can be found the assertion from miners' leaders that accidents that caused deaths and disabling injuries were higher in the last hour of work than in any other part of a shift. In addition, coalowners' representatives asserted that accident rates were higher in the earlier parts of shifts and that the faster winding of men that was necessary to ensure that no individual worked more than eight hours would increase the chances of winding accidents.[60] A ballad composed in the 1890s as part of the campaign insisted:

Yn nghanol awyr afiach	Down 'midst foul air and gases
Drwy'r dydd mae'r Glowr hy',	The Collier works all day,
Ac yn ei amgylchynu	And many are the dangers
Y mae peryglon lu;	Which ever round him stay;
Llefaru'n nghlust y *Collier*	But, hark! He hears a whisper,
Mae Iechyd teg ei wawr,	From Health it now does come:–
'Rho'r *Sledge* a'r *Mandrel* heibio	Throw down the sledge and the mandrel
Ar ben yr Wythfed Awr.'	When Eight Hours' work is done.[61]

A seven-hour day followed in 1924, but was swiftly suspended by the Coal Mines Act two years later; again, disability figured in the discussions over working hours. In this instance, opponents of the reduction in hours argued that they would cause *more* accidents and disabling injuries, since piece-rate workers would be inclined to rush their work in order to earn the same sums of money. The *Colliery Guardian*, mouthpiece of the coalowners, opined that 'it naturally follows that the last hour may indeed be the most dangerous, for in it the miner may be attempting to bring up his "darg" to the appointed standard'. An eight-hour day would allow the miner to 'work more leisurely or there will be fewer men employed; in either case, the exposure to risk will be reduced'. Their 1926 article also argued that the miner needed the first hour to 'get into his swing'.[62]

As we have seen, faceworkers were paid piece rates, and so had unconventional working patterns or did not work set hours. This meant that they were able to manage their work practices and intensity a little better than other grades of workers, who, paid flat rates, were more likely to observe set working hours. The particular organisation of work in each colliery and coalfield also influenced the working hours of other underground workers. As far as haulage workers were concerned, for example, hauliers in south Wales worked shifts of similar length to colliers, whereas haulage workers in the north-east of England were required to work a long shift to cover the two daily shifts of the hewers. The result was that they worked roughly half as much again as the hewers they served.[63] There was a certain irony in this pattern for impaired workers, since hewers who suffered an injury or an occupational disease were often moved to 'light work' (discussed in detail later in the chapter) on the surface but then faced longer working hours.[64]

Not usually included in considerations of the mining workforce but still nevertheless crucial to the functioning of the industry (and tellingly prominent in coalfields fiction) were miners' wives, mothers and other female members of their families in the home. The work of boys and men at the pit would not have been possible without a considerable amount of unpaid female labour in the home and, as V. L. Allen commented, 'Wives have been adapted to meet the needs of mining as effectively as the miners themselves.'[65] This idea was given articulation by the women's sections of the labour movement in the early decades of the twentieth century as activists attempted to raise the profile of 'women's issues' and so framed the home as a woman's workplace: as Elizabeth Andrews, the women's organiser of the Labour Party in Wales and herself the daughter of a miner and wife of a former miner, stated, 'The Home is the Woman's Workshop.'[66]

Similar to miners themselves, while the character of their work was broadly similar from place to place, the precise character of the women's workplace varied from coalfield to coalfield. This was due, in part, to the housing forms utilised in different coalfields, but also, more importantly, due to the age of the housing stock. A large proportion of the houses inhabited by miners' families in the north-east of England, for example, were built in the first half of the nineteenth century, when the coal industry was developing at a rapid rate. The later development of coal communities in south Wales meant that larger numbers of houses were built in an era when bye-laws stipulated certain minimum standards of quality and when sanitary technology was more effective, though the incredible rate of in-migration placed enormous strain on the housing stock and created a housing crisis in the years before 1914 that was not matched in other coalfields.[67] The experience of Scottish coalfields was different again and, while there was variation from one place to another, housing there reflected the inferior quality of housing in Scotland relative to other parts of Britain generally, and was of a very low standard.[68]

Too often, miners' houses were small and cramped, with too little room for the large families that inhabited them. Miners' families tended to be larger than average, since the possibility of men earning relatively high wages by their early twenties encouraged early household formation and resulted in higher fertility rates.[69] In addition, many mining families looked to ease the burden on household resources by taking in lodgers, while other families sub-let part of the house to another family in the form of 'apartments', which served to increase the overcrowding; in fact, 10 per cent of all houses in the north-east of England and south Wales were sub-let in 1911, and the proportion was on the increase in south Wales at that time.[70] Indeed, the rapid development of the south Wales coalfield in this period, as well as that of the Fife coalfield in Scotland, meant that housing provision failed to keep pace with population increase in those two places in the two or three decades before 1914, with the effect that occupancy levels exceeded five persons per dwelling.[71]

Scottish MP, former miner and successful novelist, James C. Welsh, highlighted the inadequacies of miners' housing in a speech to Parliament:

> I saw a miners' row – about four or five hundred houses, all of them single apartments. There were two holes in the walls for beds. It was certainly a happy home, as happy as it could be made under the circumstances, but in one of the beds lay an injured parent, brought home from the mine, writhing and groaning in agony, and in the other bed lay a dead child, and at night time, during the period of waiting between death and burial, the dead child had to be lifted out to allow the living ones to get in.
>
> It was not because they were thriftless or drunken people, but because economic circumstances were such that they created conditions of that kind, that made it absolutely impossible for human lives to be lived.[72]

Welsh forcefully contrasts this tragic scene with the 'Aladdin's cave of riches'[73] on display in Parliament to argue that such a wide discrepancy is immoral and unjustifiable. Jack Jones, another miner-writer, blamed the poor housing conditions faced by miners in south Wales on the control the 'Company' had over every aspect of coalfields life:

> Everything was 'Company' owned and controlled. Schools, houses, doctors, teachers, clergymen of the Church of England, canal, railways, banks, souls. So the Company doctors [visiting cholera cases in Company homes] didn't dare open their mouths too wide about the housing conditions of the place.[74]

Both men foreground the health impact of inadequate accommodation and frame poor housing as a political issue.

Individual testimony provides another window on the experiences of individual families of poor housing well into the twentieth century. One of the Durham miners' wives who featured in the Women's Health Enquiry Committee in the 1930s, for example, lived in a cottage that was described in the survey as 'atrocious'. The cottage had two bedrooms, one of which had only a skylight while the other had one small window, the roof was in a poor condition and let in water when it rained, the oven was defective, there was no gas, no bath, no electricity and all water for the baths of her husband and working son had to be lifted onto an open fire for heating before being decanted into a tin bath.[75] This was not very different to the experience of a large proportion of miners' wives, since colliery houses were rarely equipped with baths; Dot Jones noted, for example, that 'as late as 1920 only 2.4% of the 26,822 working-class homes in the Rhondda had baths'.[76] It was not until 1926 that pithead baths became a legislated provision, covered by the Miners' Welfare Fund and funded by a levy on royalties, and so the majority of miners continued to bath at home well into the 1930s.[77]

These houses were the workplace of the majority of women living in the coalfields, and though the age and quality of buildings varied from coalfield to coalfield, the character of the work carried out within the home by wives and other female members of the family was broadly similar across the coalfields. This work, of course, involved servicing the various needs of the colliery workers in the family, and such was the onerous nature of the tasks involved that it was described by one contemporary authority on women's health as 'domestic slavery'.[78] The preparation of food, the raising of children, the washing of miners' bodies, clothes and boots and the constant cleaning and tidying of the home environment were the daily lot of the miner's wife. Indeed, some historians have noted that the domestic responsibilities of miners' wives, due to the high volume of dirt brought into the home, the larger families and the poor standard of housing, were greater than those of the wives of other types of workers.[79] In a powerful short story from 1942, in which a miner's wife and mother of five strapping sons is gradually worked to death, the beleaguered woman complains, 'one collier's more work in the house than four clean-job men'.[80]

The preparation of the miner's bath was the domestic activity most linked to women's disability by feminist and labour women campaigners in the early decades of the century. This was because the mere act of drawing a bath involved the woman in considerable heavy labour, starting, in many cases, with a walk to a communal standpipe, then the transportation of sufficient water to the home, the lifting of heavy pans of water onto open fires, and then the decanting of those heavy pans into the bath ready for the miner to be washed.[81] Possibly repeated a number of times a day, depending on the number of miners in the family, this activity placed enormous strains on women's bodies and, added to the effects of numerous pregnancies and poor obstetric care, resulted in a significant level of female reproductive impairment. In her testimony to the Sankey Commission in 1919, Elizabeth Andrews, the Labour Party's women's organiser for Wales, stated that:

> A midwife of 23 years' experience … in the Rhondda stated to me that the majority of cases she has had of premature births and extreme female ailments are due to the physical strain of lifting heavy tubs and boilers in their homes which they had to do under the present housing conditions.[82]

Pithead baths, she argued elsewhere, would mean:

> shorter hours, less drudgery, dirty work for the women. More rest. More leisure. Less physical strain on mothers. No need for handling and lifting heavy tubs and boilers. Healthier mothers, brighter mothers, cleaner and brighter homes.[83]

The working lives of mining women in the home were, in their ways, just as hard, if not more so, as those of their male family members. In her study of late nineteenth-century Rhondda, historian Dot Jones claimed: 'the mortality rates of women who worked in the home were higher than those of their menfolk who worked in the pit, in direct contrast to national mortality trends'.[84] And yet, such women continued to perform their domestic roles despite suffering debilitating conditions and ailments, and had few means by which to lessen the strain on their bodies.

While the power of the British labour movement, with miners at the heart of matters, was harnessed to bring about statutory limits to working hours, no such campaigns were waged to limit the working hours of miners' wives in the home, despite those wives often working twice as many hours in a day as their husbands underground. One campaigner, the author of the 'Women's Column' in the *Rhondda Socialist* newspaper in south Wales, pointed out in 1912 that while miners had won their long-sought aim of an eight-hour working day, and that while legislation had been passed to limit the working hours of women in factories and workshops, no such amelioration of the working hours of women in the home was likely. Freedom from 'tiring drudgery' and such 'glaring inequality' was to be achieved only if women themselves took the issue up and if their husbands came to realise that they needed to strive on behalf of their wives as much as themselves.[85]

Part of the problem faced by women labouring in the home can be found in the shift systems of male workers. Since mining households might have two, three or more miners (for example, a man, perhaps his brother, working sons and lodgers), a woman might have been confronted with having to service the needs of a number of male workers starting and finishing shifts at different times of the day. In such a situation, the onerous burden of sending the male worker off to his shift and then later preparing a bath, cleaning clothes and tidying the house of the resultant mess and disorder would have been repeated a number of times in the day, with considerable strain on a woman's body. The Women's Health Enquiry Committee found that while the wives of most workers rose at 6:30am, those of miners and bakers were often required to rise at 4am to see their husbands and sons off to work in the morning; some such wives never had a period of more than four continuous hours of unbroken sleep in any twenty-four hour period.[86] One Durham woman mentioned in the Enquiry rose at 3am to get her eldest son off to work, went back to bed and rose again at 7am to see to the needs of the household and then did not turn in again until 11pm.[87] The pattern of shifts was crucial and could cause a multiplication of the workload for any individual woman: Elizabeth Andrews, in her testimony to the Sankey Commission, noted that while there were two shifts in south Wales there was also a third shift for repairers (i.e. 7am to 3pm, 3pm to 11pm and, for the repairers, 11pm to 7am), so that 'It means for a woman who has two sons and a husband working that if they work on different shifts, her life is nothing but slavery. She gets neither rest nor leisure under those conditions.'[88]

Mining disabilities

Work in and related to the coal industry impaired large numbers of individuals and the industry gained a reputation for its considerable dangers and the extensive toll in lives, injuries and ill-health. The dangers posed to mineworkers by large-scale disasters received the most attention within the media and were treated in a melodramatic and sensationalist manner, but, in many ways, it was the more mundane, everyday risks that brought about the greatest amount of impairment. In the first place, most accidents happened underground rather than on the surface. In 1920, for example, of the 117,302 individual miners across the entire industry who were injured sufficiently to necessitate seven or more days off work, 91 per cent were injured in accidents underground. Of these 106,730 individuals, fully 41,358 (35 per cent) were injured in accidents involving the fall of materials from the roof or sides underground.[89] These might have entailed falls involving a few tons of material that had the capacity to kill or maim, or the fall of a single rock that was no less dangerous to any individual miner in its way.[90] Throughout the interwar period almost a half of all fatalities and 'injuries' (i.e. injuries sufficient to disable a man from working for seven days or more before 1924, or three days or more after 1924) came as a result of falls of the roof or sides.[91] All underground workers, to a greater or lesser degree, faced the risks posed by the possibility of falls of rock and coal, but faceworkers were subject to the greatest risk, since the task of opening faces or 'dropping' the coal increased the instability of the rock and coal strata before the roof and the sides could be supported adequately. Furthermore, geological characteristics underground varied from one coalfield to another, and so the risks faced by miners in various coalfields differed; in 1920, for example, 3,767 miners from Scottish coalfields, 5,875 in Durham and Northumberland and 7,975 in south Wales were injured.[92] These regional variations are reflected in coalfields literature to a certain extent: mining disasters involving floods are more commonly found in novels set in Scotland and north-east England,[93] whereas those involving gas explosions tend to be set in Wales.[94] Specific regional geological features are also central to the plot of certain novels, such as the dangers of a weak blue-shale roof under the longwall system in Harold Heslop's *Last Cage Down* (1935), or the investigation into the high incidence of lung disease among anthracite miners in A. J. Cronin's *The Citadel* (1937).[95]

Apart from falls, the other large classification of underground accidents that led to injury and disabling conditions was related to haulage. Whether powered by horses, by hand or by mechanical means, impact and crush injuries caused by trams and tubs were the cause of a great deal of disablement. In the early 1920s roughly 30,000 underground workers were injured every year to such a degree as to be off work for seven days or more, amounting to 26 per cent of all mineworkers injured for seven days or more in each year.[96] Shaft accidents were less important but still injured and killed large numbers of workers, while the movement of coal on the surface similarly brought workers into contact with fast-moving and heavy machinery and trams that damaged bodies with ease.

Falls of rock and haulage accidents, whether underground or on the surface, caused impact and crush injuries, largely to limbs – with arms, legs, hands and feet broken – but sometimes to the head and the body. Before the better management of fracture and other orthopaedic cases from about the 1930s, such injuries might have led to recovery, but often resulted in malformed fractures, amputation, permanent spinal injuries or a range of other, less serious but nevertheless debilitating injuries.

In addition to such impact or crush injuries, miners also suffered 'beat' diseases, such as 'beat hand', 'beat knee' and 'beat elbow'. These conditions developed as a result of constant pressure, such as when kneeling or pressing against a hard surface, or through repeated impacts, as when using a pick, and involved inflammation that caused that part of the body to become swollen and tender to touch. The affected part of the body would also throb, or 'beat' in the north-east of England, thus giving the condition its name.[97] The long-term nature of 'beat' diseases made them less visible than other impairments but affected miners' ability to continue their work, their mobility and their quality of life. These occupational diseases, at least as they affected coalminers, were scheduled as compensatable under the Workmen's Compensation system from 1906 onwards, and it is evident from the statistics that there was a constant increase in the numbers of notified cases in the decades that followed, so that, by the late 1930s, there were approximately 6,000 new cases across the industry every year, roughly three-quarters of which were 'beat knee'.[98] One medical authority noted in 1914 that most cases recovered within a relatively short space of time but that some ended in permanent impairment.[99]

Another occupational disease that affected miners and that was scheduled within the compensation system alongside the 'beat' conditions under the measure passed in 1906 was miners' nystagmus. Nystagmus is a condition of the eye caused by work in low light conditions in which the main symptoms are an involuntary oscillation of the eyeball, with resultant vertigo, headaches and nausea, night blindness and sensitivity to bright light.[100] Bert Coombes suggested that sufferers were marked by their particular behaviour:

> I have watched them waiting near the pit mouth until someone comes along who will read the wording on a new notice to them; they fumble their way about the village streets when twilight comes; they rely on their hearing to help their uncertain eyes.[101]

The condition was not curable, nor even treatable, in the period up to the 1940s, but symptoms would often abate with the removal of the sufferer from the circumstances that brought on the condition in the first place. For miners, of course, this meant that the individual was removed from underground work and re-employed on the surface; some were able to continue to work underground after a period in better light conditions, but a greater number were transferred to work on the surface, while others were forced to leave the industry altogether.[102] Again, similar to the case with the various 'beat' diseases, the number of cases of nystagmus in the coal industry increased after notification was made compulsory in 1906, so that there were roughly 10,000 ongoing cases at any time in the interwar period.[103] Ascertaining the relative numbers of sufferers in each coalfield is impossible, since the policies adopted by employers and their mutual indemnity organisations or insurance companies determined the numbers of cases certified each year.[104] Contemporary medical authorities insisted that the disease disproportionately affected faceworkers: of the 685 cases discussed by T. Lister Llewellyn in his review in 1913, 81 per cent were employed at the coalface and only small numbers of other grades of workers were found to suffer the condition.[105]

Perhaps the most notorious of occupational diseases that affected miners, and one that caused massive levels of impairment, was chest disease. A study of miners' chest disease has described it as the 'largest occupational health disaster in British history', and the period from 1880 to 1948 witnessed a transformation in the understanding of and responses to this condition.[106] Referred to as 'miners' asthma' or 'miners' lung' at the start of this period, classified as 'silicosis' in the early decades of the twentieth century and distinguished as 'coal workers' pneumoconiosis' by the 1940s, the condition was the subject of intense industrial struggles, pioneering scientific and medical research and, ultimately, successful political lobbying that saw it recognised within the compensation system and as a matter of significant government intervention.[107] Quite simply, the inhalation of coal dust caused the lungs to become congested and damage to be done to the delicate structure of the lungs. The miner himself, at least initially, would become breathless, would suffer coughing fits and would become increasingly fatigued as his aerobic capacity was compromised. As the disease took hold a sufferer would be unable to complete even light manual tasks. He lost weight and assumed an emaciated look, and eventually died from heart disease as a result of the strain placed on the heart.

It is not easy to assess the extent of chest disease among coalminers in the first half of the twentieth century. The changing nature of scientific understanding and medical knowledge, and the changing compensation landscape, meant that statistics are not particularly accurate for the period before 1948. It is also important to note that union, medical and official attention to the condition, at least in the period up to 1948, was concentrated in south Wales, where the majority of cases emanated from the anthracite district in the western part of the coalfield, despite the incidence of the disease in all British coalfields to varying degrees. According to official statistics, pneumoconiosis caused the deaths of 1,334 south Wales miners between 1937 and 1948, and the permanent disablement of 18,297 others, but the miners' union for the region put the figures at 2,088 and 38,449, respectively.[108]

All those working within the coal industry inhaled some amount of coal dust – the coal-trimmers who loaded the coal into ships at the docks were even found to suffer pneumoconiosis in research carried out in the 1940s – but, again, it was the hewer who suffered this condition more than other grades of workmen.[109] Despite the presence of dust at all points in the process of raising coal, it was at the coalface that the highest concentrations were found, both because of the dust produced by the work there and also because the ventilation underground tended to be less effective at the extremities of the workings.[110]

Moreover, as a piece worker, the hewer was perhaps incentivised to work faster than other grades of worker and, due to the nature of the mining workforce and the character of the occupational trajectory in the industry, he also tended to be younger than most other workers. The effect was that not only were faceworkers affected to a greater degree but the sufferers of pneumoconiosis also tended to be young in age. It was found, for example, that 33 per cent of all sufferers in the Cynon Valley in south Wales in the 1950s were under the age of forty, while the proportion for the neighbouring Rhondda valleys was 26 per cent.[111] Men in their forties, thirties and even twenties contracted pneumoconiosis and were aged prematurely by the ravages of the disease.[112] Though hewers faced the greatest risks, Enid Williams found that other categories of worker were also vulnerable. Although an underground labourer's job was lighter than that of a hewer, the work was often dustier.[113] Williams also found that old and infirm miners, perhaps moved from underground work to work on the screens as a result of impairment, could often face greater dust levels than in any other part of the colliery.[114] Mechanisation increased dust levels more generally, so that miners in the 1930s and 1940s faced greater dust levels than their predecessors.[115]

While miners were subject to a great many risks and experienced a variety of impairments as a result, they were not the only members of the mining community who faced impairment as a result of the coal industry. The wives and other female family members they left at home each morning to go to work also paid a price for the winning of coal. A great deal of attention in the 1920s and, especially, 1930s, in addition to the focus of historians since that time, was focused on the matter of maternal mortality, but a much greater number of women suffered maternal morbidity and were impaired by the injuries and complications of childbirth; in this sense, the experience of miners' wives mirrors that of their husbands, whose injuries and impairments far outnumbered the more newsworthy fatalities that received the lion's share of the attention. Observers were clear that there existed a large amount of reproductive injury and impairment, even if only a small proportion of it came within the notice of doctors and other health workers. In her important report into maternal mortality published in 1924, for example, Dame Janet Campbell found that ante- and post-natal clinics had begun to reveal the true extent of women's ill-health and debility: 'We find that the expectant mother is often ill-nourished; she is frequently anaemic; indigestion and constipation are accepted as a matter of course; varicose veins and dental caries pass almost unnoticed except perhaps when pregnancy accentuates the aching and weariness of her legs, or causes a more rapid decay of defective teeth.'[116] By the 1930s, when increased attention was being focused on maternal mortality, one 'follow-up' survey of 2,000

Edinburgh mothers found that 30 per cent of them 'were found to be suffering from various complaints and disabilities which required treatment'. It was noted that such a proportion meant that 'for every mother who dies there are sixty-five others who suffer some impairment of health as a result of pregnancy and childbirth'.[117] Even official investigations were noting the significant toll of impairment that followed on from pregnancy and childbirth: 'But for the relatively few women who die, many are seriously ill, some suffer permanent damage while others are left with some former weakness aggravated and with a shorter expectation of life.'[118]

The Women's Health Enquiry Committee of the 1930s, the results of which were reported in *Working-Class Wives* by Margery Spring Rice in 1939, similarly noted that attention had been focused on maternal mortality rather maternal morbidity. Through the completion of a questionnaires by 1,250 women in different parts of Britain, including miners' wives from Durham and south Wales, the Enquiry set out to offer a more complete picture of the character and extent of reproductive impairment.[119] Spring Rice wrote that maternal morbidity was 'extremely widespread and enduring, so that a woman tends to become progressively less fit with the birth of each child'.[120] Of the 1,250 women who responded as part of the Enquiry, 'gynaecological trouble' occurred definitely in 191 cases and evidence of it appeared in a further 203, but, Spring Rice reported, 'for various reasons no professional diagnosis has been made – the woman herself is ignorant of the cause of her pain or discomfort'.[121] Partly as a sign of this fact, the women themselves described such gynaecological impairments in lay rather than medical ways, as 'uterine trouble', 'womb trouble' or 'internal trouble'. Similarly, an official investigation into the matter in Scotland in the 1920s found that in 10,000 gynaecological cases studied that were admitted to hospital, 65 per cent of women had given birth previously and 28 per cent suffered impairments caused by those previous deliveries.[122]

Miners' wives featured prominently in these accounts of the 'toll of motherhood'. One of the respondents to the Women's Health Enquiry Committee was a thirty-two-year-old miner's wife from Durham. She had been married for fifteen years and had seven children, the eldest of whom was fourteen. Her family lived in a colliery house with an open ash-privy at the back, a damp back bedroom, no sink under the tap, and a coal-house and an ash-pit at the back of the house. Ashes and coals had to be carried through the sitting room, which was itself used as a bedroom and did not have windows that opened. She rose from bed at 4am and then retired to bed at the end of the day between 10pm and midnight. Her home was described as clean, her children had never been ill, their diet was varied and good and the health visitor described her as 'an amazing woman, with indomitable pluck'. All this effort, in such conditions, came at a cost to her health; she suffered: neuritis as a result of the heavy work of 'possing' (i.e. washing clothes in a tub with a 'poss stick') and mangling clothes; pyorrhoea, for which she had had all her teeth extracted; problems with her kidneys as a result of Bright's Disease; headaches and biliousness; cystitis as a result of pregnancy; and pain in her right side as a result of menstrual periods, 'due to ovarian trouble'.[123]

Another miner's wife in the same coalfield, 'Mrs. D. of Durham', had six children and faced terrible housing conditions, with no bathroom or scullery or indoor sink. She suffered from inflamed eye, 'bad rheumatism', decayed teeth and a prolapsed uterus.[124] In south Wales, 'Mrs. Y... has five children of whom the eldest is 4½. As her only difficulty she says, "I have had children too quickly after each other and with young children they take up all my time. Am unable to breast feed". The Health Visitor says "Mrs. Y. looks in very poor condition, she says she always feels tired and disinclined to do anything. I think she was probably anaemic before marriage and five pregnancies in five years have drained her vitality."'[125] Thus, the unsatisfactory working condition of miners' wives, the strain of attempting to cope with such onerous burdens and the effects of numerous pregnancies in quick succession resulted in a high toll of impairment for miners' wives, perhaps a higher toll than their husbands experienced in the notoriously dangerous coal industry.

Employment of disabled people

The impairments of mineworkers were many and varied, but it would be a mistake to think that these necessarily caused their exclusion from the industry. Throughout the period, impaired individuals found work both underground and on the surface. Certainly, large numbers of such people were excluded from work in the coal industry in a variety of ways both deliberate and systematic, especially when the state of the economy or other factors gave the employers an advantage in the labour market. Nevertheless, large numbers of people were not disabled from working in the industry as a result of their impairment and remained an important part of the labour force, with opportunities, even if they were limited, for work in certain parts of the industry.

Disabled individuals were employed in the coal industry in a variety of ways throughout the nineteenth century, but the systems of statutory compensation which emerged in the late nineteenth century, and which form much of the discussion of the second chapter of this book, were crucially important. The first of these was the Employers' Liability Act in 1880, which recognised employers' responsibility for accidents in the workplace and was superseded by the more encompassing Workmen's Compensation Act of

1897, which led to the first major system of state compensation for injury and disease. However, in the first place not every disabled person in employment after 1897 came within the remit of the compensation system. While not typical of the experience of most disabled people in the coalfields, many miners completed lifetimes of work underground with a congenital disability, or one which did not arise from their work. An example of the former was Thomas Sharrock, a blind miner who worked in Pemberton, Wigan. His story made it to the Dundee *Evening Telegraph*, which honoured Sharrock for his thirty-year career as a 'hooker-on' and 'putter', key underground jobs. The story used the 'overcoming' trope that 'his infirmity has not debarred him from participating in some life', including being Grand Master of his local Oddfellows.[126]

In other instances, miners hid the fact or extent of their impairment in order to avoid the unwanted attentions of a manager, or else to convince a potential employer of their employability. One miner, described as a 'cripple with a stiff leg', remembered how he attempted to conceal his impairment: 'Well, if you walk along the top of the P. D. "Pit" with your hands in your pockets they will make you pull them out, and look at them and when they see me walk stiff they won't give me a start.' Miners with hidden impairments also cropped up in accounts of accidents in Inspectors of Mines' reports. For example, the 1913 reports of W. Walker, Inspector of Mines for the Scotland division, noted a series of deaths that year from railways, sidings and tramways. 'Three of the persons killed suffered from physical disabilities', his report noted, 'one being very deaf, one blind in one eye, and the other old and infirm.' The report concluded by relating their disability to their area of employment: 'Such persons should not be employed in places where there are moving wagons.'[127] Whether these workers concealed their impairments from the colliery company or whether the company itself employed these men in contravention of the rules, a certain deception had taken place in these instances, and disabled miners passed as non-disabled.

Apart from miners with congenital impairments, and apart from those who concealed an impairment from colliery officials or the mines inspectors, another group of workers were perceived as impaired and were disabled by the attitudes others held of them. This attitude was summarised by Henry Barnett in his 1909 work, *Accidental Injuries to Workmen*:

> The workman may be physically fit to earn the same wages as before the accident, but may not be able to obtain employment in consequence, say, of the loss of two or three fingers. The disinclination of employers to give work to maimed and mutilated men is well known. There is here a loss of wage-earning power if the inability to work is due to the injuries.[128]

Instances involving congenital or concealed impairments are, by their nature, impossible to quantify, but they clearly existed in the industry and were the experience of a certain number of the inhabitants of coalfield communities. Far more visible, industrially, politically and medically, were the workers who came within the remit of the workmen's compensation legislation first passed in 1897. Indeed, that piece of legislation and the numerous subsequent amendments to it were crucial in determining the attitudes of employers, government and the medical establishment and, more importantly, the experiences of disabled miners. It might even be argued that while the First World War and the fate of disabled veterans were crucial to changes in the understanding of and responses to impairment in British society more generally, it was the workmen's compensation legislation passed a number of decades earlier that was transformative for the inhabitants of industrial communities.[129] The legislation shaped experiences, helped to define notions of normalcy and disability and determined the industrial relations of impairment.

Both before and after the 1897 Act, some workers adjusted their working practices upon becoming impaired, came to rely on the support of workmates a little more or else accepted the reductions in their productivity and income that the impairment entailed. Such workers did not often come within view of employers, unions or any other agency but were present in the industry. More obvious were those individuals so impaired that a more significant change needed to be made to their working lives. Under the regime of the compensation legislation such men were termed 'partial compensation men' and 'partially disabled', since they were sufficiently impaired to be prevented from continuing their previous roles, but not so impaired as to be prevented from working altogether, and were shifted to 'light work' in the colliery. In such 'light work', they earned an income, albeit less than the one earned in their previous role, but were also paid a sum of compensation to reflect, at least partially, their reduced earning capacity. Each miner was unique in the character of the impairment they experienced and the subsequent employment trajectory they followed as attempts were made to match their 'light work' to their particular impairments (though, of course, employers had varying degrees of flexibility, or indeed none at all). This provision is evident in the miners who came within the remit of the Scottish Coal Workers' Compensation Scheme. For example, James Dalrymple, who had contracted miners' nystagmus, was considered 'fit for work on the surface', but anything underground would have caused 'aggravation' of his condition.[130] Another miner, Charles Robertson, with a strained back, was deemed by the medical referee to 'never be fit for face work' again and 'not fit to walk far underground'. Robertson was instead posted to work at the 'picking tables', sorting coal, while also receiving partial compensation.[131]

Sometimes light work could be provided after an extended period away from the mine. Samuel Edmunds, a miner from Penrhiw-Fer, Rhondda, recalled the situation of his father:

> Dad had his hand off, left hand, in the mines with the tram. He was a haulier and lost his hand. There was no compensation as such in those days, but he did get twenty-five pounds for the loss of his hand. He was brought home. I was in the house at the time, this was around 1901. They took him to hospital to have it off. As he couldn't go back down the pit at that time, he bought two horses and a brake and after getting a licence from the Council he started as a brake-driver, out all day collecting people from the train station. Take them home he would, Dinas Station to Pen-y-graig. Then he'd take boozers home from the pubs. Fridays, Saturdays, he always got paid, he always got his fare even if they were laugh-drunk. When the trams came about 1910, his business was done away with. He had to go back to the mine. They gave him a light job underground.[132]

That job was to help put dust alongside the roads underground, intended to help prevent explosions. The father died at fifty-seven, 'they said it was asthma then, but now they know it's silicosis.'[133]

The numbers of men employed on 'light work' demonstrate the continued and active participation of disabled people in the workplace; but, while the retention of work in the industry would have been welcomed in many cases as the best option for the individual from an economic point of view, it also brought problems for many men and they faced new difficulties in their altered situation. Most of these problems came from the scrutiny of employers and their medical appointees in the compensation system, and the pressure they applied to these 'partial compensation' men. Thus, when the Scottish brusher Kenneth Sparling started his new job at the picking tables, his doctor thought 'he might be able to do a little more if he were trying, and if he were forcibly extending and moving the contracted fingers'.[134] In another example, Matthew Glass, a hewer at Hetton Colliery near Durham, had his left leg amputated after being knocked down and run over by a set of tubs at work. He took up 'light work' sorting coal on the belts, but when he 'could not manage' the colliery management refused to pay full compensation.[135] Medical Referees certified that he was able to work as long as his artificial limb was of sufficient quality. Though he was not able to work at the conveyor belts sorting coal, the Referee suggested that 'he could … carry on such work if he were provided with a seat or he could undertake a gate man's job or work in the lamp cabin.'[136] In such instances, therefore, the transition to 'light work' could involve real difficulty and new problems that had to be negotiated. Some attempt was occasionally made to ease an injured man's return to work, but the nature of these industrial workplaces proved disabling in many instances.[137]

Undoubtedly, the question of returning to work was a complex experience for recently impaired miners and some were quite clear that they did not wish to return to their former jobs but, instead, would prefer some other employment of 'light work' or else the payment of full compensation. The interplay of these factors was seen in 1926, when the Ocean Coal Company won a case at Pontypridd County Court against a miner who had lost his eye in the pit. The miner was fighting for the right to refuse to return to work 'on the ground that he had a genuine fear that if he went underground to work at the face, he would lose the sight of the remaining eye and thus become totally blind'. The court ruled in favour of the company, thus denying the miner compensation and forcing his return to the coalface, and the judge noted that 'a one-eyed man is not prevented from following his ordinary occupation below ground'.[138] A former faceworker in Fife who had lost the vision in his left eye took up a job as a roadsman and repairer in 1926, having been 'unwilling to work at the face':

> he had been able to adjust himself fairly well to his altered circumstances and to do that work, but ... he found difficulty in judging distances, particularly in low places, and had not the same confidence in moving about, or the same readiness in his work as formerly ... that his main reason for declining to return to the face was that injuries to the eyes were more liable to occur than at roadsman's or repairer's work, which was the case, and if he received an injury to his right eye such as he sustained to his left, he would be practically blind for life.[139]

The miner fought against the decision of face work as 'suitable employment', which was eventually agreed. Yet, overall, the *Colliery Guardian* article argued that 'as a rule [the one-eyed miner] is able sooner or later to return to his work at the face, providing the remaining eye is sound and its vision normal'.[140] In another case, a miner with a crushed middle finger was declared 'fit for his former work as a miner' but 'refuse[d] to start' at his old position underground and has 'caused the greatest possible trouble in this case'; the company proceeded to 'terminate the right to compensation'.[141] Bert Coombes describes the experience of returning to work too soon after dislocating his knee joint trying to free it from under a collapsed pit roof, due to the inadequacy of the compensation he received: 'They had a way of assessing our earnings and paying an amount that was roughly about half of what I would have earned if working. So to add to my suffering I had the misery of knowing that we were going behind financially; therefore I could not afford to stay in the house until I had recovered.' He was injured in the same, vulnerable knee in the first week back: 'That caused me to have another seven weeks at home, and the insurance people were quite convinced that I enjoyed getting knocked about.'[142] These examples show the complexity of any return to work for impaired miners. On the one hand, they show that some injured miners had the opportunity and the desire to return to their former jobs or to other roles in the industry, but they also demonstrate the fears, risks and difficulties that a return to work sometimes involved.

Such illustrative examples are instructive, but they conceal the broader factors that influenced the likelihood of success in gaining 'light work'. The extent to which impaired individuals were able to find work or to retain employment in the coal industry was determined by a number of broader considerations far beyond their control. Two factors in particular conditioned attitudes towards the employment of impaired workers and influenced their chances of gaining or retaining employment: the workings of the statutory system of workmen's compensation and changes to it over time, on the one hand, and the state of the economy and the fortunes of the coal industry, on the other hand. Notwithstanding the responsibility, and economic sense, of companies providing 'light work' to men impaired in their own employment, the system of workmen's compensation instituted by the legislation passed in 1897 made the employment of impaired workers far less attractive to new employers, since it was believed that such workers posed a higher risk of accidents. It was feared that old, unfit and impaired workers would serve to increase compensation liabilities because of their greater likelihood of suffering or causing accidents.[143] This belief was clearly evident in the decisions of many employers to discard 'old and infirm' miners in the wake of the passage of the 1897 Act. The legislation was implemented in July 1898 and, almost immediately, something like a thousand workers in the south Wales coalfield lost their employment.[144] One trade union official in the region described the employers' action as 'tyrannical' and maintained that 'These men had spent their strength, their substance, and their lives in the service of the company, and now they were cast adrift on the mercy of the world.'[145]

This action on the part of the coalowners in south Wales does not seem to have been replicated in the other coalfields at this time. Industrial relations were particularly poor in south Wales, far more so than in the north-east of England, where a joint Arbitration Committee was established by coalowners and trade union representatives to hear and decide cases that would otherwise have been submitted to the county courts.[146] That is not to argue that this pressure on the employment of impaired workers was absent from regions other than south Wales. In 1912, for example, managers at the Consett Iron Company in Durham wrote to the under-manager of its colliery at Chopwell to inform him that he needed to dismiss a certain number of workmen and it was old and impaired workers who were to be selected for dismissal: 'There is a decision made to retire men that are considered "useless" – taken mainly from the aged or infirm working at the Pits, in an attempt to reduce the number of employed in "off-hand" labour.'[147]

Nevertheless, despite such instances, and despite the variations in practice between coalfields, the generally buoyant state of the coal industry in the period up to 1914 meant that opportunities for impaired miners were not completely absent. The precise number of opportunities, and the character of the work that was available to them, varied from place to place and over time. The daily working requirements of a colliery determined the numbers and grades of workmen required to produce coal, and there was perhaps a finite number of 'light employment' positions to be had at any one colliery. Angela V. John has found, for example, that women surface workers were seen to be 'usurping the rightful jobs of [disabled] men'.[148]

The situation in the decades after 1914 was far more complex. The workings of the compensation system, in addition to a more difficult economic context and strained industrial relations, all had a bearing on the experiences of disabled workers in the coal industry. This complexity was evident in the First World War. Upon the outbreak of war, large numbers of men left the coal industry to enlist in the army, with 313,000 miners signed up by February 1916.[149] Despite some initial uncertainty in the industry as it adjusted to different market conditions, the demand for coal grew during the course of the war and was crucial to the war effort. Indeed, the coal industry became a reserved occupation and miners, especially faceworkers, were discouraged from enlistment and, later, exempted from conscription. There was no official policy within the industry, or emanating from government, to replace workers in the industry with impaired ex-miners, and so very little direct reference to the practice can be found. Nevertheless, the pressure of labour shortages led employers to draw upon the reserve army of disabled workers, as they did in other times of labour shortage, and offered the prospect of increased opportunity for employment to men who would have struggled to gain work otherwise. One of the few to articulate the practice was Frederick Mills, managing director of the Ebbw Vale Steel, Iron and Coal Company in south Wales, who stated at a recruiting meeting that 'There was a large number of men available from the surface labour class whose places could be taken by older men, wounded men, and men who had gone into retirement, but who had come out to take their share.'[150]

With military conscription in 1916 and, more especially, 'comb-outs'[151] of the coal industry from 1917 onwards, the opportunities for impaired workers increased and larger numbers were absorbed by the industry. A comb-out of the coal industry in the early part of 1917, for example, focused on three classes of workmen, one of which was unskilled surface workers, which would have multiplied the opportunities for employment for impaired workers since these were typically the types of jobs done as 'light work' under the workmen's compensation system.[152] Another of the three categories of workers that were to be subject to this comb-out were workers who had entered the industry since August 1915. The military authorities were convinced that many men had entered the coal industry, as a protected industry, in order to avoid being conscripted, but trade union officials pointed out that this group of workmen also included former miners who, suffering the effects of an injury or an occupational disease, had left the industry for some time in order to recover or else had pursued another calling as a result of impairment but had been forced back after their ventures had failed. William Brace, representing the Home Department in a meeting with members of the executive committee of the Miners' Federation of Great Britain (MFGB) in February 1917, but drawing upon his own mining background, pointed out the ways in which such men returned to the industry in this period:

> a man may have nystagmus, or he may have asthma, and instead of going on light employment, or working on the surface of the pit, he may go to a little shop, say a barber's shop, or something like that, and give himself a chance to recover. That is the type of man I have in mind. You and I know scores of men of that character.[153]

In that same meeting Williams Abraham, representing south Wales on the MFGB deputation, and William Straker, from Northumberland, also mentioned men who worked as insurance agents. Such movement out of and then back into the coal industry would have been true of other periods of time, but the dislocation caused to the economy by the First World War might have been sufficient to force or entice such individuals to return to the industry in greater numbers at that time.

Comb-outs of the coal industry were focused on particular classes of workmen and avoided the conscription of faceworkers, who were crucial to hopes of increasing production, but, in doing so, faced the law of diminishing returns. This was, of course, because such surface work tended to be filled increasingly by disabled workers during this period. Indeed, by April 1917 James Winstone, a miners' leader from south Wales, opined that a further comb-out of surface workers would have been futile and that something approximating 70 per cent of all such surface workers in south Wales were medically unfit for service in the armed forces.[154] Robert Smillie, president of the MFGB, estimated that only one in four of all men returned to the military as a result of comb-outs were fit to serve, thereby again demonstrating the extent to which impaired workers had entered the industry in large numbers during and as a result of the war.[155] Apart from impaired workers who came back into the industry during the war years, some injured soldiers were also placed in the coal industry after a period of convalescence so as to free up other men to join the armed forces.

This, according to the Northumberland representative on the Executive Committee of the MFGB, J. Cairns, was the practice in his district, and he estimated that there were as many as twenty such individuals in some pits in the area.[156] Therefore, there seems to be good reason to believe that the opportunities available to impaired workers for employment in the coal industry increased during the First World War and that large numbers either returned after being invalided out of the industry previously or else remained after a point when they would have been forced to leave the industry at any other period.

The interwar economic depression, however, changed the context in which disabled workers sought to retain or gain employment and, generally, served to make the retention of work more difficult. The large ranks of the unemployed meant that employers were given an advantage in the labour market and were able to actively choose between workers rather than merely accept the men that were available to them. In the context of the workmen's compensation legislation and contemporary ideas about efficiency and productivity, impaired workers found it difficult to defend their place in the labour market. In addition, economic depression lessened the numbers of possible vacancies for partially disabled men to fill, since not only did many collieries close, but many others worked short time, possibly two or three days in the week, or else witnessed the closure of one or two districts underground, with a resultant decrease in the labour force. As the labour market contracted, so the opportunities for 'light work' suitable for partially disabled men lessened. This was also exacerbated by the process of mechanisation, since it greatly altered the working practices on the surface and reduced the need for labour relative to the amount of work done.[157] In a discussion in the House of Commons in 1938, for example,

> Mr George Hall asks Minister of Labour whether he is aware of the large number of unemployed miners who are partially disabled owing to accidents received in the course of their employment, and who are now, owing to the prolonged depression, unable to obtain employment in the coal-mining industry.[158]

While disabled miners all faced difficulties during this period of economic depression, the situation was especially marked for miners with nystagmus, since four-fifths of all colliery labour worked underground and these positions were unsuitable for such men; the smaller number of surface jobs offered the only opportunities available to these men. If a nystagmus sufferer was unable to get a job on the surface at his own colliery, the chances of gaining employment on the surface of another colliery were virtually non-existent, since employers tended to reserve such positions for 'light employment men' from their existing workforces.

More than that, the particular character of nystagmus as a condition meant that sufferers were further disadvantaged, even relative to other impaired men. Some employers, often pressured by their mutual indemnity or insurance companies, adopted an unofficial policy of refusing to re-employ sufferers from nystagmus – certainly this was the approach taken by Lanarkshire coal companies in the interwar period.[159] The effect was that in September 1936 a greater proportion of miners certified with nystagmus and eligible for partial compensation were unemployed in Lanarkshire than in any other coalfield in Britain. At that time 56.9 per cent of all miners with nystagmus were unemployed, while 37.2 per cent were in light employment on the surface and only 5.9 per cent were employed underground. The figures for Scotland were 83.3, 16.7 and 0 per cent, respectively. In fact, the other two case study coalfields also had relatively poor records as far as finding employment for partial compensation men was concerned (south Wales: 76.2 per cent out of work, 18.9 per cent employed on the surface and 4.9 per cent underground; the north-east of England: 81.8 per cent, 14.2 per cent and 4 per cent, respectively). The three coalfields were the three worst in Britain in this regard and stood far behind Lancashire and Cheshire, Derbyshire and Nottinghamshire, where between three-quarters and two-thirds of all sufferers of nystagmus were re-engaged.[160]

The case of Lanarkshire demonstrates the particular ways in which the implementation of the compensation legislation and the effects of the economic depression combined to create distinct problems for this group of disabled miners relative to miners with other impairments. By the terms of the legislation, 'nystagmic' miners were eligible for full or partial compensation, depending on the severity of their impairment, and a responsibility was placed on employers to provide light employment for those paid partial compensation. This was not a binding commitment, however, and employers, driven by self-interest or else concerned at perceived abuses, often looked to minimise any such responsibility. Employers in Lanarkshire were keen to avoid the employment of miners previously certified with nystagmus in underground work, since they found that a reoccurrence of the condition was quite possible, and so required that miners taken on should sign a declaration that they had not previously been certified with nystagmus.[161] Thus, a great deal of hardship was caused to sufferers of nystagmus by the workings of the compensation system and the economic depression. The effects on the individuals concerned were significant: a judge at the Pontypridd County Court who heard the case of such a nystagmus sufferer in 1924 described such men as 'human derelicts', devoid of any hope of employment and treated poorly by a compensation system that could not meet the particular needs of individuals in a period of mass unemployment.[162] Labour

MP Jack Lawson remarks on the difficulty for men with nystagmus to find work, in his novel *Under the Wheels* (1934):

> Harry Rew was the victim of nystagmus. 'Eyestagmus,' he calls it, unconscious that he had murdered a strictly scientific word, and at the same time given a lesson to medical science in scientific accuracy, for nystagmus is a disease of the eyes. Harry Rew had looked at coal so long that it made his eyes jump to look at it in the pit. If he had kept on looking at it he would have gone blind. So they gave him the 'caller's' job at bank. Lucky Harry! To-day he would have been given a few shillings a week, scrapped and lost among the statistics in the Minister of Mines' Report. But in those slow, unprogressive days he was given a job in the lamp cabin and a hammer to disturb the sleepers of Westburn.[163]

Lawson is clearly making a pointed remark about the contrast between the 'slow, unprogressive' past, where men nevertheless had opportunities that are no longer available now that so many are 'scrapped and lost among the statistics in the Minister of Mines' Report'. A positive view of the economic opportunities of the past is not uncommon in coalfields literature of the 1930s, when unemployment was so high and the writers want to emphasise the contrast between a fully employed, productive industrial area and an unproductive and declining industrial community. As in the example above, the inclusion of both older and disabled miners in the colliery workforce is used as a positive emblem of the idealised past, as compared to the present situation of high unemployment among all men, with almost no opportunities for older or disabled workers.

The presence of large numbers of disabled former miners in the ranks of the unemployed showed up in various social surveys on unemployment as greater attention was paid to the social characteristics of the unemployed and to the factors that led to joblessness in the first place. One survey carried out in Merthyr Tydfil in 1929, for example, found that 60 per cent of the unemployed men in the town were over the age of forty and noted that a large proportion of them were 'physically unfit'.[164] This seems to have been a particular problem in south Wales, relative to other coalfields. The social survey on unemployment conducted on behalf of the Pilgrim Trust in the 1930s, for example, found that a high proportion of the unemployed men in the Rhondda valleys sample suffered some form of physical impairment, largely as a result of nystagmus and 'silicosis'. Indeed, the report suggested both that the proportion was greater than might be expected in the working population generally and also that it was higher than was the case in other depressed areas. Indeed, another of the report's six case study areas was Crook, a mining community in Durham, and the report found that the physical condition of unemployed men was 'higher than elswhere' and that 'there is appreciably less of the physical disability (including industrial disease)' than was the case in the south Wales case study.[165] This suggests, perhaps, that injury, disease and impairment were greater in south Wales than in other coalfields, which, given the higher accident rates and greater levels of occupational disease, is not wholly unreasonable. In addition, the higher level of disability revealed in the Rhondda relative to Crook might also have been due to the greater severity of the economic depression in south Wales – larger proportions of men were made unemployed and thereby became a problem as they came within sight of such investigations into long-term unemployment. Another factor was possibly the more settled industrial relations in the north-east of England, where the Arbitration Committee took some of the heat out of the issue of disabled miners and where more paternalistic employers continued to recognise their responsibilities to men injured in their employ.

The return of better conditions from the mid- to late 1930s, and especially the boost given to the industry with the build-up to, and the start of, the Second World War allowed greater numbers of older or disabled men to be reabsorbed into the industry. In an article on the south Wales coalfield in the *Spectator* published in 1945, for example, it was pointed out that unemployment had fallen from quarter of a million in 1933 to barely 15,000 by 1945 and that something like 10,000 individuals 'pronounced unfit for industrial work (some hadn't had a job for 15 years) have worked again as watchmen, sweepers-up, and on odd light jobs in factories'.[166] A great many of these worked outside the coal industry, of course, and certainly the Miners' Federation in south Wales noted the difficulty experienced in getting light employment for all those who required it.[167] In addition, where it was not possible to find light employment for impaired former miners in the coal industry, Regional Controllers for the Ministry of Labour and National Service would place the individual in appropriate work in another industry.[168] Nevertheless, labour shortages in the coal industry and the particular circumstances in the industry during war conditions were still responsible for a large part of this increase in employment for impaired individuals. A miners' leader in south Wales suggested that disabled men continued to be employed underground where previously they would have finished work: 'It's only the Essential Works Order which keeps a lot of those anthracite miners down the pit at all,' he stated.[169]

A complicating factor in the employment of impaired miners in the war years, at least in south Wales, were changes to the compensation rules relative to pneumoconiosis. By the Coal Mining Industry (Pneumoconiosis) Compensation measure of 1943, those miners certified as suffering from the disease were stopped from working in industry.[170] The effects on pneumoconiotic miners and their families were devastating. By end of 1945, 12,000 men in south Wales had been certified with the disease, and they were being certified at rate of 100 a week by that time. Of this number, it was found that two-thirds were under fifty years of age and one quarter under forty and therefore still of working age and, quite likely, had families to support.[171] This 'exodus' from the industry in mono-industrial communities in south Wales, where little alternative employment was available, caused considerable hardship and 'thousands of families' were forced to rely on compensation payments and unemployment benefits.[172] Whereas something like 70 per cent of the certified pneumoconiotics found alternative employment outside the coal industry in the period of full employment during the latter years of the war, the figure was as low as 30–40 per cent in the late 1930s, and again by 1946 when Royal Ordinance Factories started closing.[173] It is little wonder that one of these 'forgotten men' was able to characterise himself and his fellow sufferers as 'the living dead' of the coalfield, 'forgotten after a lifetime of service', 'sentenced to a hopeless, destitute and empty future'.[174]

Nevertheless, a major change in the employment prospects of pneumoconiotic miners came with the passage of a measure in 1948 that allowed some certified men to return to work in the pits. This meant that 'seriously incapacitated' pneumoconiotics were permitted by the legislation to return to work in 'approved dust condition' on the surface, while men with lesser degrees of incapacitation were allowed to return to underground work.[175] In the absence of alternative sources of employment, and perhaps for a number of cultural reasons relating to work in a solidaristic and mutualistic work environment, large numbers of impaired men returned to the coal industry in the late 1940s and 1950s, so that by 1960 20,000 pneumoconiotic miners were employed in the coal industry.[176]

The miners' unions had campaigned for the nationalisation of the coal industry for many decades before this was finally achieved in 1947, and had always argued that a nationalised industry would replace the profit motive of private owners with a commitment both to the well-being of the nation and to the industry's workers.[177] This change in ownership was also accompanied by a serious shortage of labour and an energy crisis which caused serious political difficulties to the Labour government, so that efforts were made to recruit as many workers into the industry as possible.[178] More than that, while it was not perfect, trade union leaders nevertheless discerned a different atmosphere in the early months of nationalisation and a better prospect for disabled workers. Not only were there fewer disputes over compensation rights and payments to disabled workers, but there was also a greater commitment to finding employment for partially disabled men within the industry. The National Union of Mineworkers (NUM) was encouraged by the 'increasing efforts' of the National Coal Board (NCB) to find employment for such men and, indeed, the commitment at some collieries to find them as well-paid work as possible. The South Wales

Area of the NUM, for example, noted the case of James Morgan, Gelli Colliery, Rhondda, who, having lost his sight as a result of an accident, was provided with training and given employment as a telephone operator.[179] This commitment on the part of the NCB also extended to efforts to provide employment in ancillary industries connected to the coal industry, such as in the production of mining machinery.[180]

Nevertheless, this commitment on the part of the newly nationalised industry came up against the finite number of 'light employment' positions in the industry, as it always did, and many impaired miners continued to face unemployment as a result of their situation, much to the chagrin of trade union leaders. In 1947 an MP asked the Minster of Fuel and Power about the fate of unemployed ex-miners suffering minor impairments but fit for surface work, and was told rather vaguely that 'an effort [will be] made to find work for them of a character suitable to their conditions'. He noted the rejection of many on medical grounds, there being 'considerable difficulty … because in the main, these persons are suitable only for work on the surface and, as we are not in need of more workpeople for surface work, it is not easy to re-employ them'.[181]

The effects of the wartime labour shortage and the dire need to increase production focused attention on the recruitment of young and fit men for face work, but part of this strategy involved the recruitment of 'older or unfit men' in order to free up 'on-cost' workers (i.e. underground workers who did not work at the face) to move to face work. A large proportion of the 'unfit' workers would have been former miners still being demobilised from the armed forces and, more importantly, former miners recruited from other industries: in 1947 alone, 41,000 ex-miners returned to the industry in answer to the desperate call for workers.[182] More tellingly, the NCB changed its approach to former miners who had applied to return to the coal industry but who were rejected by colliery doctors as being unfit. Such men had claimed compensation for industrial disease or injuries previously but had commuted their claims for lump-sum settlements and, such was the desperate need for workers, the NCB advised its doctors to now accept them, despite continued impairments.[183]

Therefore, the fortunes of disabled miners varied with those of the industry itself from 1880 to 1948 and with changes to the system of workmen's compensation. These broader factors determined the context in which such miners attempted to retain their employment after becoming impaired, and decided the labour market in which the value of their labour to employers increased or decreased over time. More generally, the extent and character of the labour of disabled workers, while not uncomplicated, demonstrates that while the coal industry created impairment on a massive scale, and in a variety of ways, it did not necessarily disable impaired workers from employment. Impaired workers were indeed marginalised in this particular area of the industrial economy, and faced economic hardship, prejudice and a loss of status, but they were not driven out of the industry completely and continued to constitute a prominent and visible presence in the workforce.

Conclusion

Disabled workers have largely been either left out of economic history or discussed only in terms of their exclusion. Histories of industrial Britain have largely ignored the interaction of impairment with the economic process of industrialisation, and the nuances of the economic position of disabled workers are very often overlooked. This period of late industrialisation, from the late nineteenth century through to the mid-twentieth century, was an eventful one for disabled people, as welfare innovations, fluctuations in economic circumstances and levels of employment, as well as changes in attitudes to accidents and safety, constantly changed the context in which disabled workers attempted to make their way in life. Furthermore, variations between regions and industries, and over time, ensured that there was no homogeneous experience of industrialisation for disabled people in the British coalfields, but that experiences were influenced by an array of factors and considerations. The experiences of disabled workers in the coal industry also demonstrate that, while their lives were subject to quite severe restrictions and difficulties, they were not wholly without agency and that they continued to aspire to a decent standard of living, a comfortable family life, and a degree of self-respect and consideration from others.

Notes

1. For example, see Michael Oliver, *The Politics of Disablement: A Sociological Approach* (Basingstoke: Palgrave Macmillan, 1990); Victor Finkelstein, *Attitudes and Disabled People: Issues for Discussion* (New York: International Exchange of Information in Rehabilitation, 1980).
2. N. K. Buxton, *The Economic Development of the British Coal Industry from Industrial Revolution to the Present Day* (London: Batsford Academic, 1978), p. 98.
3. John Benson, *British Coalminers in the Nineteenth Century: A Social History* (Dublin: Gill and Macmillan, 1980).
4. Benson, *British Coalminers in the Nineteenth Century*, p. 7.
5. Benson, *British Coalminers in the Nineteenth Century*, pp. 9–12.
6. Benson, *British Coalminers in the Nineteenth Century*, pp. 216–17.
7. Benson, *British Coalminers in the Nineteenth Century*, pp. 17, 216–17.
8. Buxton, *The Economic Development of the British Coal Industry*, p. 85.

9 Benson, *British Coalminers in the Nineteenth Century*, pp. 22–5.
10 Barry Supple, *The History of the British Coal Industry, Volume 4. 1913–1946: The Political Economy of Decline* (Oxford: Clarendon Press, 1987), p. 10.
11 John Stevenson and Chris Cook, *Britain in the Depression: Society and Politics 1929–39* (Harlow: Longman Group, 1994 edition), pp. 66–70; *Report of the Commissioner for the Special Areas in England and Wales* [Cmd. 5896], 1938–39, xii, pp. 95–6.
12 Sidney Pollard, *The Development of the British Economy 1914–1990* (London: Arnold, 1997 edition), pp. 35–6, 49–52, 140–2, 168–9.
13 An overview of coalfields literature in the period 1880–1948 is given in Chapter 6.
14 Such as Joseph Skipsey, or Thomas 'Tommy' Armstrong.
15 There were a number of Methodist ministers who were also novelists who wrote about the coalfields, such as Ramsay Guthrie (pseudonym Rev. J. G. Bowran, Primitive Methodist), Hugh Gilmore (Primitive Methodist), Harry Lindsay (pseudonym of Henry Lindsay Hudson, Wesleyan Methodist), Samuel Horton (Primitive Methodist), W. M Patterson (Primitive Methodist) and John Thomas (Calvinist and later Independent, and Welsh-language novelist).
16 For example, Richard Cope Morgan's biography *The Life of Richard Weaver, the Converted Collier* (London: Morgan & Chase, 1861), Howard Peases's *The White-Faced Priest and Other Northumbrian Episodes* (London: Gay & Bird, 1896) and Owd Mo's *From Coal-Pit to Joyful News Mission* (Rochdale: Joyful New Book Depot, c.1890).
17 For example, Thomas Mitchell, W. A. Hammond, Joseph Johnson and Charles H. Kelly.
18 For example, Independent Labour Party Publications, Lawrence and Wishart (initially associated with the Communist Party), Gollancz, and Michael Joseph Ltd.
19 Jack Jones, *Unfinished Journey* (London: Hamish Hamilton, 1938), p. 282.
20 Jones, *Unfinished Journey*, p. 291.
21 Roy A. Church, *The History of the British Coal Industry Volume 3: 1830–1913: Victorian Pre-Eminence* (Oxford: Clarendon Press, 1986), p. 209.
22 The following treatment of mining occupations is dependent on Benson, *British Coalminers in the Nineteenth Century*, pp. 28–63; Church, *The History of the British Coal Industry, Volume 3*, pp. 201–15; information extracted from the *Reports of the Inspectors of (Coal) Mines, 1894*, [C. 7667], 1895, xxii, presented on 'Mining Occupations', Durham Mining Museum website, http://www.dmm.org.uk/educate/mineocc.htm, accessed 21 October 2016; and James Barrowman, *Glossary of Scotch Mining Terms* (Hamilton, 1886), available at Scottish Mining Website, www.scottishmining.co.uk/Indexes/Barrowman.html, accessed 21 October 2016.
23 Martin Daunton, 'Down the Pit: Work in the Great Northern and South Wales Coalfields, 1870–1914', *Economic History Review*, 34:4 (1981), p. 585; Church, *The History of the British Coal Industry, Volume 3*, pp. 211–13.

24 Daunton, 'Down the Pit', p. 585; Church, *The History of the British Coal Industry, Volume 3*, pp. 207–8; Alan Campbell, *The Scottish Miners, 1874–1939. Volume One: Industry, Work and Community* (Aldershot: Ashgate, 2000), pp. 78–9.
25 Benson, *British Coalminers in the Nineteenth Century*, p. 29.
26 Tom Hanlin, *Yesterday Will Return* (New York: The Viking Press, 1946), p. 78.
27 N. K. Buxton, *The Economic Development of the British Coal Industry from Industrial Revolution to the Present Day* (London: Batsford Academic, 1978), pp. 109, 112; David Greasley, 'Fifty Years of Coal-Mining Productivity: The Record of the British Coal Industry before 1939', *Journal of Economic History*, 50:4 (1990), p. 883.
28 Greasley, 'Fifty Years of Coal-Mining Productivity', p. 896.
29 Buxton, *The Economic Development of the British Coal Industry*, p. 114–15.
30 Buxton, *The Economic Development of the British Coal Industry*, p. 115.
31 Supple, *The History of the British Coal Industry, Volume 4. 1913–1946: The Political Economy of Decline*, p. 27.
32 *Report of the Royal Commission on the Coal Industry (1925)* (London, HMSO, 1926), p. 192.
33 *News Chronicle*, 18 February 1936.
34 B. L. Coombes, *These Poor Hands: The Autobiography of a Miner Working in South Wales, with an Introduction by Bill Jones and Chris Williams* (Cardiff: University of Wales Press, 2002), p. 74.
35 Coombes, *These Poor Hands*, p. 82.
36 Coombes, *These Poor Hands*, p. 82.
37 Coombes, *These Poor Hands*, p. 82.
38 Coombes, *These Poor Hands*, p. 84.
39 Coombes, *These Poor Hands*, p. 84.
40 Lewis Jones, *Cwmardy* (London: Lawrence & Wishart, 1937), pp. 397–8; Sid Chaplin, *The Thin Seam* (London: Phoenix House, 1950), pp. 141–9.
41 Gwyn Jones, *Times Like These* (London: Victor Gollancz, 1979 [1936]), p. 287.
42 Chaplin, *The Thin Seam*, p. 89.
43 See pages 35–6.
44 Chaplin, *The Thin Seam*, p. 92.
45 Daunton, 'Down the Pit'.
46 *South Wales Worker*, 30 May 1914, p. 6.
47 'Cavil' was the word used in the north-east of England for the working area allocated to hewers underground and drawn for by lots.
48 John Swan, *The Mad Miner* (London: Houghton Publishing Co, 1933), pp. 171–2.
49 See, for example, Miners' Federation of Great Britain, *Annual Conference held at the Central Hall, Bath Street, Glasgow, on Tuesday, July 24th, 1917, and following days*, pp. 43–6, 87. In this instance, the resolution was moved by a south Wales delegate and seconded by a colleague from Scotland.
50 Benson, *British Coalminers in the Nineteenth Century*, pp. 55–6.
51 Quoted in Campbell, *The Scottish Miners, 1874–1939. Volume One*, p. 82.
52 Benson, *British Coalminers in the Nineteenth Century*, pp. 58–9; Campbell, *The Scottish Miners, 1874–1939. Volume One*, pp. 82–3.

53 B. L. Coombes, *Those Clouded Hills* (London: Cobbett Publishing Co., 1944), p. 27, also p. 29; see also Benson, *British Coalminers in the Nineteenth Century*, p. 59.
54 Daunton, 'Down the Pit', p. 587; see also Benson, *British Coalminers in the Nineteenth Century*, p. 56.
55 Daunton, 'Down the Pit', pp. 587–8.
56 Church, *The History of the British Coal Industry, Volume 3*, p. 257.
57 Benson, *British Coalminers in the Nineteenth Century*, p. 56; Campbell, *The Scottish Miners, 1874–1939. Volume One*, p. 83.
58 Daunton, 'Down the Pit', p. 589.
59 M. W. Kirby, *The British Coalmining Industry, 1870–1946: A Political and Economic History* (London: Macmillan, 1977), pp. 68, 24.
60 See for example, *The Eight Hours Movement (Coal Mines): Proceedings at a Joint Conference of Representative Coal Owners and the Miners' Federation of Great Britain held at the Westminster Palace Hotel, London, S.W., on the 21st Jnuary, and the 11th February, 1891* (1891), esp. pp. 10–11, 42–3.
61 *Mesur yr wyth awr / The Eight Hours Bill* (s.l., s.n., between 1894 and 1899).
62 *Colliery Guardian*, 30 July 1926; see also the letter on this matter in *The Times*, 3 July 1926.
63 Daunton, 'Down the Pit', pp. 588–9.
64 Miners' Federation of Great Britain, *Annual Conference held at the Central Hall, Central Hall, Westminster, London, on Thursday and Friday, November 7th and 8th, 1918*, p. 73.
65 V. L. Allen, *The Militancy of British Miners* (Shipley: Moor Press, 1981), p. 74. Elizabeth Andrews, the Labour Party's women organiser for Wales, also noted in 1923 how 'it is not only the men who are employed by the Mineowners, but their wives are also employed (without pay) to clear up the dirt in the homes that ought to have been left at the pit top'; *Colliery Workers Magazine*, September 1923, in Elizabeth Andrews, *A Woman's Work is Never Done and Political Articles*, edited by Ursula Masson (Dinas Powys: Honno, 2006), p. 65.
66 Andrews, *A Woman's Work is Never Done*, p. 71.
67 Church, *The History of the British Coal Industry, Volume 3*, pp. 608–9.
68 See, for example, *Report of the Royal Commission on the Housing of the Industrial Population of Scotland*, Cd. 8731 (Edinburgh: HMSO, 1917), xiv. Indeed, this Royal Commission was largely initiated as a result of political pressure from the Scottish Miners' Federation and conducted careful investigation into housing conditions in the country's mining regions.
69 M. R. Haines, 'Fertility, Nuptiality, and Occupation: A Study of Coal Mining Populations and Regions in England and Wales in the Mid-Nineteenth Century', *Journal of Interdisciplinary History*, 8:2 (1977), pp. 259–62; also Valerie Gordon Hall, 'Contrasting Female Identities: Women in Coal Mining Communities in Northumberland, England, 1900–1939', *Journal of Women's History*, 13:2 (2001), pp. 110–11; Benson, *British Coalminers in the Nineteenth Century*, p. 121.
70 On lodgers, see Dot Jones, 'Counting the Cost of Coal: Women's Lives in the Rhondda, 1881–1911', in Angela V. John (ed.), *Our Mothers' Land: Chapters*

in *Welsh Women's History 1830–1939* (Cardiff: University of Wales Press, 1991), pp. 119–20; Church, *The History of the British Coal Industry, Volume 3*, p. 602.
71 Church, *The History of the British Coal Industry, Volume 3*, p. 608.
72 James C. Welsh, *The King and the Miner: A Contrast* (London: ILP Publication Department, 1923), p. 6.
73 Welsh, *The King and the Miner*, p. 6.
74 Jack Jones, *Bidden to the Feast* (London: Corgi Books 1968 [1938]), p. 51. This novel was set mid- to late nineteenth century.
75 This woman also suffered anaemia, 'whiteleg' (i.e. phlegmasia alba dolens, a form of deep vein thrombosis with sympotoms of edema, pain and a characteristic white colouration of the leg), constipation and piles, bad dental caries, headaches, palpitations, faintness, and experienced a period of facial paralysis; Margery Spring Rice, *Working-Class Wives: Their Health and Condition* (London: Virago, 1981 edition; originally published in 1939), p. 122.
76 Jones, 'Counting the Cost of Coal', p. 116.
77 W. John Morgan, 'The Miners' Welfare Fund in Britain 1920–1952', *Social Policy & Administration*, 24:3 (1990), p. 205.
78 Dame Janet Campbell, 'Introduction', in Spring Rice, *Working-Class Wives*, p. xv.
79 Gordon Hall, 'Contrasting Female Identities', p. 112.
80 Rhys Davies, 'Nightgown', in *Collected Stories*: Volume 1, edited by Meic Stephens (Llandysul: Gomer 1996), p. 238.
81 For portayals of this process, see Margaret Llewleyn Davies (ed.), *Life as We Have Known It* (London: Virago, 1977 [1931]), pp. 67–72; Coombes, *These Poor Hands*, p. 41.
82 Coal Industry Commission, *Vol. II: Reports and Minutes of Evidence on the Second Stage of the Inquiry*, Cmd. 360 (London: HMSO, 1919), xii, p. 1019.
83 Andrews, *A Woman's Work Is Never Done*, p. 66.
84 Jones, 'Counting the Cost of Coal', p. 109.
85 *Rhondda Socialist*, 11 April 1912, in Jane Aaron and Ursula Masson (eds), *The Very Salt of Life: Welsh Women's Political Writings from Chartism to Suffrage* (Dinas Powys: Honno, 2007), pp. 220–2.
86 Spring Rice, *Working-Class Wives*, pp. 96–7, 108.
87 Spring Rice, *Working-Class Wives*, p. 122.
88 Coal Industry Commission, *Vol. II: Reports and Minutes of Evidence*, p. 1020; see also the testimony of Agnes Brown from Bellshill, Lanarkshire (pp. 1022–25).
89 H.M. Chief Inspector of Mines, *Mines and Quarries: General Report, with Statistics, for 1920, Part II. Labour*, 1921 (239), xli, p. 61.
90 B. L. Coombes, *Miners Day* (Harmondsworth: Penguin Books, 1945), p. 8.
91 *Report of the Royal Commission on Safety in Coal Mines*, Cmd. 5890 (London: HMSO, 1938), xiii, p. 65.

92 H.M. Chief Inspector of Mines, *Mines and Quarries: Part II. Labour*, p. 61; H.M. Chief Inspector of Mines, *Mines and Quarries: General Report, with Statistics, for 1920, Part I. Divisional Statistics*, 1921 (115), xli, p. 17.
93 For example, flood disasters are included in Scotland-set literature such as James C. Welsh's *The Underworld, The Story of Robert Sinclair, Miner* (London: Herbert Jenkins, 1920) and Tom Hanlin's *Miracle at Cardenrigg* (London: Random House, 1949); also in Durham-set novels Harold Heslop's *The Gate of a Strange Field* (London: D. Appleton and Company, 1929) and A. J. Cronin's *The Stars Look Down* (London: Gollancz, 1935).
94 For example, gas explosions, reports of unsafe levels of gas and survivors with burn-scarred bodies are variously portrayed in Wales-set literature including: Harry Lindsay's *Rhoda Roberts* (London: Chatto & Windus, 1895), Joseph Keating's *Son of Judith* (London: G. Allen, 1900), Allen Raine's *A Welsh Witch* (London: Hutchinson & Co., 1902), Ellis Lloyd's *Scarlet Nest* (London: Hodder & Stoughton, 1919), Lewis Jones's *Cwmardy* (London: Lawrence & Wishart, 1937), Jack Jones's *Black Parade* (London: Faber & Faber, 1935), Susan Buchan's *The Scent of Water* (London: Hodder & Stoughton, 1937) and Glyn Jones's 'Explosion' in *The Water Music* (London: G. Routledge & Sons, 1944).
95 Harold Heslop, *Last Cage Down* (London: Lawrence Wishart Books, 1984 [1935]); A. J. Cronin, *The Citadel* (London: Vista, 1996 [1937]).
96 H.M. Chief Inspector of Mines, *Mines and Quarries: Part II. Labour*, p. 61.
97 Frank Shufflebotham, 'The Hygienic Aspect of the Coal-Mining Industry in the United Kingdom: Lecture V. Beat Hand, Knee, Elbow and Buttock', *British Medical Jounal*, 4 April 1914, p. 755.
98 *Statistics of Compensation and Proceedings under the Workmen's Compensation Acts, and the Employers' Liability Act, 1880, in Great Britain*, 1908–38 (annual series).
99 Shufflebotham, 'The Hygienic Aspect of the Coal-Mining Industry in the United Kingdom', p. 756.
100 T. Lister Llewellyn, 'A Lecture on Miners' Nystagmus', *British Medical Journal*, 28 June 1913, p. 1359; see also, *Report of the Royal Commission on the Coal Industry (1925)* (London, HMSO, 1926), p. 195.
101 B. L. Coombes, *I Am a Miner* (London: Fact, 1939), pp. 72–3.
102 An official report claimed in the late 1930s that 'Work is the salvation of "nystagmic" workmen, and surface employment plays as great a role in the treatment of the disease as underground work does in its production'; *Report of the Departmental Committee on Certain Questions Arising under the Workmen's Compensation Acts*, Cmd. 5657, (London: HMSO, 1938), xv, p. 4.
103 Statistics of compensation and proceedings under the Workmen's Compensation Acts, and the Employers' Liability Act, 1880, in Great Britain, 1908–38 (annual series).
104 See, for example, the fall in certified cases recorded in the Lanarkshire coalfield from 1931 to 1932; *Report by the Departmental Committee on Certain Questions Arising under the Workmen's Compensation Acts*, pp. 6, 45–6.

105　Llewellyn, 'A Lecture on Miners' Nystagmus', p. 1360.
106　Arthur McIvor and Ronald Johnston, *Miners' Lung: A History of Dust Disease in British Coal Mining* (Aldershot: Ashgate, 2007), p. 2.
107　In addition to McIvor and Johnston, *Miners' Lung*, see Mark W. Bufton and Joseph Melling, '"A Mere Matter of Rock": Organized Labour, Scientific Evidence and British Government Schemes for Compensation of Silicosis and Pneumoconiosis among Coalminers, 1926–1940', *Medical History*, 49:2 (2005), pp. 155–78; Mark W. Bufton and Joseph Melling, 'Coming up for Air: Experts, Employers, and Workers in Campaigns to Compensate Silicosis Sufferers in Britain, 1918–1939', *Social History of Medicine*, 18:1 (2005), pp. 63–86.
108　*NUM (South Wales Area) Executive Council Annual Report, 1948–9*, p. 93.
109　On the incidence of pneumoconiosis among coal-trimmers, see McIvor and Johnston, *Miners' Lung*, p. 85.
110　On the variable risks of dust exposure in different parts of the underground workings, see Enid M. Williams, *The Health of Old and Retired Coalminers in South Wales* (Cardiff: University of Wales Press Board, 1933), pp. 17–20.
111　McIvor and Johnston, *Miners' Lung*, p. 56.
112　See Ben Curtis and Steven Thompson, '"This Is the Country of Premature Old Men": Ageing and Aged Miners in the South Wales Coalfield, c.1880–1947', *Cultural and Social History*, 12:4 (2015), pp. 587–606.
113　Williams, *The Health of Old and Retired Coalminers*, p. 19.
114　Williams, *The Health of Old and Retired Coalminers*, pp. 19–20.
115　Williams, *The Health of Old and Retired Coalminers*, p. 45.
116　Janet M. Campbell, *Maternal Mortality* (London: HMSO, 1924), p. xvi.
117　Standing Joint Committee of Industrial Women's Organisations, Report on *"Protect the Nation's Mothers"* (London: Labour Party, 1936) presented to the National Conference of Labour Women, Sheffield, May 1935, p. 6.
118　Ministry of Health, *Report on an Investigation into Maternal Mortality*, Cmd. 5422, 1936–37, xi, p. 12.
119　On the methodology utilised, see Spring Rice, *Working-Class Wives*, pp. 21–7.
120　Spring Rice, *Working-Class Wives*, p. 20.
121　Spring Rice, *Working-Class Wives*, p. 37.
122　Scottish Board of Health, *Report of the Scottish Departmental Committee on Puerperal Morbidity and Mortality* (Edinburgh: HMSO, 1924), p. 10.
123　Spring Rice, *Working-Class Wives*, pp. 85–6; interestingly, Spring Rice maintained that the women who faced these difficulties but who still maintained a positive attitude and continued to cope with their domestic responsibilities most effectively were more numerous in the north of England and Scotland than in the 'south'; Spring Rice, *Working-Class Wives*, p. 85.
124　Spring Rice, *Working-Class Wives*, p. 164.
125　Spring Rice, *Working-Class Wives*, p. 53.
126　*Evening Telegraph*, 24 February 1889.

127 Reports of W. Walker, H.M. Inspector of Mines for the Scotland Division, p. 37 in *Reports of the Inspectors of Mines for the Year 1913*.
128 Henry Norman Barnett, *Accidental Injuries to Workmen, with Reference to Workmen's Compensation Act, 1906. With Article on Injuries to the Organs of Special Sense* (London: Rebman, 1909), p. 33.
129 On the significant role of the First World War, see Mike Mantin, 'Coalmining and the National Scheme for Disabled Ex-Servicemen after the First World War', *Social History*, 41:2 (2016), pp. 155–70; Joanna Bourke, *Dismembering the Male: Men's Bodies, Britain, and the Great War* (London: Reaktion Books, 1996).
130 National Archives of Scotland (hereafter NAS), CB 19/1, 14704/12, Scottish Coal Workers' Compensation Scheme, Directors' Minute Books, 1912–1914, James Dalrymple v The Fife Coal Company Ltd.
131 NAS, CB 19/1, 2056/12, Scottish Workers' Compensation Scheme, Directors' Minute Books, 1912–1914, Charles Robertson v The Fife Coal Co. Ltd.
132 Jeffrey Grenfell-Hill (ed.) *Growing up in Wales: Collected Memories of Childhood in Wales 1895–1939* (Llandysul: Gomer, 1996), p. 50.
133 Grenfell-Hill, *Growing Up in Wales*, p. 52.
134 NAS, CB 19/1, F.2561/14, Scottish Workers' Compensation Scheme, Directors' Minute Books, 1912–1914, Kenneth Sparling v The Fife Coal Co. Ltd.
135 Durham County Record Office (hereafter DCRO), C47, Durham Miners' Association Compensation Department, Minutes of the Arbitration Committee, January to December 1925, 21 December 1925.
136 DCRO, C47, Durham Miners' Association Compensation Department, Minutes of the Arbitration Committee, January to December 1925, 29 December 1925.
137 Ashington Coal Company in the north-east of England consulted a doctor over the appropriate form of light work for disabled miners on their return to work; Griselda Carr, *Pit Women: Coal Communities in Northern England in the Early Twentieth Century* (London: Merlin Press, 2001), p. 63.
138 Glamorgan Archives, DPD/2/5/6/160, Powell Duffryn Collection Papers concerning compensation, 1925–1926, 14 December 1926.
139 *Colliery Guardian*, 27 August 1926.
140 *Colliery Guardian*, 27 August 1926.
141 NAS, CB 19/4, Scottish Coal Workers' Compensation Scheme, Directors' Minute Books, 1919–1921, F831/18 Hetherington v The Fife Coal Co. Ltd.
142 Coombes, *These Poor Hands*, pp. 63–4.
143 This is exactly how workmen's compensation legislation worked in other countries too; see Sarah F. Rose, *No Right to be Idle: The Invention of Disability, 1840s–1930s* (Chapel Hill: University of North Carolina Press, 2017).
144 *Cardiff Times*, 10 December 1898, p. 1. Indeed, the south Wales miners' leader William Abraham ('Mabon') anticipated that this would be the immediate outcome of the legislation; *Cardiff Times*, 22 May 1897, p. 1.
145 *Evening Express*, 18 November 1898, p. 2.

146 DCRO, D/DCOMPA 235, Durham Coal Owners' Mutual Protection Association, Agreements with Durham Miners' Association concerning compensation for non-fatal accidents, 29 June 1898; see also Departmental Committee on Workmen's Compensation, *Report by the Departmental Committee Appointed to Inquire into the System of Compensation for Injuries to Workmen*, Cmd. 816 (London: HMSO, 1920), xxvi, p. 57.
147 DCRO, D/X 1005/21, Correspondence to let aged or infirm men go at Chopwell Colliery, 10 September 1912.
148 Angela V. John. *By the Sweat of Their Brow* (London: Croom Helm, 1980), p. 200.
149 J. M. Winter, 'Britain's "Lost Generation" of the First World War', *Population Studies*, 31:3 (1977), p. 452; Mike Mantin, 'Coalmining and the National Scheme for Disabled Ex-Servicemen after the First World War', *Social History*, 41:2 (2016), p. 158.
150 *Monmouth Guardian*, 5 November 1915, p. 3. It was often suggested that older men, which might have included men with disabilities, might be taken on to release other men for the front; see, for example, *Llais Llafur*, 1 April 1916, p. 1; *Cambrian Daily Leader*, 7 March 1916, p. 6.
151 Selection criteria were used to 'comb out' eligible men from the workforce for conscription into the army.
152 Miners' Federation of Great Britain, *Recruiting of Miners. Deputation of the Executive Committee of the Miners' Federation of Great Britain to the Right Hon. Sir George Cave, K.C., M.P. (Secretary of State for the Home Department), Thursday, February 1st, 1917* (Manchester, 1917), pp. 4–9.
153 Miners' Federation of Great Britain, *Recruiting of Miners*, pp. 26, 28.
154 Miners' Federation of Great Britain, *Special Conference held at the Central Hall, Westminster, London, on Thursday and Friday, April 19th and 20th, 1917*, p. 12.
155 Miners' Federation of Great Britain, *Special Conference held at the Central Hall, Westminster, London, on Wednesday, June 20th 1917*, p. 27.
156 Miners' Federation of Great Britain, *Special Conference held at the Westminster Palace Hotel, London, on Tuesday and Wednesday, May 9th and 10th, 1916*, pp. 17–18.
157 *Report of the Departmental Committee on Certain Questions Arising under the Workmen's Compensation Acts*, Cmd. 5657 (London: HMSO, 1938), xv, p. 20.
158 *Hansard*, 12 May 1938.
159 *Report by the Departmental Committee on Certain Questions Arising under the Workmen's Compensation Acts*, p. 6.
160 *Report by the Departmental Committee on Certain Questions Arising under the Workmen's Compensation Acts*, p. 48.
161 *Report by the Departmental Committee on Certain Questions Arising under the Workmen's Compensation Acts*, pp. 6–8, 21–3. The same practices were employed in south Wales; South Wales Miners' Federation, *Annual Report of Executive Council, 1935–1936*, pp. 34–5.

162 *Western Mail*, 21 June 1924, p. 9.
163 Jack Lawson, *Under the Wheels* (London: Hodder & Stoughton, 1934), p. 26.
164 National Library of Wales, Thomas Jones C. H. papers, John Davies and David E. Evans, 'Report on Merthyr Tydfil', 11 July 1929, p. 5.
165 *Men Without Work: A Report made to the Pilgrim Trust* (Cambridge: Cambridge University Press, 1938), pp. 66–7, 72, 81, 424.
166 *The Spectator*, 23 February 1945, p. 7.
167 South Wales Miners' Federation, *Report of Compensation Department, 1943–1944*, p. 47.
168 Miners' Federation of Great Britain, Minutes of the Executive Committee Meeting, 8 June 1944.
169 *The Spectator*, 23 February 1945, p. 7.
170 McIvor and Johnston, *Miners' Lung*, pp. 86–7.
171 C. M. Fletcher, 'Pneumoconiosis of Coal-Miners', *British Medical Journal*, 5 June 1948, p. 1065.
172 'Report of Compensation Department, 1945–1946', in *NUM South Wales Area Council Annual Report, 1945–1946*, p. 61.
173 Fletcher, 'Pneumoconiosis of Coal-Miners', p. 1066.
174 *The Miner*, 1:4 (January, 1945), p. 14.
175 McIvor and Johnston, *Miners' Lung*, pp. 87–8.
176 McIvor and Johnston, *Miners' Lung*, pp. 148–9.
177 For an example of the variety of arguments made in favour of nationalisation, see Independent Labour Party, *The Mineowners in the Dock: A Summary of the Evidence Given before the Coal Industry Commission* (London: Independent Labour Party, 1919).
178 National Coal Board, *Annual Report and Statement of Accounts for the Year Ended 31st December 1947*, pp. 1–5.
179 *NUM South Wales Area Council Annual Report, 1948–1949*, p. 81.
180 Fletcher, 'Pneumoconiosis of Coal-Miners', p. 1067.
181 Hansard, 1 May 1947.
182 National Coal Board, *Annual Report and Statement of Accounts for the Year Ended 31st December 1947*, pp. 46–7.
183 Ministry of Labour and National Service, *Report for the Year 1948*, Cmd. 7822, 1948–49, xvii, p. 32.

2

MEDICALISING MINERS? MEDICINE, CARE AND REHABILITATION

In a lecture to the Oxford Ophthalmological Congress in July 1915, Dr Frank Shufflebotham, a doctor and medical referee in the workmen's compensation system, pressed the case for increased interest on the part of the medical establishment in the causes and consequences of illness and injury among coalminers:

> I venture to think that never was there a time in the history either of medicine, or of this country, when it was more important to consider from a medical point of view the amount of damage done to the workers by accident and disease in ordinary course of their employment ... I do not think that sufficient attention has been paid by the medical profession as a whole to the conditions of employment in this country, at all events, by those whom we have regarded as the leaders of the profession.[1]

The speech, though focusing mostly on eye diseases, encapsulated an intensifying medical scrutiny of workers, and especially miners, in the first half of the twentieth century. Shufflebotham was himself a major figure in medical research into coalminers, one of the growing number of experts who delivered lectures, participated in debates and published research articles in specialised journals about industrial injuries and diseases in this period.[2] The 'medical profession' displayed ever greater interest in the bodies of miners, in their sickness, injuries and disabilities, and in efforts to return them to work as soon and as far as possible.

This chapter examines the role of healthcare services, medicine and the medical profession in relation to disabled people in coalfield communities. Members of the medical profession had an important role to play in coalfield communities and, while the extent of their involvement in the lives of disabled people varied from one type of disability to another, it nevertheless increased over time from the late nineteenth to the mid-twentieth century.

This attention to medical services and this idea of medicalisation is not unproblematic from a disability studies perspective, and the ways in which medical history and disability history differ require careful consideration. Ever since the development of the 'social model' of disability from the 1970s onwards, and its use to challenge and replace the 'medical model' in explanations of disability, medicine's role in the lives of disabled people has been profoundly controversial and has given rise to significant criticism and suspicion. According to its critics, the medical model locates disability in the biology of individuals with congenital or chronic illness, bodily impairments or other departures from 'normal' bodily functions. The model defines such bodily states as pathological problems that require medical interventions in order to correct deviant bodies and return the impaired individual to normalcy, or else as close to it as possible.[3] In this model, medical professionals are implicated in a system that marginalises and oppresses disabled people because diagnosis involves a judgement of deviation from the norm, while the increasing commitment to a concept of cure in modern medicine also reconfigured people with incurable impairments as aberrant.[4]

Crucial here, too, is the concept of medicalisation. As used in medical sociology and medical history, medicalisation refers to the process by which medicine increased in influence and authority in the nineteenth and twentieth centuries. It refers to the extension of medical authority over more aspects of daily life and the reconceptualisation of previously social issues as medical problems that necessitated medical interventions.[5] Such medicalisation privileged 'objective' medical expertise at the expense of lay, patient illness narratives. This led to the creation of significant power differentials as the autonomy of the sick or injured individual was subordinated and they were forced into a passive, dependent sick role that necessitated the unquestioning acceptance of the doctor's opinion.[6] Disability scholars share many of these critiques of medicine within their conception of the 'medical model' and extend this analysis to assert that medicine performed an important role in capitalist society in the modern period. It did this through the institutionalisation of impaired people in hospitals, workhouses, prisons and asylums, thereby freeing more people to engage in capital modes of production, and by assisting the categorisation of bodily ability for the needs of a capitalist economy through welfare and compensation systems.[7]

For these various reasons, as Beth Linker has noted, disability studies scholars and disability historians have been reluctant to give too much prominence to medicine in their work for fear of reinstating a medical model in place of the social model that emphasised prejudice, stigma, social and economic structures, the design of buildings and spaces, and other factors in the disabling of people with impairments.[8] In addition, many disability histories have focused on 'healthy disabled' people or the 'predictably impaired', whose impairments were fixed, permanent, in no need of medical treatment. This approach, however, neglects a large proportion of disabled people and, as Linker states, 'More historical attention should be paid to the unhealthy disabled, those who because of chronic pain, deteriorating health, and threat of death may need, experience, and even seek out frequent medical interventions.'[9] The history of healthcare and medical provision has its place in the history of disabled people, therefore, since sickness and injury that were secondary to the particular impairment were common experiences, and disabled people consulted doctors, were admitted into hospitals and underwent treatment or rehabilitation.

In the context of coalmining communities, the process of medicalisation was underpinned by the development of medical understandings of coalminers' health and bodies, the creation and dissemination of a body of expert knowledge and the emergence of a group of specialists who came to assume a degree of authority and power in the field. This movement did not carry all before it, and medical authority continued to be partial, contested and subject to lay influences, even by the end of the 1940s; but there is little doubt that the medical profession took greater interest in miners' well-being during the period and that it succeeded in gaining some power and authority over their bodies. This was reflected in literary depictions of medical examinations and in portrayals of doctors as heroes or, more negatively, as gatekeepers in the pay of the colliery owners in compensation disputes. By the 1930s and, especially, the 1940s, medical, rehabilitation and convalescent facilities dedicated to the needs and well-being of disabled miners were established across Britain's coalfields, though provision was patchy and on a small scale. However, the treatment of disabled miners within such services was not an unalloyed blessing and tended to infringe on the autonomy and well-being of such men.

The miner's body

By the turn of the twentieth century coalmining had long held a real fascination for the British public. From the mid-nineteenth century countless human-interest articles or more technical studies, published in the flourishing popular periodical press of that period, attempted to explain the nature of the work underground to an interested British public. Apart from the rather macabre fascination with colliery disasters and other accidents that imperiled life and limb, attention to the perceived distinctive character of the miner's body was notable in these studies and helped to establish the miner and his community as people and places apart. The miner's body was sculpted, it seemed, by the conditions in which he laboured, and allowed him to operate in the unique working environment found underground. Writing in the early 1860s, for example, J. R. Leifchild opined that 'his stature is rather diminutive, his figure disproportionate, his legs more or less bowed, his chest protrudes, and his arms are oddly suspended ... In all these particulars we note the hereditary features of a class working in darkness and in constrained positions.'[10] Almost a century later, Ferdynand Zweig observed that miners constituted 'a physical type of their own' and offered a similar description to that advanced by Leifchild. The miner, he wrote, is 'strongly built, broad-shouldered, and short', with 'a tendency to bow-shaped legs', all of which were 'a sort of adaptation for the mines.'[11]

This interest in physical distinctiveness was often taken a step further in the racialised discourse of the period in which, as Anne McClintock has argued, miners were represented 'as a "race" apart, figured as racial outcasts, historically abandoned, isolated and primitive.'[12] This specialisation is reflected in coalfields novels such as the suggestively titled *The Underworld* (1920) and *The Morlocks* (1924), an allusion to H. G. Wells' new species of workers evolved to exist wholly in subterranean conditions in *The Time Machine* (1895).[13] The clearest sense of the miner as a breed apart can be found in a Welsh term, used by and about miners during the nineteenth century, that understood coal workers as 'tanddaearolion bethau' (literally, 'underground things', or 'underground beings') and distinguished miners from all other individuals, who were classed as 'daearolion bethau' ('ground things', or 'overground things').[14] The miner's body was no less objectified by more sympathetic observers: George Orwell's description of these 'splendid men' with 'wide shoulders tapering to slender supple waists' and 'small pronounced buttocks and sinewy thighs' is perhaps the most famous example.[15] Miners, and their bodies, therefore, were considered distinct and unique, both in the popular perception and by the professional groups who came to study them to an increasing degree. A short, curved, bowed-legged figure becomes a recognisable 'stock' feature, particularly in literature of the late nineteenth and early twentieth centuries: 'an auld pitman, if thee legs is a guide', remarks one observer in *Kitty Fagan* (1900).[16] While bodily curvature is sometimes treated as an advantage (even an evolutionary advantage) to the miner for his work in small spaces, it is also seen as a 'grotesque' class- or race-related body type: 'the width of his shoulders and chest conveyed some idea of his enormous strength, but, like a wedge, his body dwindled grotesquely to the short, thin, bowed legs of the typical pitman.'[17]

For their part, miners viewed their own bodies in a rather functional manner and the idea that his body was the miner's capital was commonplace in the nineteenth and twentieth centuries. Again and again, the productive capacity of his body, and the extent to which it could allow him to make a living and support a family, were emphasised by the miner and his representatives. Harold

Heslop a miner, author and activist, shows how making money is tied to strength in *The Gate of a Strange Field* (1929), where the central character: 'had learned the greatest lesson of the mines – the lesson of strength. In the mines the weaklings are at a discount.'[18] The muscular body of the collier can also represent wider industrial wealth: 'their strength will be turned into coal. Yes. Black lumps of coal which will be turned into gold at the docks ... It is the flesh and brains of our people that gives life to the world. Without them the world is dead.'[19] In this example from Lewis Jones's 1939 novel *We Live*, the workers' bodies are fuel for 'the world' and 'gold' for the capitalists, but at the expense of the miner's body in both injuries and long-term health impairments. Even the archetypal 'big hewer', such as Big Jim of *Cwmardy* (1937) and *We Live*, cannot earn enough in the long term to provide for age-related impairments, or illness in the family. Jim's son Len, who has been out of work with pneumonia, argues that his father has no financial stability even after decades of work in which he has 'given [his] wonderful body to the pit', because 'when I lose a month's work because I'm too bad to go to the pit, we get in arrears with the rent and have to owe money for food'.[20] Scottish miner Tom Hanlin, who started writing coalfields fiction while in hospital, convalescing from a mining accident, similarly focuses on the precarious nature of work dependent on muscular strength, in which 'the world had hired [the miner's] muscles for the day':[21]

> The fear of work that would be beyond your physical capacity, the meeting of conditions that would defeat you, expose you as unfit for this, the only work you knew in order to survive ... This is the fear that gets brutal work done, that breaks up the unity of the common man, this is his surrender to the greed and ignorance that builds glittering cities and demands a good life for itself.[22]

As in the above example from Jones's *We Live*, Hanlin contrasts the wealth generated by coal for owners and, more broadly, for the British Empire's 'glittering cities' against the cost to the miner's body and disruption to political solidarity when faced with the fear of falling into poverty.

Importantly, the miner's body came to be politicised during the nineteenth century, and figured as a central concern in the industrial politics of the coal industry, perhaps as much as wages and hours.[23] At a general level, the 'toll of the mine' on the lives and limbs of colliery workers served as an important rhetorical weapon, wielded by miners and their representatives to exert pressure on a particularly *laissez-faire* group of employers who did little to improve the working or community lives of their workers.[24] More specifically, material relating to injury, occupational disease and disability was employed in detailed and technical debates on working hours, underground safety and, of course, workmen's compensation.

This politicisation of the miner's body reached its apogee in the 1940s as state-funded rehabilitation services, government-instituted research into miners' pulmonary disease, the nationalisation of the coal industry, the passage of a generous Industrial Injuries Act and the creation of the National Health Service effectively nationalised the miner's body and thereby gave it a status it had never previously possessed.

Medical encounters

Of all the various medical professionals and health services with which disabled miners came into contact, it was the general practitioner who was the most significant in terms of medical engagement with disability. On a prosaic level, it was significant because daily consultations with 'works surgeons' or 'colliery doctors' were far more numerous than any other type of medical encounter. This was perhaps inevitably the case, given that the doctor was the first point of call in any health-related situation, but it was exacerbated in coalfield communities by the relative paucity of medical specialists and institutional provision. Numerous surveys and investigations in the late nineteenth and twentieth centuries found that coalfields tended to be the least well-provided-for regions in terms of the numbers of general practitioners, specialists, hospital beds and specialised services.[25] In his semi-autobiographical novel, *The Citadel* (1937), A. J. Cronin, who worked in the south Wales coalfield as a doctor and was very bitter about the lack of facilities, has Dr Denny make a rather exaggerated speech:

> Look here, Manson! I realise you're just passing through on your way to Harley Street, but in the meantime there are one or two things about this place you ought to know. You won't find it conforms to the best traditions of romantic practice. There's no hospital, no ambulance, no X-rays, no anything. If you want to operate you use the kitchen table. You wash up afterwards at the scullery bosh. The sanitation won't bear looking at.[26]

Of crucial importance was the form of organisation that made provision for general practitioner services in industrial districts in Britain. A variety of different methods of 'contract medical practice' were utilised in industrial communities, including friendly societies, works clubs, medical aid societies, trade unions, private clubs set up by general practitioners and provident dispensaries.[27] Most schemes were based on a particular workplace or else covered a single community or a relatively small district, and so the defining feature was a proliferation of organisations and considerable variation in terms of the provision made by each scheme. The level of payments that brought eligibility (and whether those payments were flat rate or graduated according to income), the inclusion of dependent wives and children, the numbers of doctors, the presence of paramedical personnel in the schemes, access to hospitals or other secondary services and a number of other areas of provision varied from one organisation to the next.[28]

The characteristic form in the south Wales coalfield was the medical aid society, which was universal across the region, to the extent that friendly societies were benefit societies alone and did not provide general practitioner care as they did in other coalfields.[29] The medical aid societies were among the most robust and sophisticated of workers' medical schemes and involved lay committees of workmen's representatives – including, at times, disabled workers – which, in many instances, wrested control of the finances of the schemes from their employers during the late nineteenth and early twentieth centuries. Such control, in the instances where it was secured, was then exercised to engage medical personnel on fixed salaries, much to their chagrin and that of the British Medical Association, and to use excess funds to develop the provision made to members. The Tredegar Workmen's Medical Aid Society was the most famous example of the schemes in south Wales. It succeeded in enlisting almost the entire community in membership and providing members with general practitioner, physiotherapy, massage, dentistry and nursing services, in addition to access to the Society's own cottage hospital and a range of other, larger hospitals to which the society subscribed and a broad array of other medicines, medical comforts and surgical appliances.[30] In these organisations any process of medicalisation was driven by workers, their families and their representatives as much as by members of the medical profession.

In his autobiography, *Adventures in Two Worlds* (1952), A. J. Cronin claims that the Tredegar society influenced Aneurin Bevan and 'can definitely be regarded as the foundation of the plan of socialised medicine which was eventually adopted by Great Britain'.[31] For Cronin's part, contemporaries widely regarded his novel, *The Citadel*, as helping to promote the socialist ideology that led to the founding of the National Health Service (NHS), but this has been disputed in more recent criticism which highlights the novel's pessimistic attitude to social systems and its idealisation of the individual.[32]

Cronin's concern with nationalised medicine and the medical aid society model is not unique among coalfields literature of south Wales. Rhys Davies comments on both the advantages and disadvantages of the medical aid society (though it is not specifically named), mediated through the perspective of the middle-class political agitator Dr Tudor Morris, in *A Time to Laugh* (1937). Morris is wary about the influence of the mine manager over the panel doctors, believing that 'someone must stand unpurchased and unowned',[33] and yet he also sees the advantages of the medical aid society and speaks at a Miners' Federation-organised event:

> he nobly explained at length the advantages of the scheme. Everybody knew of families crippled through illness, physically and financially, in this place where disease and destruction were very active; and who knew what misfortune waited for the healthiest, going down the pit ... [34]

Some miners in the audience are critics of the scheme, concerned that 'Several someones' going to get fat on it, doctors mostly ... 'specially those that's shareholders in the pits' and that 'the women will be running to the doctor every day, enjoying themselves and inventing bad things wrong with them.'[35] The emphasis on the risk of malingering is similar to Cronin's *The Citadel*, but Davies also highlights the suspicion of collusion between owners and doctors who may have a vested financial interest. In both novels the doctor is a heroic individual, trying to put their principles above financial interest.[36] The medical aid society is critiqued as worthy in principle, but potentially flawed because of the loss of the doctor's independence and a changed dynamic of entitlement that may encourage increased demands on the doctor's services, or even malingering.

In English and Scottish coalfields, other forms of organisation were more common. In Durham and Northumberland, for example, works clubs involved flat-rate payments of 6d. each fortnight (which the medical practitioners in the region pushed up to 9d. in 1899). Similar to their counterparts in south Wales, coverage included dependent family members.[37] Friendly societies also provided medical attendance in Durham as individual societies appointed medical officers or else groups of societies made joint provision; again, lay committees, elected by members, carried out the routine administrative work of these organisations.[38] John D. Milne, a doctor who graduated in 1944 and began practice in the mining community of Ormiston, East Lothian in 1946, remembered how insured workers in the community were all covered for panel practice[39] under the National Health Insurance system and miners paid an additional 6d. a week, for which they gained a free choice of doctor and coverage for their wives and children.[40] Indeed, the Scottish miners were covered under the National Health Insurance scheme through their trade union, as the Scottish Miners' Federation, similar to the Durham Miners' Association, became an 'approved society' for the administration of the scheme.[41] Such club practices were able to provide a level of care that compared quite favourably with that secured by more affluent or even middle-class sections of the population. The MacAlister Report, which reported on Scottish health services in 1920, claimed that the 'the system provides for the miner and his family many, though of course not all, of the benefits of continuous medical guardianship ... an able and energetic colliery doctor may assume a freedom of initiative and control in relation to the family health of his contract patients' not enjoyed by a counterpart who tended to private, fee-paying patients.[42] Nevertheless, despite variations, each scheme had general practitioner services at its heart and it was from this particular medical professional that most disabled people obtained medical care.

Unsurprisingly, the patient lists of medical practices in mining communities were dominated by miners, and surviving practice records for colliery districts indicate that their injuries, illnesses and ailments formed the bulk of the daily work of doctors in these districts.[43] In her study of general practice in the century up to 1948, Anne Digby found that the vast majority of the cases that presented in colliery surgeries in coalfield districts consisted of chronic chest complaints and accident cases.[44] Doctors suffered excessive workloads in industrial districts and were not able to do much more than deal with the majority of cases in a perfunctory manner, in the shortest time possible: case histories were not taken, physical examinations were rare and the majority of patients were rapidly ushered out of the surgery with a prescription of stock medicines.[45] One doctor, who practised at Ebbw Vale, south Wales in the interwar period, stated in his autobiography that 'no-one was sent away without a bottle of medicine, whether they needed it or not'.[46] There were exceptions: Digby argued that the doctors in the Cresswell practice at Dowlais, south Wales retained 'their medical curiosity' and kept abreast of 'modern methods of diagnosis and treatment'. Fast patient throughput on routine cases allowed greater time for more complicated or more interesting cases, and higher standards of clinical care.[47]

With the large workloads faced by colliery doctors and the short duration of consultations, not to mention the medical-model perspectives adopted by doctors, it is unsurprising that many disabled miners found a visit to the doctor to be a rather cold and impersonal experience. Will Arthur, a miner who worked in Mountain Ash, south Wales, contracted miner's nystagmus, such that his 'eyes were going around like saucers'. Interviewed in 1973, he described having to go to see two doctors in Cardiff and being

> told to strip, taken in before these two doctors, one of them said 'Bend', so I 'Bent'. 'Up, up', and he called the other doctor and he said, 'Bend again', and I bent and he said, 'Up, up' and he said, 'Put your clothes on'. So I thought, that's that, and it was. He looked at what I had said, my name and all that, and he said, 'Miner', 'Yes'. 'Miners' nystagmus', he said, 'Oh', I said, 'Just a mild attack'. 'No good my boy', he said, so that was that.[48]

That, indeed, was that. This particular consultation was for the purposes of an assessment to determine eligibility for compensation payments, but it is evident that dissatisfaction with the quality of care received by miner patients was widespread and persistent.[49] Cronin's *The Citadel* argues from the other side that the colliery doctor had such a large caseload that it was 'impossible'[50] to fully examine every patient, especially the men coming in for certificates:

> Andrew examined him, found him suffering from beat knee, gave him the certificate of incapacity for work.
> The second case came in. He also demanded his certificate, nystagmus. The third case: certificate, bronchitis. The fourth case: certificate, beat elbow.[51]

The conveyor-belt nature of the consultations here dehumanises the doctor, while the patients are transformed into mere cases requiring 'certificates'. On the other hand, the relationship between a doctor and his patient could be an intensely personal one, and a kindness shown by a dedicated and sympathetic doctor could provoke intense gratitude and loyalty. Certainly a great many miners and members of their families valued the care and attention given to them by colliery doctors, and such doctors were considered important members of their communities and assigned a status similar to the local minister. Bert Coombes, never shy in his criticism of employers and others who exploited the labour of his fellow workmen, maintained that while there were doctors who were 'brutal and overbearing' in manner, these were only a minority, and that for the most part 'no praise could be overdone' for the majority of doctors in mining regions. Coombes claimed that doctors acted as 'confessor, clerk and general adviser to his people' and likened them to 'guardian angels'.[52]

More than bedside manner, however, it was the effectiveness of therapeutic interventions that stood to have the greatest impact on the lives of disabled people, and here the medical story is, for the most part, one of failure. Nystagmus was 'treated' through removing the miner from the low light conditions that caused the condition in the first place. While symptoms lessened or cleared with that removal from underground work, miners were not 'cured', and would suffer a return of the symptoms if they returned to work in poor light conditions.[53] Nor did the treatments available for the care of miners with chest diseases make a material difference to the lives of these men. The absence of effective therapeutics lay behind Shufflebotham's assertion in 1914 that 'There is no disease to which the saying "Prevention is better than cure" is more applicable', and his advice was that the suppression of dust and the removal of the miner from the dusty atmosphere were the most important preventives, though he did mention pharmacological responses, particularly potassium iodide, nux vomica and ammonium carbonate, largely intended to ease respiration.[54] Little had changed by the mid-1940s, despite the considerable amount of research that had been conducted by that time, and C. M. Fletcher was forced to concede that

'With regard to therapeutic as opposed to prophylactic measures, we cannot offer cure'; palliative measures were all that could be offered by that time.[55] In the absence of effective treatments, miners with pulmonary disease were often sent for periods of convalescence in one of the many homes that came to be established from the second half of the nineteenth century. Coal companies, trade union branches, friendly societies and other organisations all subscribed to convalescent homes and sent miners diagnosed with 'silicosis', 'emphysema' or other complaints for a period of recuperation.[56] As such, convalescent homes were, until about the 1930s, more social than medical institutions, and did not involve much in the way of medical supervision or treatment. Another response was merely for the miner to absent himself from work on a regular basis in an attempt to manage his condition. Bert Coombes found in the 1940s that miners with chest disease absented themselves from work, perhaps for a day each week, in the 'hope to stave off the disease by losing time frequently and so clearing the lungs'.[57] Even in the early twenty-first century, chronic obstructive pulmonary disease is managed, rather than cured, through the use of inhalers, medicines and steroids intended to ease the symptoms and make breathing easier.

Therapeutic interventions were more numerous in relation to other disabling conditions of miners, but there is little reason to think that they were more effective. Fractures and crush injuries, especially to limbs, were common; while rest and recovery were sufficient for minor instances, others led to medical or surgical responses by doctors. In the opinion of some, amputation was far too common a response to the damage done to limbs in accidents. Welsh miner Jack Jones conveys this fear in his historical novel *Black Parade* (1935) when a miner remarks sceptically on the new hospital that: 'anything the matter – off it comes, that's why there's so many on crutches everywhere. A week last Tuesday I helped to carry Tom Roderick from the pit into that accident ward, and the next I heard was that they had taken his leg off.'[58] A short sequence of the records of the Highfield Public Assistance Institution at Sunderland reveals miners such as 'William L.', a 39-year-old miner from Shotton, diagnosed with 'necrosis' of the tibia as a result of a compound fracture a number of years previously, who was 'cured' through the amputation of the leg. The same fate befell a twenty-nine-year-old miner named John Nixon, who was 'cured' of a compound fracture of the ankle by the amputation of his leg, while Samuel Adlam, forty-two years old, was treated for a crushed hand through the amputation of his first finger.[59] The limited skills of some colliery surgeons, and the more general inability of orthopaedics to carry out the complex repairs to limbs that came in the post-war period, meant that amputation was often the easiest or, indeed, the only option. The medical view, which did not extend beyond the immediate situation to consider the personal and social consequences of amputation, could conceive of such cases as 'cured'.

Miners' medical schemes were crucial in the provision of general practitioner services, but they were also important to disabled workers in a variety of other ways; indeed, it might be argued that they assisted impaired miners in more practical ways than did the practitioners who treated them on a day-to-day basis, though the extent to which this assistance was medical in character varied. In the first place, many workmen's schemes and organisations subscribed to a variety of institutions in order to gain access to the services in those places for their members. Many of the early grants from the Ebbw Vale Workmen's Doctors' Fund, for example, were to send patients for specialised treatment outside south Wales. Train fares to Bristol Royal Infirmary, Bristol Eye Hospital and Bath Mineral Hospital were all provided for those that needed them.[60] In the north-east of England, lodges of the Durham Miners' Association, similar to lodges in coalfield unions across Britain, subscribed to large voluntary hospitals and smaller cottage hospitals so as to secure letters of recommendation to allow members to be admitted, while their counterparts in the Mid and East Lothian Miners' Association subscribed to the Edinburgh Royal Infirmary to meet their members' medical needs.[61] Again, medicalisation was as much driven by workers and their organisations as by doctors and the medical profession.

The workmen's medical funds were also active in the provision of prostheses and, given the large numbers of injuries to limbs, especially legs, and in view of the tendency for surgeons to 'treat' many injuries through amputation, artificial limbs were a particularly crucial area of provision. These were rarely provided by employers or hospitals directly, though some examples can be found: the Dowlais Iron Company (which also employed coalminers) kept an extensive 'Truss and Wooden Leg Register' between 1891 and 1902.[62] At the same time the generosity of coal companies was limited, and instances arose where the company refused to pay for repairs or corrections to the limb.[63] More often, workers obtained artificial limbs through mutual aid, whether by means of friendly societies, medical schemes or merely ad hoc collections to enable an injured miner to purchase his own limb, rather than from the employer. In the short story 'The Benefit Concert' (1946) by Rhys Davies, Jenkin loses a leg to an infected mining-related wound but he receives no compensation from the colliery and is too fearful of the courts to pursue his claim. Consequently the local chapel offers to organise a benefit concert to raise money to buy an expensive prosthetic leg in steel and leather. However, the story is hardly to the credit of the chapel deacons, who, having raised in excess of what is needed, refuse to allow Jenkin to use the additional money to open a small shop, and instead refurbish the chapel, forcing him back into the mine.[64] In south Wales the medical aid societies were important in supplying prosthetics to their members, and the societies' minute books are filled with instances of miners, and indeed members of their families, being provided with prosthetics.[65] Crucially, they were provided upon application by the members themselves rather than imposed on them by doctors, though, following a Foucauldian perspective, such instances of medicalisation from below were perhaps more total than any imposition by doctors from above.[66]

The supply of an artificial limb did not end the schemes' involvement in the matter and it is clear that a degree of after-care was generally offered to impaired miners; the schemes often assisted the impaired individual with the fit of the artificial limb and with its maintenance in subsequent years. Some of the better schemes paid for members to travel to the workshops of artificial-limb makers to be measured properly for their limbs, arranged as many subsequent visits as were necessary to achieve the best fit, paid for repairs to older or damaged limbs and generally represented the disabled member in any dealings with the artificial-limb maker.[67] That is not to say that the generosity of miners' schemes was limitless: the finite resources of the societies necessitated attention to eligibility and to the adoption of a certain cost-consciousness in the choice of limb. In March 1897, for example, three applications were made to the Ebbw Vale Workmen's Medical Society, by two workmen and a woman. While one applicant was provided with a 'foot and socket leg' costing around £6 6s. 0d., the other workman and the female applicant were each recommended wooden legs costing £1 1s. 0d. each.[68]

Medical aid societies did not limit themselves to providing artificial limbs. Other prosthetics and assistive devices were available, most commonly trusses, but also orthopaedic boots, surgical belts, spectacles and a range of 'invalid chairs'.[69] At the same time, new technology could be rejected for questionable reliability. The committee of the Ebbw Vale scheme refused to grant the full amount for an 'ear apparatus' for the wife of a miner 'who was very deaf' in October 1943. In addition to its being too expensive, the committee reported that 'these aural instruments were very rarely successful, and were more often than not discarded by the patients after a short time'.[70] Hearing aids were rejected several times by the Tredegar Workmen's Medical Aid Society, suggesting further scepticism of certain types of technology for deaf workers and perhaps a discerning attitude towards such aids that accepted only those devices that brought about an improvement in the everyday lives of disabled people.[71] This perhaps suggests a potential dialogue between deaf miners about the wildly varying quality of contemporary hearing aids, much as the pages of the *Deaf Chronicle* and *British Deaf-Mute* separated useful technology from 'Swindles on Deaf people' by 'Quack doctors who profess power to cure deafness' with new gadgets.[72]

Prosthetics are a crucial material piece of disability labour history. Many miners continued to work after being fitted with them, such as John Burt of the Fife Coal Company, who wore his 'pin and bucket' artificial limb while working on the motor haulage engine underground.[73] There are several references in coalfields fiction to miners with 'peg legs' working at the colliery, including underground, before the First World War.[74] These generally occur in novels of the 1930s and 1940s as a way of contrasting the pre-war buoyancy of the industry, which could 'even' find employment for the partially impaired, with conditions during the Depression. In these novels a high level of unemployment is also shown to allow a system where workers are easily replaceable by younger men, to the detriment of veteran miners with mining-related injuries and impairments. Clearly, a permanent disability did not necessarily mean ending work. Medical aid societies used the ability to work as a means to determine financial priorities and the amount to be paid for the acquisition of an artificial limb. In 1898 a rule was passed at the Ebbw Vale society to set the maximum cost of an artificial limb at £4, but to spend more if it would enable the worker to follow their employment.[75] Later that year an applicant was informed that the grants were 'not intended for cases of long standing but only related to cases of a workman who having received an injury necessitating amputation required an artificial limb to enable him to resume work'.[76] On the one hand, it might be argued that medical aid societies thus emphasised the moral and, perhaps, therapeutic benefits of work. On the other hand, they also worked to lessen the disabling impacts of impairment and attempted to enable disabled miners to continue with their working lives.

Membership of mutualist organisations could be quite strictly controlled, but they remained important to disabled people. Through such organisations, disabled people were recognised as central to the community and their particular needs were prioritised and, as far as possible, met. The Tredegar society resolved that 'a member, whilst disabled, is entitled to full benefits'.[77] More than that, disabled members were able to play a role in the administration of these democratic organisations and, in many instances, served on the committees that made decisions and set priorities. One member of the Tredegar Workmen's Medical Aid Society in the late 1930s, for example, utilised his own personal experience of wearing a prosthetic leg to offer informed advice on the limbs provided to members of the Society and his 'expertise' was drawn upon in other cases.[78] In these mutualist organisations, quite extensive levels of lay control, including the involvement of disabled individuals, were exercised over medical authority, and doctors were required to conduct themselves and their practices according to the strictures set down by workmen's committees.

At the same time, however, it is clear that these mutualist organisations were instrumental in the process of medicalisation as they looked to extend the reach of medical expertise over more aspects of the lives of greater numbers of people. Efforts were constantly made to increase the numbers of doctors who served on these schemes, to extend the types of paramedical services offered to members and to increase the number and types of medical comforts provided to disabled members. Such policy initiatives were guided by insights provided by disabled committee members and impaired ordinary members, and the medicalisation that occurred was driven by an informed view of the value of these initiatives in people's everyday lives. Doctors did not play a central role in these activities. They were involved only in the amputation of a limb; there was no medical management of stumps, nor medical intervention to assist with the fit of prostheses, which was done by the lay committee in negotiation with the artificial-limb company. Impairment in such instances was conceived in terms of a medical model by which prostheses replaced missing limbs and gave the impression of normalcy, but this was done through the agency of impaired people and under their own volition, arguably suggesting an internalised cultural pressure to 'pass' as able bodied.

While the medical interventions of general practitioners were of only limited value to the disabled miner or his disabled family members, primary care was still the most important medical arena in which impairment was addressed by medicine and where medicalisation took place. Nevertheless, it was not the only context in which disabled people were treated medically, and hospitals became an important institution in which disability was 'treated'. Voluntary hospitals, first initiated in the eighteenth century, grew in number and size from the latter decades of the nineteenth century, and individual institutions diversified as new departments were established and various specialist consultants were appointed to the honorary staffs.[79] Dependent as they were on voluntary support, hospitals tended to be founded first in more affluent or larger communities, and coalfields tended to lag behind in terms of hospital provision, despite the massive levels of need that existed as a result of injuries and occupational disease. Nevertheless, institutions, many of them cottage hospitals, came to be established in British coalfields during the second half of the nineteenth century and into the twentieth century, and disabled miners were treated in greater numbers.[80]

Geographical factors, local cultures of paternalism and philanthropy and the strength and attitudes of regional labour movements all influenced the particular character of hospital provision in different coalfields. South Wales possessed sizeable voluntary hospitals in the larger, more socially heterogeneous towns in the region, such as Swansea, Cardiff and Newport, in addition to a large number of smaller cottage hospitals in individual mining communities that were, to all intents and purposes, 'miners' hospitals'. Miners in the region utilised the smaller, local hospitals as accident centres and were referred to the larger infirmaries on the coast when more specialist care was required.[81]

In contrast, both the north-east of England and the coalfields in Scotland were more dependent on the larger infirmaries in nearby cities, especially Newcastle, Durham and Middlesbrough, and Edinburgh and Glasgow, respectively, for accident and consultant services, and workers were much less involved in the provision and management of their own cottage hospitals in those regions. The *British Medical Journal* noted in 1942, for example, that mining communities in Lanarkshire 'depended mainly on Glasgow for all hospital and outpatient treatment',[82] while the Accident Report Book of the Scottish Mine Owners' Defence and Mutual Insurance Association, also relating to Lanarkshire, demonstrates that the majority of injured miners recorded were either taken to the infirmary at Glasgow or sent home.[83]

These coalfields were not completely devoid of cottage hospitals, of course, and institutions such as Ashington Hospital and Ellison Hall Infirmary in the north-east and Blantyre Cottage Hospital and Randolph Wemyss Memorial Hospital in Scotland might be considered 'miners' hospitals'.[84] Indeed, the small Ashington Hospital, equipped with forty-four beds by the 1940s, was taken over by the miners and managers of the Ashington Coal Company in the interwar period and was staffed by a single medical superintendent, the company's surgeon, whom the company lent to the hospital on a part-time basis. The hospital was intended for the treatment of accidents and illnesses that afflicted the contributors and their families, and, with the exception of emergency accident cases, did not take cases from outside the ranks of its contributors until a handful of cases were admitted during the 1940s. Another small hospital was the Horden Cottage Hospital in Durham, which was initiated by the local coal company to offer rapid treatment in accident cases arising in the company's concerns; the institution possessed only six beds and later became a clearing station for accident cases that were sent on to larger hospitals, primarily the Sunderland Royal Infirmary.[85] Nevertheless, despite the existence of such small miners' hospitals in the north-east of England and in the Scottish coalfields, it remained the case that there were far fewer small or cottage hospitals than in south Wales, and injured miners in those other coalfields tended to end up in the larger voluntary hospitals in the major towns and cities of their respective regions. Whatever the precise character of hospital provision in each case, however, coalfields were nevertheless marked by a paucity of institutional provision relative to other regions, and a considerable amount of unmet need existed in this period.[86]

Whatever the organisation of hospital services in each coalfield, it is clear that miners' organisations gained increasing power and influence in the management and, even, control of medical services in the late nineteenth and early twentieth centuries and were able to have at least some influence over the ways in which these services attempted to meet their particular needs. Firstly, through subscriptions and donations, miners contributed to the finances of local hospitals; such payments were made either individually, through hospital contributory schemes, or collectively, through pit committees or union lodges.[87] Workmen's contributions had come to form an increasingly important element of voluntary hospital finances in the second half of the nineteenth century, and attempts had been made, with varying degrees of success, to secure and increase working-class representation on the hospitals' board of management.[88] In these important ways medicine was not just something that did things to miners' bodies, as a crude vision of medicalisation might have it; rather, miners themselves were crucial to the development of medical services and, arguably, to the extension of medical expertise over their own bodies.

A little surprisingly, perhaps, given the absence of effective medical treatments, some occupational disease cases were admitted into hospitals in mining regions in the late nineteenth and early twentieth centuries. Miners were admitted into Sunderland Infirmary suffering from 'Miners' Phthisis' and 'Miners' Nystagmus', and it is difficult not to conclude that the hospital acted as a place of convalescence in such cases.[89] Indeed, such cases were often transferred from the medical wards to convalescent homes as hospitals came to provide such facilities from the late nineteenth century onwards, as was the case with the Schaw Home, attached to Glasgow Royal Infirmary and opened in 1895–96.[90]

More numerous than the cases of chronic occupational disease were the many accident cases admitted. By their nature, emergency accident cases necessitated immediate care and attention in a way that chronic afflictions did not, and large numbers of miners were transported directly to hospital after an accident, even if that meant a long journey from pit-head to sick-bed.[91] Many such accident cases came under the care of consultant surgeons, and surgical responses were more numerous than medical.[92] Many of the operations performed on injured miners were quite mundane in character and involved little more than procedures intended to clean a wound, drain an abscess or manage a hernia.[93] More complicated procedures were also performed, of course, and the degree of long-term impairment was greater in these cases. In the 1890s, W. E. Harker, surgeon at the Royal Victoria Infirmary, Newcastle, performed laminectomies on miners with spinal injuries, wired compound fractures and amputated limbs with crush injuries. These all involved greater or lesser degrees of permanent impairment for the miner involved.[94]

Miners supported a range of other medical institutions also and, of all the specialist institutions to which support was given, it was ophthalmic hospitals and blind charities that most benefited from the funding supplied by miners' organisations. This was undoubtedly because of the large amount of occupational blindness, eye injuries and diseases suffered by miners.[95] Large numbers of workplaces, most notably collieries, contributed towards the funds of the Glasgow Ophthalmic Institution, for example, and, by the early 1880s, the Institution received almost two-thirds of its income from workplaces.[96] In return, it admitted large numbers of miners with eye injuries for surgical treatment.[97]

Impaired miners and medical knowledge: lung diseases, miners' nystagmus and orthopaedics

The period between 1880 and 1948 saw considerable changes in the medical profession's understanding of the miner's body. The dust diseases silicosis and pneumoconiosis and the eye condition nystagmus were two major areas of change in medical knowledge. Their histories provide clear insights into the consequences of medical and scientific research, not to mention the development of medical services, for disabled people in the modern period. In addition, the development of orthopaedics and its uses in the treatment and rehabilitation of injured miners, similarly had considerable implications for the lives and experiences of disabled people. Nevertheless, these three areas, pulmonary disease, nystagmus and injuries to limbs, here taken in turn, illustrate the varied and complicated nature of that process of medicalisation that is so important to the history of medicine and disability in the twentieth century.

The aspect of mining health most studied by historians, by far, has been the dust diseases that ravaged mining communities and which continue to have an effect in the twenty-first century, even after the closure of almost all British collieries.[98] Pneumoconiosis, caused by inhalation of the dust produced in the working of coal, has been recognised by historians as 'the most deadly and disabling of coal miners' chronic occupational diseases', and, indeed, 'the largest occupational health disaster in British history'.[99] Historians have studied the development of medical and scientific understanding of the disease, on the one hand, and the interactions between trade unions, employers and the state in the registration, control and management of the disease, on the other, but there has been little attention to the medical aspects of the disease in terms of miners' experiences or their interactions with medicine.

Dust diseases were slow to be recognised, or to be attributed to working conditions and acted upon by government and the medical establishment. In the nineteenth century many members of the medical profession were sceptical even of the diseases' existence. Dr Andrew Smart, a researcher into dust diseases based in Edinburgh, for example, told the 1885 Annual Meeting of the British

Medical Association that two years previously he had 'express[ed] the view that anthracosis, or "miner's [sic] consumption," had but a doubtful, if any existence'. Although now recognising anthracosis' existence, Smart still refuted the link between coal dust and disease, even suggesting that 'there must be some special protective feature in coal-mining operations not shared in by the rest of the dusty trades'.[100] Even by the early twentieth century doctors could be found who insisted that coal dust was beneficial to miners, and even that it was the dust that gave Welsh miners their excellent singing voices.[101] These erroneous views reached the popular imagination. In 1902 the bestselling novelist Allen Raine remarked: 'Fortunately for the colliers it [coal dust] is not unwholesome, or their lives would be seriously endangered by the clogging of their skin.'[102] McIvor and Johnston note that miners' chest diseases had appeared in medical journals in the 1830s, had disappeared by the late nineteenth century and then reappeared in the early twentieth century.[103]

Research into miners' dust diseases gathered pace from the second decade of the twentieth century onwards, often as a result of the pressure exerted by miners' trade unions, and it resulted in official recognition through inclusion in the statutory workmen's compensation system. An Act passed in 1918 instituted compensation payments for workers suffering chest disease as a result of work underground in which silica was present in the rock to a high degree and this was extended to miners engaged in drilling and blasting in 1928. Further research and political pressure by the trade unions resulted in a further amendment in 1935, when the need to prove the silica content was removed and all underground workers became eligible for compensation payments.[104] Silicosis in coalminers came to dominate all silicosis claims: by 1938, 51 per cent of disablement cases and 78 per cent of new disablement cases in Britain were attributed to the coalmining industry.[105] As recognition of the issue increased, and support grew for the idea that dust was harmful, employers intensified their resistance and many refused claims.[106] Coalminers' pneumoconiosis, finally recognised as a distinct and compensatable disease, was scheduled in 1942.[107]

In an official sense, miners' chest diseases were a problem confined to the south Wales coalfield in the 1930s and 1940s as disproportionately greater numbers of cases were notified in the region and as major research projects were carried out to ascertain the causes and character of the disease. In the years 1931 to 1937, for example, 5.23 in every 1,000 underground workers in anthracite mines in south Wales were certified with silicosis, compared to 0.06 in 1,000 in other British coalmines combined.[108] Official statistics put the death toll of silicosis and pneumoconiosis for south Wales miners at 1,334 between 1937 and 1948, while a further 18,297 were classed as permanent disablement cases; in contrast, the South Wales Area of the NUM contended that the figures should be 2,088 and 38,449, respectively.[109] Whatever the true extent of the pneumoconiosis problem, it was clear that south Wales bore a heavy burden relative to other coalfields: in comparison, only eighty pneumoconiotics were found in collieries across the north-east of England in 1943.[110] A memo from the Ministry of Fuel and Power in 1944 stated that south Wales possessed 'the "black spots" of the mining industry' for industrial pulmonary disease.[111]

Thus, miners' chest diseases underwent a process of medicalisation as they came to be defined as a medical rather than occupational problem, as medical and scientific research was carried out to discover the aetiology of the disease and as medical diagnoses allowed access to compensation payments. In this process, the miners' trade union was an important agent, as it encouraged scientists and medics with an interest in this matter to come to south Wales to conduct their research and encouraged miners to allow themselves to undergo medical examination and X-rays in order to develop knowledge and understanding of the disease.[112] The trade union's role in the medicalisation of miners' chest disease is best demonstrated in the adversarial nature of the compensation system. As Michael Bloor has noted, the union adopted an 'instrumental use of expertise', by which it countered the medical advice procured by employers in compensation cases by securing its own medical expertise to support impaired miners' claims to compensation.[113] Dai Dan Evans, a miners' leader in south Wales, was quite clear that medical expertise was purchased by the union on behalf of the impaired miner:

> So they [the company] sent him to a specialist, one employed by the coalowners, and he'd say this man is fit to go back to his normal work. The other man employed by us would say he's not fit to go back to his normal work ... Now. Both men have studied the same problem. They've studied medicine. And they've examined the same person: they've examined the same incapacity. And yet these two men will come to different conclusions ... Now. Is that because of ...? Not because of the condition of the man, but because of the difference between the person that employs them, the two classes that employ them.[114]

In these circumstances, impaired miners were not merely the objects of medical scrutiny and authority but, through their trade unions, were able to direct medical expertise to their advantage.

While progress was slow, fitful and contested, medical and scientific understanding of miners' pulmonary disease nevertheless increased in the first half of the twentieth century. Another major development in medical knowledge of miners' diseases, almost entirely overlooked by modern historians, concerned

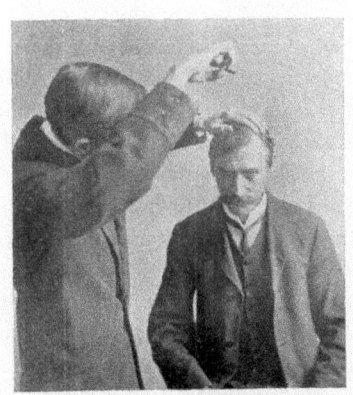
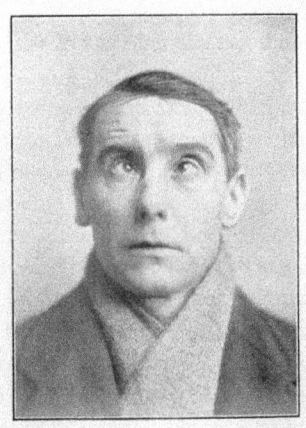

1 A miner is tested for nystagmus using 'the head test'. From the First Report of the Miners' Nystagmus Committee, 1922.

the eye condition nystagmus, characterised by the uncontrollable oscillation of the eyeball (Figure 1). Nystagmus was prevalent across the country's coalmines – McIvor and Johnston estimate that over 10,000 miners had developed the condition by the 1920s – but it continued to be 'poorly understood before the Second World War'.[115] Nystagmus was scheduled under the workmen's compensation legislation earlier than many of the other occupational diseases associated with miners: it was scheduled as an industrial disease under the 1906 Act, and clarified as 'nystagmus in the process of mining' in 1913. Much like the discourses on dust diseases, the causation of nystagmus was the subject of fierce medical debate. Two narratives dominated explanations of its primary cause. The first was that it was a consequence of the position of the miner at work, primarily as a result of the miner's lying on his side while working, while the second explanation attributed the disease to poor illumination, made worse by the safety lamps used underground.[116]

The latter explanation came to be accepted within the medical profession. Dr Josiah Court, who carried out research into the disease in Derbyshire, the Forest of Dean and Durham, proclaimed in 1919 that he had 'entirely demolished the received theory that Nystagmus was due to the strain on the eyes caused by the cramped position in which the men work'.[117] In the Durham collieries which Court inspected, he found that 'nearly a third of those using the safety lamp were affected, and yet they never lie upon their sides to work, they never turned obliquely upwards'.[118] Nevertheless, this did not end the alternate view being propagated in medical and trade journals: the *Colliery Guardian* continued to publish articles refuting the illumination theory well into the 1920s and 1930s.[119] Much like pneumoconiosis, the medical debate surrounding nystagmus was long, complex and full of uncertainty, and this had consequences for impaired miners' experiences of the compensation system.

The medical discourses surrounding dust diseases and miners' nystagmus demonstrate the complexity and contested nature of medical knowledge. More than that, medical or professional understandings differed from lay attitudes and miners and their families made sense of impairment in distinctive ways. Nowhere was this clearer than in lay attitudes towards the efficacy of medical science's ability to 'cure' or ameliorate impairments and the use of patent medicines, 'quack' cures and alternative systems of medicine. Ointments, embrocations and liniments were concocted by family members or individuals in the community and utilised to ease the aches and pains of work and everyday life. One doctor who practised in the Aberdare region, south Wales, before the First World War remembered a 'Mrs. Scott' of 'Gwynfa Terrace' who prepared her famous linseed poultices whenever anyone became ill and patients apparently saw no need to consult a doctor after seeing her.[120] In Ernest Rhys' collection of interconnected tales, *Black Horse Pit* (1925), set in the north-east of England where he had worked as a young mining engineer in the 1880s, a cure-all known as 'Hollover's "White Bottle"' looms large:

> In its magic powers and strange efficacy Black Horse Pit believed to a man – all save the pit-doctor, Dr. Smith, who made a grimace as if he were chewing bitter aloes when it was mentioned. It always was mentioned, for the recognised thing to do when a man was brought out of the pit disabled by a runaway tub or fall of stone was to set him down at Hollover's cabin door. Then, with an air of immense assurance, Hollover [who worked at the foot of the mineshaft] brought out the white bottle, and gave the damaged man a delicate douche on the joint affected, or, if it was a cut or wound, on a dirty rag fetched out of his rag-bag, which he applied *secundum artem*.
>
> 'It's enough to poison any man he puts it on,' said the doctor; 'rotten eggs, turps, lamp-oil, I shouldn't wonder; and a beastly dirty clarty clout to make it worse.'
>
> But what is science against faith? If the management had suppressed Hollover's white bottle there would have been a strike.[121]

In these 'reminiscent tales',[122] published four decades after Rhys left the mines, the White Bottle *does* wield a restorative power.

Patent medicines, usually obtained from pharmacists or else through advertisements in newspapers, were also popular. One of the best known was Dr William's Pink Pills for Pale People, one of those cure-all patent medicines that seemingly cured more complaints than was credible. Advertisements for such products were tailored for the various readerships of the newspapers in which they appeared and one such advertisement, aimed at miners, included a testimonial from a miner breaking both legs from a falling roof who had 'three doctors attending me off and on, and although they were exceptionally kind and did all they possibly could for me, I never got relief'. Had the pale person not received the pink pills, he '[did] not think I would now be alive'.[123]

More significant as far as impairment is concerned, miners, similar to many other manual workers, patronised bone-setters for a range of physical injuries and complaints.[124] Such untrained practitioners, whose skills were often passed down from generation to generation, attempted to give relief to stiff joints, dislocations, sprains and fractures by the manipulation of limbs or the body. Belief in these men was said to be implicit, and bonesetters were highly regarded in the communities in which they practised; two bonesetters in south Wales, William Price of Merthyr and Albert Whittle of Aberdare, even advertised their services in a local directory.[125] Another bonesetter, William Rae from Blantyre in the Lanarkshire coalfield, became famous beyond his mining community in 1904 as the local, national and medical press picked up his story and publicised his activities in 'bloodless surgery'.[126] After he treated a famous footballer in 1904, hundreds of injured and impaired individuals starting flocking to Blantyre each day to be treated by this 'miner healer', this 'collier surgeon', and Blantyre came to be described in the sensationalist tabloid treatment of the story as a 'Scottish Lourdes' and a 'Cripples' Mecca'.[127]

Despite the scorn of the medical establishment, bonesetters were not as far removed from mainstream medicine as other alternative practitioners, and certainly the techniques of bonesetters informed the development of orthopaedics, at least to some extent. It is indicative, for example, that David Rocyn Jones, the Monmouthshire county medical officer, was the descendant of three generations of bonesetters, and had one brother who continued the family tradition during the interwar period and another brother who became an orthopaedic surgeon, as did one of his sons.[128] The crucial point here, though, is that miners and their families looked beyond organised biomedicine for their health and well-being, and rejected the methods and techniques of professional doctors, preferring to follow their own sense of what worked and what brought relief.

While a great deal of scientific and medical research was carried out into nystagmus and pulmonary disease in the first half of the twentieth century, there was very little development in effective medical treatments and this partly explains the popularity of self-treatment and alternative systems of medical care. These two conditions were largely managed through removing the disabled worker from the conditions in which he had contracted the complaints in the first place. Sufferers from nystagmus were moved to lower-paid, lower-status work on the surface in better light conditions, if they did not leave the industry altogether, while pneumoconiotics faced considerable social and economic dislocation, particularly between 1943 and 1948, when they were required to leave the industry altogether if diagnosed with the disease.[129] In this sense, nystagmus and pneumoconiosis were medicalised to the extent that sufferers were subject to medical scrutiny and were required to undergo medical examination to prove eligibility for compensation payments, but they did not undergo any new, invasive or, indeed, effective medical interventions, nor were they institutionalised in hospitals or homes to any large degree.

In contrast, the development of orthopaedics in the same period witnessed not only developments in knowledge and understanding but also more extensive provision of medical and rehabilitation services that impacted in more direct and intimate ways on miners' bodies and had greater consequences for the experiences of impaired miners. Roger Cooter has shown how the development of orthopaedics in Britain in the 1920s was far more concerned with wounded veterans of the First World War and 'crippled' children than with the more numerous casualties of industry, as well as the ways in which the context changed in the 1930s and 1940s.[130] As orthopaedists sought new areas of influence for their particular skills and expertise, so the political and industrial context also changed to create more favourable conditions for the rehabilitation of injured workers and, as one of the most hazardous of industries, coal was central to the developments that took place in these years.[131]

A great deal of the work of rehabilitation was carried out in former convalescent homes that came to be medicalised in the 1930s and 1940s as orthopaedic techniques and treatments were increasingly applied. Convalescence, as an idea and a practice, had long been established in the industrial districts of Britain, none more so than the coalfields. In south Wales, the Rest Convalescent Home at Porthcawl was founded in the 1860s, largely through the charitable donations and subscriptions of the region's elites, and was intended for the working poor. By the late nineteenth century funding was received from a broad array of bodies and organisations, including miners' friendly societies, medical schemes and trade union lodges, so that miners and members of their families came to form the greater part of the home's clientele.[132] This change in the funding basis and patient base was reflected in developments in other coalfields in the same period as friendly societies and the Co-operative movement came to provide access to convalescent care for their respective constituencies, both of which might have included at least some miners, and as a right rather than as a charitable bounty.[133] Many of the larger voluntary hospitals also established convalescent homes in the latter part of the nineteenth century, in part to manage the pressure that was being placed on bed resources as more patients experienced longer stays in these institutions.[134]

The sources of income of convalescent homes underwent further significant change in the 1920s and 1930s as the Miners' Welfare Fund – a statutory body funded by a 1d. levy on each ton of coal raised in Britain and intended to improve the recreational facilities and health services in mining districts – came to make large grants to convalescent institutions.[135] Ayrshire District Miners' Convalescent Home in Kirkmichael and Talygarn Rehabilitation Centre in south Wales were both opened in 1923, for example, in spacious, healthy locations, to provide convalescence for injured and aged miners and their families. However, these were, by and large, social rather than medical institutions, and they focused more on the management of the regimen of the 'patient' than on any therapeutic interventions. Rest, good diet, light recreation and fresh air were intended as the main means by which the injured and sick would recuperate and be fit enough again to resume their former lives. In addition, the massive demand for places meant that long stays and extensive therapy were simply impossible and periods spent at the institutions were often envisaged as more akin to holidays than any medical experience.[136] The years during and just after the First World War witnessed a greater use of physiotherapy (i.e. physical, occupational and recreational therapy) as medical personnel came to play a more important role in convalescence, but it was the development of orthopaedics in the 1930s that led to greater medicalisation in convalescent homes as surgical interventions, greater medical supervision and efforts at physical rehabilitation changed regimes for miners to a greater degree than at any point previously.[137]

Such developments were evident from the 1930s onwards. A residential rehabilitation centre at Uddingston, near Glasgow and out-patients' orthopaedic clinics in the mining areas, were initiated in 1935 by the Lanarkshire Orthopaedic Association, a body with representatives from the miners' trade union, the employers' association and the local medical practitioners, while a residential orthopaedic centre at Berry Hill Hall, Mansfield and an out-patient centre at Wigan were both started in 1940. All three were initiated by the coalowners' associations or mutual indemnity companies (i.e. companies created by groups of employers to pool the insurance risks posed by injury and disability) in their respective areas and received significant financial assistance from them. The rationale for employer support was both to lessen the financial liabilities caused by serious impairment and to prevent collieries being clogged up with difficult 'light work' cases.[138] In the late 1930s a joint statement submitted by the senior surgeons of the Royal and Western infirmaries, Glasgow, to the Inter-Departmental Committee on the Rehabilitation of Persons Injured by Accidents stated quite explicitly that it was employers' organisations, friendly societies and the insurance companies, which dealt with workmen's compensation payments, that should fund rehabilitation centres, since 'money laid out for this purpose would give a good economic return'.[139]

Such was the utility of fracture clinics and residential rehabilitation centres that the Miners' Welfare Fund, managed by joint committees of employers' and union representatives, provided financial assistance to extend these types of medical interventions, just as it had supported convalescent homes. In 1933, for example, £25,000 was granted to the Sheffield Royal Infirmary to build a fracture unit in the Miners' Welfare ward, while £13,000 was given to the Manchester Royal Infirmary in 1938 when the fracture clinic was incorporated into a new orthopaedic and physiotherapy building.[140] The government White Paper on Coal in 1942 recommended 50 per cent grants for rehabilitation centres from the Miners' Welfare Fund.[141] By 1944, eight centres had been built, and several were converted convalescent homes, including Talygarn.[142] An Inter-Departmental Committee was formed to report on rehabilitation of disabled miners, and praised the cooperation of institutions for realising the medical ideal of rehabilitation, arguing that it should set a precedent for further collaboration in rehabilitation work between the Medical Service of the Ministry for Fuel and Power and the departments responsible for the rehabilitation scheme.[143] The Tomlinson Report, the blueprint for the Disabled Persons (Employment) Act of 1944, singled out the rehabilitation centres for particular praise.[144]

These various fracture clinics and residential rehabilitation centres involved quite significant medical interventions in relation to the bodies of impaired miners. Orthopaedists were convinced that the management of disability through surgery and rehabilitation was superior to the vocational training that merely taught the miner to cope with his impairment and trained him to undertake new forms of work.[145] This specialised, orthopaedic approach to impairment can be clearly seen in operation at the Western Infirmary, Glasgow. All fracture cases were seen by a member of the permanent staff within three hours of arrival and each case was overseen until the individual was able to leave the institution, so that the fracture healed correctly and any joint functioned as well as possible.[146] This involved ensuring that the fractured limb was managed so as to minimise the amount of atrophy and contraction of the surrounding muscle through the particular ways in which any limb was immobilised and the various exercises that could still be done while the limb was immobilised.[147] A great deal of the success or failure of any case was placed on the shoulders of the miner himself: 'recovery can only come by the unremitting hard work of the patient himself', opined E. A. Nicholls, surgeon at the Berry Hill Hall Miners' Rehabilitation Centre, '[i]gnorance, stupidity, apathy, and sheer laziness must all be overcome'.[148] This is a perfect illustration of the idea inherent in the medicalisation critique that the patient was required to put aside his own autonomy, assume the sick role and accept the expert authority of the surgeon over his health and his body. It also coincides with the idea that disability can be overcome through individual effort and determination.[149]

Rehabilitation followed such surgical intervention. Cooter notes that the definition of rehabilitation was a little uncertain in the 1930s and 1940s and variously included physical training, vocational education, surgical interventions and psychotherapy.[150] This was certainly evident in those rehabilitation facilities intended for miners. The Miners' Welfare Fund was clear in its estimation of the transformative role of rehabilitation:

> Besides treating the actual injury or affliction, rehabilitation aims at restoring general muscle tone, full function of body and limbs, general health, strength and self-confidence, and then re-settling the individual in industry in his old occupation or retraining him and settling him in some other occupation more suited to his physical capacity if altered.[151]

The restoration of function, health and strength, as close as possible to the miner's former state, was thus crucial. At the residential rehabilitation centres, treatment consisted of a regime of exercise in the gymnasium, physiotherapy (including the use of massage and heat treatment, and electricity to stimulate muscles), team games, handicrafts and outdoor work.[152] (Figures 2 and 3) Orthopaedists also hoped to extend their influence over the return to work of impaired miners, with input on the selection and supervision of the type of work to which each miner returned, or else the employment of 'medico-social workers as a link between the centre, the surgeon, the patients and the industry', but this ambition does not seem to have progressed beyond conceptions of the idealised role of the surgeon in the rehabilitation process.[153] As far as the Durham Miners' Rehabilitation Centre at Chester-le-Street was concerned, the 'surgeon-in-charge' examined each miner referred to him by the miner's general practitioner or the surgeon at the fracture clinic and hospital, to see if he was an appropriate object for the care of the Centre. He would then decide the miner's course of treatment during the stay at the Centre and, interestingly, would discharge the miner according to one of four classifications: that he was fit for immediate return to full employment, that he was fit for light work leading

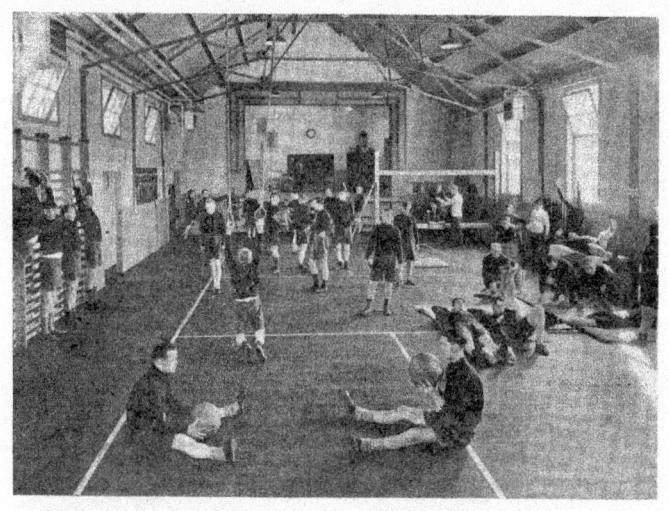

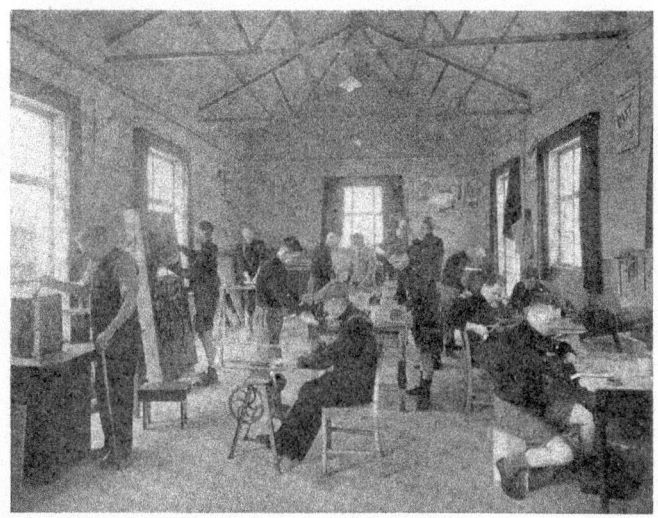

2 Miners partaking in exercises and handicraft at a rehabilitation centre, 1940s

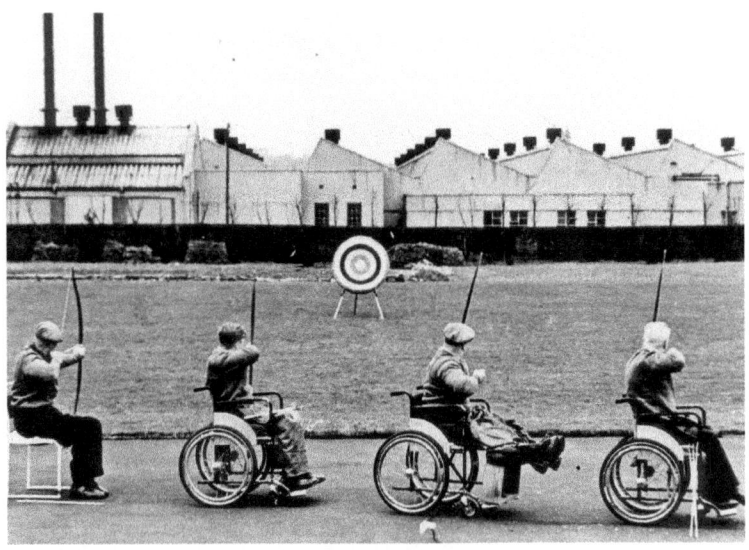

3 Miners practise archery at Uddingston Rehabilitation Centre, near Glasgow. Courtesy of the National Mining Museum Scotland Trust.

to full employment, that he was 'fit permanently for light work adapted to some residual incurable disability', or discharged 'unfit for further employment in mines but recommended for vocational re-training'. In the case of this centre, the surgeon also undertook to make occasional visits after discharge to ascertain the miner's progress and would then make a report to the miner's doctor, who could then refer the miner back to the Centre.[154]

If orthopaedists are to be believed, the miner patients were initially suspicious of the work carried out at fracture clinics and rehabilitation centres, but largely because they feared that the aim was merely to get them back to work in order to swell the employers' profits. Once this misconception was overcome and the orthopaedists' independence from the employers was established, it was claimed, disabled patients then accepted the clinics and centres 'purely as a treatment centre' and were more open and more cooperative in their responses to the medical professionals with whom they came into contact.[155]

Conclusion

In the years following the installation of a majority Labour government in 1945 the coal industry was nationalised and a national health service was created. Both were the culmination of long struggles or campaigns, or else the product of a great deal of discussion, disagreement and development in the years before the 1940s. Aneurin Bevan's awareness of the conditions in coalmining communities and, indeed, his involvement in a working-class mutualist organisation, the Tredegar Workmen's Medical Aid Society, were important influences in the decisions he took in the period from 1945 to 1948. At the same time, and despite such influences, occupational health, industrial medicine and the medical responses to disability continued to be partial, fragmentary and uncoordinated, and medicine continued to fail disabled miners and to subject them to a medical model that disregarded the factors that caused their disablement.

Not even the obligation placed upon the new NCB to safeguard the health of all employees, manifest in a new Mines Medical Service, could address these failings, and the coal industry continued to lag behind other industries in the quality of medical care extended to its workers. C. G. Vickers, Legal Advisor to the NCB and later a member of the Board, argued that:

> Before nationalisation, there were a few isolated examples of colliery medical services which included surgeries, state-registered nurse, central X-ray plant, physiotherapy, and other services. In general, however, coalmining had no such service, and the doctors attached to mines were mainly there to deal with serious accidents, and for compensation cases. By contrast, good medical services, first class clinics, doctors, state registered nurses, physiotherapy, x-ray, dentistry, chiropody and other facilities are by now fairly general in other large industrial undertakings. It is, in fact, becoming accepted that any large industrial undertaking should be regarded not only as a business concern, but as a social unit and, as such, it will be expected to provide certain social services of which a medical service will be one. In return for providing an adequate medical service, industry can expect certain benefits such as, for example, the raising of morale, the increase of working efficiency, and the reduction of wastage and time lost through sickness and accidents which are, in the coalmining industry, at present very considerable.[156]

The seventy or so years before the creation of the NHS and the NCB certainly witnessed a great deal of development in understandings of the miner's body, health and well-being, and various aspects of the impairment caused by the coal industry were much better understood than ever before. The efforts made to better understand chest diseases, nystagmus and injuries were considerable, and it would be no exaggeration to claim that the miner's well-being was given greater importance by the 1940s. Considerable scientific and medical research had been carried out, various injuries, diseases and complaints had been registered as compensatable and a range of services had been developed to treat mining disabilities – miners' bodies were valued like at no other time in history, either before or since.

Crucially, however, very little of this attention or research had resulted in the development of effective therapeutics, nor indeed a view of mining impairment as being anything other than pathological and, indeed, a medical problem. Nevertheless, it is evident that medical science continued to play only a very limited role in miners' impairments. Greater medicalisation was evident in other health experiences in the first half of the century, such as childbirth, infectious disease, children's health or mental health, but continued to be quite stunted in relation to the types of ailments and injuries that afflicted miners. Despite their role in initial treatment or diagnosis, and then subsequent interventions in the compensation system, doctors had only a very limited role to play in relation to miners' disability, and a crude reading of the medicalisation critique cannot be applied to this area of healthcare and medicine.

The medicalisation model is further complicated by the roles played by miners and disabled workers in their experiences of medicine, and, as Steve Sturdy's work reminds us, the need to recognise workers' own agency is crucial.[157] This particular 'patient group' was well organised, relatively militant and powerful in political terms, and it was able to influence the debates and discussions that went on about their health and, at least in part, to organise their own health and medical services according to their own values and priorities. While disability scholars are right to claim that 'Historically, people with disabilities have been powerless, marginalized socially, politically, and economically, and denigrated by dominant cultural values', this would not seem to describe the experiences of miners very accurately.[158] The might of organised labour was considerable when compared to the power that could be mobilised on behalf of other groups such as children, women, the poor or the mentally ill, and it was often exercised to increase the extent and reach of medical services. Any assertion of the supremacy of medical expertise over the miner's body, therefore, would be flawed in the extreme.[159]

Notes

1 *Colliery Guardian*, 5 November 1915.
2 See Roger Cooter, *Surgery and Society in Peace and War: Orthopaedics and the Organization of Modern Medicine, 1880–1948* (Basingstoke: Macmillan, 1993), p. 138; Arthur J. McIvor and Ronald Johnston *Miners' Lung: A History of Dust Disease in British Coal Mining* (Aldershot: Ashgate, 2007), p. 66; Steve Sturdy, 'The Industrial Body', in John V. Pickstone and Roger Cooter (eds), *Companion to Medicine in the Twentieth Century* (London: Routledge, 2003), pp. 217–34.
3 Beth Linker, 'On the Borderland of Medical and Disability History: A Survey of the Fields', *Bulletin of the History of Medicine*, 87:4 (2013), p. 519.

4 Catherine Kudlick, 'Comment: On the Borderland of Medical and Disability History', *Bulletin of the History of Medicine*, 87:4 (2013), p. 544; Jeanne Hayes and Elizbaeth "Lisa" M. Hannold, 'The Road to Empowerment: A Historical Perspective on the Medicalization of Disability', *Journal of Health and Human Services Administration*, 30:3 (2007), p. 357.
5 Deborah Lupton, 'Foucault and the Medicalisation Critique', in Alan R. Petersen and Robin Bunton (eds), *Foucault, Health and Medicine* (London: Routledge, 1997), p. 189.
6 Hayes and Hannold, 'The Road to Empowerment', p. 355.
7 Hayes and Hannold, 'The Road to Empowerment', p. 353.
8 Linker, 'On the Borderland of Medical and Disability History', p. 519.
9 Linker, 'On the Borderland of Medical and Disability History', p. 526.
10 'Life, Enterprise, and Peril in Coal-Mines', *Quarterly Review*, 110:220 (October 1861), p. 359, quoted in James Jaffe, 'Introduction', in John Benson (ed.), *Coal in Victorian Britain, Part II: Volume 4, Identities and Communities* (London: Pickering & Chatto, 2012), p. vii.
11 Ferdynand Zweig, *Men in the Pits* (London: Gollancz, 1948), p. 4.
12 Anne McClintock, *Imperial Leather: Race, Gender, and Sexuality in Colonial Contest* (London: Routledge, 2013), p. 115.
13 James C. Welsh, *The Underworld: The Story of Robert Sinclair, Miner* (London: H. Jenkins, 1920); James C. Welsh, *The Morlocks* (London: Herbert Jenkins, 1924); H. G. Wells, *The Time Machine* (London: William Heinemann, 1895).
14 For examples, see *Y Gwladgarwr*, 22 July 1881, p. 4; *Y Gwyliedydd*, 19 March 1908, p. 2; *Y Darian*, 23 November 1916, p. 6.
15 George Orwell, *The Road to Wigan Pier*, new edn (London: Penguin Classics, 2001), p. 13.
16 Ramsay Guthrie, *Kitty Fagan: A Romance of Pit Life* (London: Christian Commonwealth Publishing, 1900), p. 78.
17 J. C. Grant, *The Back-to-Backs* (London: Chatto and Windus, 1930), p. 18.
18 Harold Heslop, *The Gate of a Strange Field* (London: Brentano, 1929), p. 33.
19 Lewis Jones, *We Live* (1939) in Lewis Jones, *Cwmardy and We Live* (Cardigan: Parthian, 2006), p. 637.
20 Jones, *Cwmardy and We Live*, p. 169.
21 Tom Hanlin, *Yesterday Will Return* (London: Nicholas & Watson, 1946), p. 120.
22 Hanlin, *Yesterday Will Return*, pp. 119–20.
23 Sturdy, 'The Industrial Body'.
24 Perhaps the most notable instance of this rhetorical use of illness, injury and disability can be found in the discussions surrounding the Sankey Commission which reported in 1919; Independent Labour Party, *The Mineowners in the Dock: A Summary of the Evidence Given before the Coal Industry Commission* (London: Independent Labour Party, 1919); for another example of the rhetorical uses of disability in a political context, see Edward Slavishak, *Bodies of Work: Civic Display and Labor in Industrial Pittsburgh* (Durham, NC: Duke University Press, 2008).

25 Martin A. Powell, 'How Adequate was Hospital Provision before the NHS? An Examination of the 1945 South Wales Hospital Survey', *Local Population Studies*, 48 (1992), pp. 22–32; Martin A. Powell, 'Hospital Provision before the National Health Service: A Geographical Study of the 1945 Hospital Survey', *Social History of Medicine*, 5:3 (1992), pp. 483–504; Martin Gorsky, John Mohan and Martin Powell, 'British Voluntary Hospitals, 1871–1938: The Geography of Provision and Utilization', *Journal of Historical Geography*, 25:4 (1999), pp. 463–82; Martin A. Powell, 'Coasts and Coalfields: The Geographical Distribution of Doctors in England and Wales in the 1930s', *Social History of Medicine*, 18:2 (2005), pp. 245–63.

26 A. J. Cronin, *The Citadel* (London: Vista, 1996), p. 17. A bosh is a sink.

27 'An Investigation into the Economic Conditions of Contract Medical Practice in the United Kingdom', *British Medical Journal*, Supplement, 22 July 1905.

28 David G. Green, *Working-Class Patients and the Medical Establishment* (Aldershot: Gower, 2005).

29 Royal Commission on the Poor Laws and Relief of Distress. Appendix volume III. Minutes of evidence, Cd. 4755, 1909, xl, p. 426.

30 Michael Foot, *Aneurin Bevan, A Biography, vol.1* (London: MacGibbon & Kee, 1963), p. 63; Harold Finch, *Memoirs of a Bedwellty MP* (Newport: Starling Press, 1972), pp. 33–5; David G. Green, *Working Class Patients and the Medical Establishment* (Hounslow: Temple Smith, 1985), p. 174, *Picture Post*, 27 April 1946, pp. 20–1.

31 A. J. Cronin, *Adventures in Two Worlds* (London: Victor Gollancz, 1952), p. 159. A. J. Cronin drew on his personal experiences as a doctor in south Wales and as Medical Inspector of Mines to portray the work of a Scottish doctor in a south Wales mining district, fictionalising Tredegar Medical Aid Society as 'Aberalaw Medical Aid Society'.

32 Christopher Meredith, 'Cronin and the Chronotope: Place, Time and Pessimistic Individualism in *The Citadel*', *North American Journal of Welsh Studies*, 8 (2013), pp. 50–65; Alan Davies, *A. J. Cronin: The Man Who Created Dr Finlay* (London: Alma Books, 2011); S. O'Mahony, 'A. J. Cronin and *The Citadel*: Did a Work of Fiction Contribute to the Foundation of the NHS?', *Journal of the Royal College of Physicians of Edinburgh*, 42 (2012), pp. 172–8.

33 Rhys Davies, *A Time to Laugh* (Cardigan: Parthian, 2014), p. 103.

34 Davies, *A Time to Laugh*, p. 178.

35 Davies, *A Time to Laugh*, pp. 177–8.

36 Morris cannot benefit from employment by the Medical Aid Society as he has been boycotted. He has alienated chapel-going collier families on account of a scandal involving being arrested while in bed with a working-class woman; he is later acquitted of the crime of incitement to riot, but the woman's miner brother is sentenced to nine months' hard labour.

37 'An Investigation into the Economic Conditions of Contract Medical Practice in the United Kingdom', *British Medical Journal*, Supplement, 22 July 1905, p. 13.

38 *British Medical Journal*, 6 June 1903, pp. 1339–40.

39 The term 'panel patients' refers to the panels of doctors established under the 1911 Act that provided care under the National Insurance (NI) system. The patients covered were eligible on account of their NI payments and consulted a doctor from the panel.
40 Royal College of Physicians of Edinburgh website, Recollections of John S. Milne, www.rcpe.ac.uk/library-archives/general-practice-east-lothian-1946-1966, accessed 17 November 2015.
41 *List of Societies approved by the Joint Commissioners and by the Commissioners for England, Ireland, Scotland, and Wales*, Cd. 6238, 1912–12, lxxviii, p. 11; Ian MacDougall (ed.), *Mid and East Lothian Miners' Association Minutes 1894–1918* (Edinburgh: Scottish History Society, 2003), p. 19; K. Brown, 'The Lodges of the Durham Miners' Association, 1869–1926', *Northern History*, 23:1 (1987), p. 143.
42 Scottish Board of Health, *Consultative Council on Medical and Allied Services, Interim Report, A Scheme of Medical Service for Scotland*, Cmd. 1039, 1920, xvii, p. 8.
43 For examples, see South Wales Coalfield Collection, Swansea University, Alistair Wilson Collection; Glamorgan Archives, Cresswell Family Practice Records.
44 Anne Digby, *The Evolution of British General Practice, 1850–1948* (Oxford: Oxford University Press, 1999), pp. 192, 210–11.
45 Digby, *Evolution of British General Practice*, p. 198; see also her '"A Human Face to Medicine?": Encounters between Patients and General Practitioners in Britain, 1850–1950', *Medizin, Gesellschaft und Geschichte*, 21 (2002), p. 95.
46 Florance O'Sullivan, *Return to Wales* (Tenby: Five Arches Press, 1974), p. 49.
47 Digby, *The Evolution of British General Practice*, pp. 198, 210–12.
48 South Wales Miners' Library, Swansea University (hereafter SWML), AUD/317, Will Arthur interview.
49 Digby, *The Evolution of British General Practice*, pp. 319–20; Steven Thompson, 'Paying the Piper and Calling the Tune? Complaints against Doctors in Workers' Medical Schemes in the South Wales Coalfield', in Jonathan Reinarz and Rebecca Wynter (eds), *Complaints, Controversies and Grievances in Medicine: Historical and Social Science Perspectives* (London: Taylor & Francis, 2014), pp. 93–108.
50 Cronin, *The Citadel*, p. 116.
51 Cronin, *The Citadel*, pp. 115–16.
52 B. L. Coombes, *Miners Day* (Middlesex: Harmondsworth, 1945), pp. 124–5.
53 For evidence on the 'treatment' of nystagmus, see Simeon Snell, 'On Miners' Nystagmus', *British Medical Journal*, 11 July 1891, p. 66; *Colliery Guardian*, 16 January 1920, p. 170.
54 Frank Shufflebotham, 'The Hygienic Aspect of the Coal-Mining Industry in the United Kingdom', *British Medical Journal*, 14 March 1914, p. 590.
55 C. M. Fletcher, 'Pnuemoconiosis of Coal-Miners', *British Medical Journal*, 5 June 1948, p. 1073.
56 For examples, see Greater Glasgow and Clyde NHS Archives, HB52/2/1, Schaw Auxiliary Home, Register of Admissions and Discharges, Feb 1933–Jul 1936.
57 B. L. Coombes, *Those Clouded Hills* (London: Cobbett, 1944), p. 27.

58 Jack Jones, *Black Parade* (Cardigan: Parthian, 2009), p. 19.
59 Tyne and Wear Archives Service (hereafter TWAS), HO.HI/11, Highfield Public Assistance Institution (Sunderland), Surgeon's Admission and Discharge Register, 2 May 1885–30 June 1890.
60 Gwent Archives, D.2472, Ebbw Vale Workmen's Doctors' Fund, Committee Minute Book, 1896–1900, passim. By the 1920s, application was made to arrange for cars to convey members home from convalescent homes but was rejected by the committee; SWMF, Executive Council and Annual and Special Conferences minutes, Annual Conference, 14–17 June 1920.
61 Brown, 'The Lodges of the Durham Miners' Association', p. 144; MacDougall, *Mid and East Lothian Miners' Association*, p. 209.
62 Glamorgan Archives, DX 83/9/1, Dowlais Iron Company Truss and Wooden Leg Register; see Ben Curtis and Steven Thompson, '"A Plentiful Crop of Cripples Made by All this Progress": Disability, Artificial Limbs and Working-Class Mutualism in the South Wales Coalfield, 1890–1948', *Social History of Medicine*, 27:4 (2014), p. 10.
63 South Wales Coalfield Collection, Swansea University, SWCC/MNA/NUM/3/5/15, South Wales Miners' Federation, Compensation Secretary's Correspondence with Area No. 4, 1934–1941, Letter to Evan Williams (SWMF Compensation Secretary) from J. M. Williams (Bute [Merthyr] Lodge), 21 September 1934.
64 Rhys Davies, 'The Benefit Concert', in Rhys Davies, *Collected Stories: Volume II* edited by Meic Stephens (Llandysul: Gomer Press, 1996), pp. 17–25.
65 This is documented extensively in Curtis and Thompson, '"A Plentiful Crop of Cripples Made by All this Progress"'.
66 Hayes and Hannold, 'The Road to Empowerment', pp. 360, 367, note that the choice to use assistive devices such as prostheses is a different matter to the imposition of such devices on people with impairments that seeks to normalise them; on the reactions of Foucauldians to calls for the 'de-medicalisation' of everyday life, see Lupton, 'Foucault and the Medicalisation Critique', pp. 207–9.
67 Curtis and Thompson, '"A Plentiful Crop of Cripples Made by All this Progress"', pp. 722–5.
68 Gwent Archives, D.2472, Ebbw Vale Workmen's Doctors' Fund Committee, Minute Book, 24 April, 27 March 1897. The woman was listed as 'Mrs Cooper', and so it is possible she was the wife of a member.
69 Curtis and Thompson, '"A Plentiful Crop of Cripples Made by All this Progress"', pp. 718–19.
70 Gwent Archives, D.914, Ebbw Vale Workmen's Medical Society, Committee Minute Book, 16 October 1943.
71 Gwent Archives, D.3246.1, Tredegar Workmen's Medical Aid Society, Minute Book, 28 March 1929. Hearing aids would of course also have been impractical in the conditions of the mine.
72 Graeme Gooday and Karen Sayer, *Managing the Experience of Hearing Loss in Britain, 1830–1930* (London: Palgrave Pivot, 2015), e-book.

73 National Archives of Scotland, CB19/1, Scottish Coal Workers' Compensation Scheme, Director's Minute Books, 1912–1914, 906/8.
74 Examples of colliers with wooden legs include surface workers (A. J. Cronin, *The Stars Look Down* (London: New English Library, 1978 [1935]) and Jones, *Black Parade*, and underground workers such as a hewer (Harold Heslop, *The Earth Beneath* (London: T. V. Boardman, 1946)) and a roadman (Jack Jones, *Bidden to the Feast*, (London: Corgi Books, 1968 [1938])). Earlier examples include a guard for the slag-heap (Ramsay Guthrie, *Kitty Fagan: A Romance of Pit Life* (London: Christian Commonwealth Publishing, 1900)) and a 'knocker'/'caller' to wake the men for their shifts (Ramsay Guthrie, *Black Dyke* (London: Charles H. Kelly, 1904)). There are also examples of men with 'peg legs' from among the mining community who were self-employed, such as a carter-grocer (Irene Saunderson, *A Welsh Heroine* (London: Lynwood & Co., 1910)), a boot-maker (James C. Welsh, *The Morlocks* (London: Herbert Jenkins, 1924)) and a baker (Rhys Davies, *The Withered Root* (London: R. Holden, 1927)).
75 Gwent Archives, D.2472, Ebbw Vale Workmen's Doctors' Fund Committee, Minute Book, 19 March 1898.
76 Gwent Archives, D.2472, Ebbw Vale Workmen's Doctors' Fund Committee, Minute Book, 31 December 1898.
77 Gwent Archives, D.3246.1, Tredegar Workmen's Medical Aid Society, Minute Book, 17 September 1936.
78 Tredegar Workmen's Medical Aid Society, General Committee Minutes, 28 February 1929, 9 March 1933, 23 March 1933, 28 November 1935, 17 September 1936.
79 Brian Abel-Smith, *The Hospitals, 1800–1948: A Study in Social Administration in England and Wales* (London: Heinemann, 1964).
80 On cottage hospitals, see Meyrick Emrys Roberts, *The Cottage Hospitals, 1859–1990* (Motcombe: Tern, 1991); Steven Cherry, 'Change and Continuity in the Cottage Hospitals c.1859–1948: The Experience in East Anglia', *Medical History*, 36 (1992), pp. 271–89.
81 Steven Thompson, 'The Mixed Economy of Care in the South Wales Coalfield, c.1850–1950', in Donnacha Seán Lucey and Virginia Crossman (eds), *Healthcare in Ireland and Britain from 1850: Voluntary, Regional and Comparative Perspectives* (London: Institute of Historical Research, 2015), pp. 150–4.
82 Alexander Miller, 'Late Rehabilitation of the Injured', *British Medical Journal*, 22 August 1942, p. 4259.
83 Glasgow University Archives, UGD 1/34/1, Scottish Mine Owners' Defence and Mutual Insurance Association 1907–1908, Preliminary Report of Accidents.
84 Ministry of Health, *Hospital Survey: The Hospital Services of the North-Eastern Area* (London: HMSO, 1946), pp. 43, 45.
85 Ministry of Health, *Hospital Survey*, pp. 43, 62.
86 Powell, 'How Adequate was Hospital Provision before the NHS?'; Powell, 'Coasts and Coalfields'.
87 Steven Cherry, 'Accountability, Entitlement, and Control Issues and Voluntary Hospital Funding, c.1860–1939', *Social History of Medicine*, 9:2 (1996), pp. 215–33;

Steven Cherry, 'Hospital Saturday, Workplace Collections, and Issues in Late Nineteenth-Century Hospital Funding', *Medical History*, 44 (2000), pp. 461–88; Barry M. Doyle, 'Voluntary Hospitals in Edwardian Middlesbrough: A Preliminary Report', *North East History*, 34 (2001), pp. 5–33. As an example, see TWAS, HO.SRI/3/1, Sunderland Royal Infirmary, Workmen's Governors Committee Minutes, 1883–1888.

88 Cherry, 'Hospital Saturday', pp. 476–8; Cherry, 'Accountability, Entitlement, and Control Issues', pp. 225–32; Doyle, 'Voluntary Bospitals in Edwardian Middlesbrough'; Steven Thompson, '"To Relieve the Sufferings of Humanity, Irrespective of Party, Politics or Creed": Conflict, Consensus and Voluntary Hospital Provision in Edwardian South Wales', *Social History of Medicine*, 16:2 (2003), pp. 247–62.

89 TWAS, HO.SRI/45/1, Sunderland Infirmary, Register of Medical Cases, 1st July 1891–28th June 1897.

90 For examples of miners with 'emphysema' and 'silicosis', see NHS Greater Glasgow and Clyde Archives, HB52/2/1, Schaw Home, Admission and Dismissions Register, 1933–36.

91 The National Archives, Kew, London (hereafter TNA), BX 3/3, Miners' Welfare Fund: Committee of Enquiry Evidence (1932), Paper No. 24: Memorandum of Evidence from the Miners' Federation of Great Britain; Miller, 'Late Rehabilitation of the Injured', p. 4259.

92 For example, the annual report of the Mountain Ash General Hospital in south Wales for 1926 noted that of the 533 in-patients admitted during the year, 439 were surgical cases, 21 were medical and 73 were accident victims; *Second Annual Report and Financial Statement of Mountain Ash and Penrhiwceiber General Hospital, 1926* (Mountain Ash, 1927), p. 18. 'Surgical' and 'medical' cases were distinguished in hospital annual reports to indicate the type of treatment provided, surgical in the case of the former and pharmacological or some other form of non-surgical treatment for the latter.

93 For examples, see NHS Greater Glasgow and Clyde Archives, HH67/38/36, Glasgow Royal Infirmary, Ward 38, Surgical, Ward Journal, Dr McEwan, 1933–4; HH67/34/32, Glasgow Royal Infirmary, Ward 34, Mr M McIntyre Case Sheets 1934 M–W.

94 TWAS, DX1032, Newcastle Royal Victoria Infirmary, W. E. Harker, record of operations, 1894–95.

95 Arthur MacNulty, 'Industrial Eye Injuries', *British Medical Journal*, 7 February 1942, p. 175.

96 NHS Greater Glasgow Health Board Archives, HB47/2/2, Glasgow Ophthalmic Institution, Twelfth Annual Report of the Glasgow Ophthalmic Institution, 14th March 1881, p. 6.

97 NHS Greater Glasgow Health Board Archives, HB 47/4/2, Glasgow Ophthalmic Institution, Register of Indoor Patients, 1876–91; *Twenty-Fourth Annual Report of the Glasgow Ophthalmic Institution (Under the Management of the Glasgow Royal*

Infirmary), 1892, p. 6; *Thirty-Eighth Annual Report of the Glasgow Ophthalmic Institution (Under the Management of the Royal Infirmary)*, 1906, p. 15.
98 The Pneumoconiosis etc. (Workmen's Compensation) Act remains in force to offer lump-sum compensation for relatives, and the Coal Industry Social Welfare Organisation (CISWO). NHS Choices, 'Silicosis', http://www.nhs.uk/conditions/Silicosis/Pages/Introduction.aspx, accessed 8 January 2015. Coal Industry Social Welfare Organisation, *Partnership in Action* (2012), http://ciswo.org/index.php/download_file/view/108/82/, accessed 8 January 2015.
99 McIvor and Johnston, *Miners' Lung*, p. 2.
100 *British Medical Journal*, 5 September 1885, p. 439.
101 For examples, see Andrew Smart, 'Note on Anthracosis', *British Medical Journal*, 5 September 1885, p. 439; R. S. Trotter, 'The So-Called Anthracosis and Phthisis in Coal Miners', *British Medical Journal*, 23 May 1903, p. 1198.
102 Allen Raine, *A Welsh Witch: A Romance of Rough Places* (London: Hutchinson & Co., 1902), p. 248.
103 McIvor and Johnston, *Miners' Lung*, p. 309.
104 Mark W. Bufton and Joseph Melling, '"A Mere Matter of Rock": Organized Labour, Scientific Evidence and British Government Schemes for Compensation of Silicosis and Pneumoconiosis among Coalminers, 1926–1940', *Medical History*, 49:2 (2005), p. 162; McIvor and Johnston, *Miners' Lung*, p. 74.
105 Medical Research Council, 'Chronic Pulmonary Disease in South Wales Coalminers', *Medical Studies*, 1942, p. 5.
106 Bufton and Melling, '"A Mere Matter of Rock"', p. 166.
107 McIvor and Johnston, *Miners' Lung*, p. 53.
108 Medical Research Council, 'Chronic Pulmonary Disease in South Wales Coalminers'.
109 National Union of Mineworkers (South Wales Area), Executive Council Annual Report, 1948–9, p. 93.
110 Durham County Record Office (hereafter DCRO), D/DCOMPA 297, Numbers of cases of Pneumoconiosis which Have Occurred since 1 July 1943, when the Coal Mining Industry (Pneumoconiosis) Compensation Scheme 1943 came into operation, 1943–1945. This regional characteristic is reflected in coalfields fiction, with 'silicosis' appearing frequently in literature from south Wales from 1937 onwards, but not in texts from the north-east of England or Scotland.
111 TNA, POWE 10/259, Mines Medical Service: Appointment of Medical Officers, 26 August 1944.
112 A. R. Ness, L. A. Reynolds and E. M. Tansey (eds), *Population-Based Research in South Wales: The MRC Pneumoconiosis Research Unit and the MRC Epidemiology Unit* (London: Wellcome Trust Centre for the History of Medicine, 2002), pp. 4, 22; more generally on the trade unions and medical research, see McIvor and Johnston, *Miners' Lung*, pp. 186–233.
113 Michael Bloor, 'The South Wales Miners Federation, Miners' Lung and the Instrumental Use of Expertise, 1900–1950', *Social Studies of Science*, 30:1 (2000), pp. 125–40.

114 SWML, AUD 263, Interview of Dai Dan Evans by Hywel Francis, 1 January 1970.
115 McIvor and Johnston, *Miners' Lung*, p. 51.
116 Both positions were outlined in a lecture by Dr T. Lister Llewellyn in 1920, who was a major figure throughout the debate and wrote a major text on the disease. See T. Lister Llewellyn, *The Causes and Prevention of Miners' Nystagmus* (London: The Colliery Guardian Company, 1912).
117 J. Court, *Miners' Diseases: Records of the Researches of Dr. J. Court (of Staveley) into Miners' Nystagmus & Anklyostomiasis [sic]* (Staveley: Sheffield Daily Telegraph, 1919).
118 Court, *Miners' Diseases*, p. 26.
119 For example, Dr Freeland Fergus – a medical referee under the Workmen's Compensation Act – in 1926 refuted previous research which attributed miners' nystagmus to 'some unusual condition of the central nervous system'. *Colliery Guardian*, 16 April 1926.
120 Francis Maylett Smith, *The Surgery at Aberffrwd: Some Encounters of a Colliery Doctor Seventy Years Ago*, ed. Denis Hayes Croften (Hythe: Volturna Press, 1981), pp. 84–5.
121 Ernest Rhys, *Black Horse Pit* (London: Robert Holden & Co. Ltd, 1925), p. 34.
122 M. Wynn Thomas, *Transatlantic Connections: Whitman U.S., Whitman U.K.* (Iowa City: Iowa University Press, 2005), p. 232. Thomas describes Rhys as elegising the passing of the pitman in this volume.
123 *The Cambrian*, 11 June 1902.
124 On bonesetters see Roger Cooter, 'Bones of Contention? Orthodox Medicine and the Mystery of the Bone-Setter's Craft', in W. F. Bynum and Roy Porter (eds), *Medical Fringe and Medical Orthodoxy, 1750–1850* (London: Croom Helm, 1987), pp. 158–73.
125 *Kelly's Directory of Monmouthshire and South Wales* (1926), p. 1261.
126 On Rae, see G. Bovine, 'The Blantyre Bonesetter: William Rae's Rise to Fame and the Popular Press', *Scottish Medical Journal*, 57 (2012), pp. 103–6; for the medical establishment's response to Rae, see *British Medical Journal*, 25 June 1904, p. 1505; *British Medical Journal*, 2 July 1904, pp. 32–3.
127 G. Bovine, 'The Blantyre Bonesetter', pp. 103–6; also, 'William Rae – The Bloodless Surgeon', Blantyre Project website, https://blantyreproject.com/2013/08/william-rae-the-bloodless-surgeon/, accessed 31 August 2018.
128 Thomas Jones, *Rhymney Memories* (Newtown: Welsh Outlook Press, 1938), pp. 63–5; *British Medical Journal*, 9 May 1953, p. 1054; *British Medical Journal*, 26 February 1972, p. 573.
129 Philip Hugh-Jones and C. M Fletcher, *The Social Consequences of Pneumoconiosis among Coalminers in South Wales* (London: HMSO, 1951).
130 Cooter, *Surgery and Society in Peace and War*, pp. 144–51.
131 The better-developed nature of services in the coal industry relative to other industries was recognised by the Miners' Welfare Fund, which even claimed that it was the best of its kind in the world. Wellcome Library, PP/HUN/C/2/45,

Miners' Welfare Commission, *Annual Report of Consulting Surgeon for 1946* (London: HMSO).
132 Glamorgan Archives, DXEL/12, The Rest Convalescence Home, Porthcawl, Annual Reports, 1863-1892.
133 Jenny Cronin, 'The Origins and Development of Scottish Convalescent Homes, 1860-1939', unpublished Glasgow University Ph.D. thesis (2003), pp. 111-15, 142-3; DCRO, D/IOR 57 56, North Eastern Counties Friendly Societies' Convalescent Home, Newspaper Cuttings, Rules, Annual Reports, 1888-1917.
134 For example, see *Evening Express*, 18 July 1903, p. 2. Schaw Home, opened in 1895-96 to serve the Glasgow Royal Infirmary, is another such example.
135 On the Miners' Welfare Fund, see W. John Morgan, 'The Miners' Welfare Fund in Britain 1920-1952', *Social Policy & Administration*, 24:3 (1990), pp. 199-211; Barry Supple, *The History of the British Coal Industry: Volume 4. 1913-1946: The Political Economy of Decline* (Oxford: Clarendon, 1987), pp. 473-8.
136 See, for example, the complaints that long stays meant that hundreds of individuals were forced to wait for an opportunity to gain admission; *Colliery Workers' Magazine*, 26 May 1925.
137 Cronin, 'The Origins and Development of Scottish Convalescent Homes, 1860-1939', pp. 127-8, 177-225.
138 Miners' Welfare Commission, *Miners' Welfare in War-Time: Report of the Miners' Welfare Commission for 6 ½ years to June 30th 1946* (London: HMSO, 1946), p. 46; Cooter, *Surgery and Society in Peace and War*, pp. 208, 210.
139 Royal College of Physicians and Surgeons, Glasgow, RCPSG 39/6/4/1, Young Family Papers, Precis of Evidence to be submitted by the Senior Surgical Staffs of the Royal and Western Infirmaries, Glasgow, to the Inter-Departmental Committee on the Rehabilitation of Persons Injured by Accidents.
140 Cooter, *Surgery and Society in Peace and War*, pp. 215-16.
141 Miners' Welfare Commission, *Miners' Welfare in War-Time*.
142 Miners' Welfare Commission, *Miners' Welfare in War-Time*, p. 47.
143 *Report of Inter-departmental Committee on the Rehabilitation and Resettlement of Disabled Persons*, Cmd. 6415 (London: HMSO, 1943), p. 44.
144 Sue Wheatcroft, *Worth Saving: Disabled Children During the Second World War* (Manchester: Manchester University Press, 2013), p. 168.
145 See, for example, the opening paragraph of E. A. Nicholl, 'Rehabilitation of the Injured', *British Medical Journal*, 5 April 1941, p. 501.
146 Glasgow Archives, Royal Society of Physicians and Surgeons, Young Papers, RSPSG 39/6/8, Interdepartmental Committee on the Rehabilitation of Persons Injured by Accidents, 14th Meeting, London, Thursday, September 30th, 1937.
147 Nicholl, 'Rehabilitation of the Injured', p. 501.
148 Nicholl, 'Rehabilitation of the Injured', p. 501.
149 Quayson, *Aesthetic Nervousness*, p. 2.
150 Cooter, *Surgery and Society in Peace of War*, p. 200.
151 Miners' Welfare Commission, *Miners' Welfare in War-Time*, p. 45.

152 Miners' Welfare Commission, *Miners' Welfare in War-Time*, p. 52.
153 For examples, see Miners' Welfare Commission, *Miners' Welfare in War-Time*, p. 53; Nicholl, 'Rehabilitation of the Injured', p. 501.
154 DCRO, NCB 7 8 8, General Correspondence and Circulars of Durham Coal Owners' Association, Durham Miners' Rehabilitation Centre, *Rules for Admission, Treatment and Discharge of Patients* (n.d.).
155 Miller, 'Late Rehabilitation of the Injured', p. 4259.
156 TNA, COAL 43/2, National Coal Board, Mines Medical Service, Policy 1946–50.
157 Sturdy, *The Industrial Body*, p. 217.
158 Hayes and Hannold, 'The Road to Empowerment', p. 356.
159 Foucault's theory of medical governmentality is outlined most clearly in Michel Foucault, *The Birth of the Clinic*, 3rd edn (London; New York: Routledge, 2003). For more recent application of Foucault's ideas to disability studies, see Shelley Lynn Tremain, *Foucault and the Government of Disability* (Ann Arbor: University of Michigan Press, 2005).

3

SYSTEMS OF FINANCIAL SUPPORT FOR IMPAIRED MINERS AND THEIR FAMILIES

When a working miner met with an injury or contracted a disease, perhaps the most pressing concern was how to survive the financial consequences. Impairment often necessitated a period of time away from work, or possibly the end of working life altogether. The loss of a weekly wage meant that the miner needed to draw upon one or more among a range of different sources of assistance. This chapter examines the various, changing ways that financial welfare was available in the late nineteenth century and the first half of the twentieth century. It considers various providers of assistance many of which dated from before 1880, such as charities, friendly societies and the Poor Law, in addition to the major developments in statutory systems of welfare which affected miners after that date. Such statutory interventions started with the Employers' Liability Act of 1880, continued with the Workmen's Compensation Act of 1897 (and several revisions in the decades after its introduction) and ended (as far as the scope of this volume is concerned) with the Industrial Injuries Act of 1946, which enshrined a generous system of benefits to injured workmen in the welfare state.

The years from 1880 to 1948 were a crucial time in the development of welfare in Britain. There was a gradual move from staunch adherence to individualism and the free market to greater state intervention in the 1880s and 1890s, and then more significant Liberal government reforms in the Edwardian period that for the first time enshrined in law the right to provisions such as school meals, pensions and health insurance. The interwar hiatus in legislation was followed by the post-war welfare settlement, which brought universal healthcare and finally abolished the individualistic and stigmatising Poor Law. These key details have formed milestones in the extensive literature on British welfare,[1] and this narrative of progression can also be seen in the shifting depiction of welfare in coalfields literature across the time period. Broadly speaking, in the earlier Victorian and Edwardian novels there is a focus on paternalistic interventions by middle- and upper-class protagonists, framed in terms of Christian values and morally 'worthy' recipients. In the working-class realist literature of the interwar period ideas about welfare are couched in terms of rights and entitlements to fair workplace treatment and compensation, where the emphasis is more often on the (im)morality of political systems such as capitalism, rather than on the 'worthiness' of specific individuals.[2] Yet, some historians have emphasised the problems with narratives based on the linear progression from individualism to collectivism, or from a paucity of provision to a 'new Jerusalem'. Jose Harris emphasises the complexity of the development of welfare, focusing instead on the 'piecemeal and unsystematic' series of policy changes that reflected the 'many counter-vailing social forces in a highly complex and diverse society'.[3] The varied experiences of miners may present something of a challenge to traditional narratives of welfare and the emergence of the social welfare state throughout the twentieth century. It is thus essential to take into account the lives and families affected by the changing legislative landscape.

Miners and their families, similar to workers and the poor elsewhere, drew upon a range of different providers in the mixed economy of welfare. Their choices, strategies and expedients varied from place to place and over time as resources waxed and waned, as their estimation of the social and cultural costs differed and as need and family circumstances exerted more or less pressure over time. Disabled miners were assisted in a variety of ways but they also suffered want, disappointment and desperation as providers failed to meet their needs or to sufficiently ameliorate the financial effects of disability.

Family and community

If the disabled person resided at the heart of a series of overlapping and interdependent nests of familial, community and social networks, then it was the family that was the closest, most intimate and most important source of support.[4] The first thing a person did when faced with hardship, therefore, was to turn inwards and to draw upon the resources provided by the family. Savings would have been drawn upon and changes made to consumption patterns and, as is shown in the next chapter on social relations, different members of the family looked to enter the world of work in order to make good any shortfall in the income of the breadwinner. Such strategies and changes were important, but could help to only a limited degree and, sooner or later, impaired miners and their families were required to look beyond the immediate family and seek support from others.

Collections or other fund-raising activities, often initiated in workplaces but extended into the broader community, were often used to raise a sum of money to assist injured miners. This could, at times, become a little more formalised. At Llwydcoed, near Aberdare, in 1898, for example, a 'benevolent prize drawing' was held to raise funds for David Hopkin, a miner with a large family who had been unable to work for the previous eighteen months as a result of an accident and would be unlikely to work again. The drawing was arranged by a small committee of his friends and fellow workers who drew up leaflets setting out his case, inserted appeals in the local newspaper and approached local elites, including the MP, for support.[5]

These community efforts, often referred to as 'lifts', figure prominently in coalfields literature, as authors utilised them to convey the close-knit character of mining communities. In the Welsh-language novel by T. Rowland Hughes,[6] *William Jones* (1944), such a 'lift' is described by a miner visiting an ex-miner friend dying prematurely from silicosis:

> Ôdd rhai'n cal 'u dewis bob Sadwrn pae i gasglu arian i helpu rhywun tost ne' withwr 'di cal anaf yn y pwll, a fe welas i ddynon yn gwitho dyblar er mwyn rhoi arian un shifft i fachan yn ffaelu.[7]

> Some were bein' chosen ev'ry Pay Saturday to collect money to 'elp somebody 'oo was bad or a workman 'oo'd 'ad an accident in the pit, and I' seen men workin' a doubler so as to give the money for one shift to a man not able to work.[8]

In Scottish miner and Labour MP James Welsh's historical novel, *The Underworld: The Story of Robert Sinclair, Miner* (1920), a manager tries to stop 'lifts' of money because he thinks it encourages men to stay off work, so he spreads rumours that the family have plenty of money. A collection is made anyway by a miner who says he can risk losing his own job over his principles and frames his actions as a point of freedom and moral principle against the manager's accusations. He ensures that the money and some tobacco are given without infringing on the dignity and pride of the family:

> 'It disna matter ... I dinna care though they had thousan's. What I don't like is this "ye'll-no-do-this-an'-ye'll-no-do-that" sort o' thing. What the hell right has ony gaffer wi' what a man does? It's a' one to him what I do. I'm nae slave, an' forby, I dinna believe they are weel-aff. They maun be hard up.'[9]

The lift is a moral and political litmus test. In contrast to the 'the "belly-crawlers" ... who "kept in" with the management by carrying tales, and generally acting as traitors to the other men',[10] the rest of the community have defied the manager in solidarity with the injured worker. This becomes a catalyst for unionisation and is associated with Scottish pride. Providing financial support within the community for a disabled miner is therefore represented as a political act, one which looks forward to more organised welfare.

Ultimately, however, family and community resources were finite, especially so in working-class communities such as those found in the coalfields, and the financial needs of disabled miners too often went unmet. The records of voluntary agencies that existed to provide welfare in coalfield communities are full of appeals for assistance from miners who found that they could not rely on familial and community resources alone. This was recognised, for example, by the Northern Coalfields Committee for their Special Emergency Grants in 1929:

> In certain cases where a member of a family is *confined to the house* by sickness or accident, acute distress may occasionally ensue. The normal insurance and/or compensation payments received during such periods must generally be regarded as sufficient mitigation of the resulting conditions, but exceptional cases may arise where assistance from the Fund would be a very real help.[11]

The Fund, therefore, was positioned as a last resort, a source of 'very real help' to those who had exhausted other avenues of support. The mining cases relieved by the Swansea Hospital Ladies Samaritan Funds were also framed as a support for vulnerable family care. An injured Dunvant collier, who had received no compensation and 'was the sole support of his mother' received 2s. 6d. a week from the Funds.[12]

In the same way, the statutory system of workmen's compensation took family circumstances into account in setting compensation payments to disabled miners. The Scottish Coal Workers' Compensation Scheme, for example, regularly mentioned family situations in its proceedings. John Black, a 38-year-old 'one-armed man' who also had his right leg broken in the pit was awarded a lump sum of up to £250 just before the First World War, the largest compensation recorded in the minutes. This decision was undoubtedly informed by the fact that 'he is a widower without family and lives in lodgings', likely an implicit acknowledgement of women's unpaid labour.[13] Similarly, pony-putter Robert Henderson in Durham was awarded £100 after losing part of his thumb and two fingers – despite not being able to prove it was in the 'course of employment' – 'as there were some sad features connected with the case'.[14] This attests less to the generosity of compensation committees – others with 'sad features' were no doubt rejected – than to the absence of family and community support available to some miners.

The voluntary sphere: self-help, mutualism and charity

While the family and the community were the most important providers of welfare to disabled miners, in terms of both the amount of assistance provided and its place in the miner's life, it was inadequate to meet the needs of many miners and their families.[15] Considerable strain was placed on working-class families by sickness and impairment, and too often the resources at their disposal proved inadequate to meet the considerable need that existed. In such instances, miners and their families were forced to look for assistance beyond the immediate family or community in order to supplement the care provided within the home. While mining communities had fewer voluntary resources than more affluent communities, still the types of voluntary welfare available to miners were numerous and ranged from self-help and mutualist forms to charitable and paternalistic provision.

Charities were numerous and varied in character across British communities and it is possible to discern some that were crucially important to mining communities and to the support of impaired miners. Blind and deaf charities, for example, were numerous in coalfield districts. For instance, the Cambrian Institution for the Deaf and Dumb in Swansea operated a 'Wonderful Penny' fundraising scheme, starting in the 1860s, in which workers from local collieries – alongside iron, copper and tinworks – donated a penny from their wages to the institution, many of whose pupils came from mining families.[16] Another, the Rhondda Institution for the Blind, opened immediately after the 1920 Blind Persons Act which made it the duty of councils to provide welfare for blind people.[17] Enshrined in the 'Conditions of Service' was the guarantee that 'A vacant place shall always be kept in the Workshops for any emergency that might arise with blind Miners or their dependents'.[18] As it was a mining area, many of those who received accommodation and participated in the workshops – which, like many other contemporary blind institutions, were focused on employment and manufacturing objects – came from mining families.[19] Opinions regarding miners' work in the institution were clearly mixed, as seen in a letter from the National League of the Blind regarding a young blind miner in the institution who was 'anxious to be trained as a telephonist', the contents of which were 'rather scathing'.[20]

Likewise, particularly in south Wales, institutions interacted with mining organisations, and local collieries regularly donated to blind and deaf institutions. The Rhondda Institution both met with the Executive Council of the South Wales Miners' Federation and the local miners' lodge and also received money quotas from colliery companies, though these were sometimes delayed or unpaid.[21] Occasionally, this dealing with the coalfields intersected directly with the economic rehabilitation work offered in the Rhondda Institution, as is seen when the Ocean Coal Company ordered fifty coal baskets made by residents of the Institution in 1927.[22] Local blind and deaf institutions were clearly seen by many as integral parts of the coalfield community.

Friendly societies, run most often by and for miners, were as numerous as charities and were a key form of voluntary welfare for impaired miners, though their self-help and mutualist character marked them out as different to charities. The friendly society movement originated, to all intents and purposes, in the second half of the eighteenth century and, from the 1790s onwards, gained an increasing degree of legal recognition and protection as the state put aside its initial fears and recognised the important contributions that societies could make to thrift, respectability and financial self-sufficiency. The movement grew in size in the early decades of the nineteenth century, especially in the 1840s as the Poor Law Amendment Act gave a boost to efforts by working-class families to remain beyond the clutches of the hated workhouse. It was also from that decade that the affiliated orders came to prominence, and societies such as the Oddfellows, the Foresters and the Shepherds spread the actuarial risks posed by sickness and death more broadly through enlisting large numbers in membership across their numerous lodges.[23]

Miners' engagement with friendly societies came in different forms. It is possible to discern many societies or lodges the majority of whose members were employed in the coal industry, perhaps even at the same colliery, or else who all derived from the same occupational group within the industry. In an example of the latter, in the early twentieth century the Durham County Colliery Enginemen's, Boiler Minders' and Firemen's Mutual Aid Association and National Insurance Approved Society offered its members both sickness benefits for up to 26 weeks and disablement benefits after sickness benefit had finished, though only after impaired members had been insured for 104 weeks and also paid the same number of weekly contributions.[24] In other instances, miners were explicitly excluded from membership of some societies. The 1885 rules of the Tradesmen's Annual Friendly Society in Shotton, County Durham, for example, listed miners alongside 'loiterers, idle persons, soldiers or sailors' as those unable to join.[25] This perhaps reflected a certain class prejudice, as better-skilled workers or members of the petit bourgeoisie looked unfavourably on miners as an occupational group; but it also constituted a recognition of the relatively dangerous nature of coalmining and the bad risk that miners' high rates of injury and sickness posed to the actuarial soundness of friendly societies.[26]

This actuarial fragility also gave rise to a number of other distinctive features that were characteristic of friendly societies and that had particular consequences for disabled miners. In the first place, careful to protect their slender resources, friendly societies placed quite strict conditions on membership, the chief of which was that potential members were required to disclose any health issues and were denied entry into the organisation if they were considered a likely bad risk. One of the rules of the Aberaman Colliery Friendly Society, for example, stated that 'No person shall become a member of this Society who is of unsound health, or suffering from any chronic or other disease', and such conditions of membership were universal across the movement.[27] This society forced members who were found to be 'not healthy' after initiation to forfeit their money and leave the society; many others imposed fines.[28] The Llanbradach Colliery Sick Benefit Society added a new rule in 1905 that benefits to any member would cease, should it be found that the claimant was 'afflicted with any disease prior to his becoming a member'.[29] As such, miners who were already impaired, whether by injury or illness, found it impossible to join a friendly society and to protect themselves against further impairment.

Upon experiencing a disabling injury or condition, friendly society members were monitored by the lay officers or other members of the society. The Durham County Colliery Enginemen's, Boiler Minders' and Firemen's Mutual Aid Association's rules required that members of the Association drawing sickness or disablement benefits had to send a medical certificate 'or other sufficient evidence of incapacity for work' to the secretary once every two weeks and, potentially, also submit to a medical examination. The Glais Benefit Society, near Swansea, employed dedicated sick visitors whose duty was to 'visit the sick within three days after receiving notice', and at least a fortnight after that. The sick visitor faced a fine for not performing the duty, and could be replaced by stewards for repeated failure to perform. This suggests that friendly society officials wanted to demonstrate how seriously their societies took the threat of abuse of benefits or 'malingering'.[30]

In addition, benefits were disallowed if the claimant were to supposedly 'bring upon himself sickness or lameness' by 'fighting, leaping, running, footballing, or any other acts of bravado, or immorality'.[31] Any benefits paid by friendly societies as a result of impairment were therefore framed and monitored from both a medical and moral viewpoint, and observed with close attention to the financial position of the particular society. Miners on the funds were monitored closely to ensure that the impairment was genuine and that the miner was not 'malingering', and also that they behaved in a moderate and respectable manner. At the same time, it should perhaps be noted that words such as 'brotherhood', 'fraternity' and 'mutualism' littered friendly society materials and, given the numerous examples of inclusive and generous treatment, this was more than mere rhetoric. These visits served to emphasise those very values and fraternity extended to disabled miners, who were not subject to any greater scrutiny than any other individual in receipt of sickness benefits. The North Eastern Counties Friendly Societies Convalescent Home elaborated on this in 1888: 'This scheme gives to the working classes an opportunity of showing to the world that they are mindful to the weak and sick ones amongst them.'[32]

Friendly societies merged their functions as mutual aid with their position as social gatherings of miners. The annual dinner and weekly or monthly club night functioned as key social events on miners' calendars, in addition to being spaces to collect their funds. Not all approved, however. Concern about the moral implications of this form of financial aid, that is, that it promoted malingering or dependency, was expressed in the Methodist-influenced coalfields novel *Rhoda Roberts: A Welsh mining story* (1895) through the device of showing the weekly collection being held in a pub. The men go in 'clean, bright and sober, to go to pay their contributions at the [Garter Sick and Benefit Society]' and emerge 'dull-eyed, heavy, filthy, and drunken.'[33]

Friendly societies were occasionally granted moral, practical and even financial support by employers, particularly in the earlier part of the nineteenth century, but they were nevertheless working-class organisations. Committees of working men administered the movement at a local level and drew upon working-class values and priorities in the decisions they made. In contrast, many permanent provident funds similarly relieved miners on account of 'disablement' but were funded and administered through the efforts of workers and employers working in conjunction with each other. Permanent relief funds were established on a coalfield-by-coalfield basis during the second half of the nineteenth century, with constituent branches or 'agencies' at each colliery that joined the movement. They were funded by worker subscriptions and employer donations, the precise proportions varying from coalfield to coalfield, and paid death benefits to the families of miners killed in workplace accidents.[34]

The first society, the Northumberland and Durham Miners' Permanent Relief Fund, was initiated in 1862 after the Hartley Colliery disaster of the same year which killed 204 people.[35] Other coalfields emulated Northumberland and Durham and founded their own permanent relief funds in the decades that followed: a society for North Staffordshire was founded in 1869, Lancashire and Cheshire in 1873, followed by Yorkshire in 1877 and south Wales in 1881.[36] The critical role of Hartley in the history of relief funds is recorded in Durham miner Harold Heslop's historical novel *The Earth Beneath* (1946), in which he dedicates a chapter to the Hartley disaster. Heslop argues that Hartley was the event that changed the way that miners portrayed themselves, a great catalyst for political discourse in which miners 'were beginning to dramatise themselves and their surroundings; their role was that of the maligned creature of injustice.'[37]

While the first such permanent relief society was established in the wake of this large disaster, the movement as a whole came to place attention not on large-scale losses of life but, rather, on the smaller incidents that took one or two lives at a time. As supporters of the movement pointed out, the numbers of lives lost to small-scale accidents in which no more than a few men were killed at a time far outstripped the death tolls caused by explosions, falls and inundations in which hundreds were killed.[38] Such 'disasters by instalment', as the small accidents were characterised in the permanent provident fund movement, did not elicit the same public sympathy or, crucially, donations as the larger disasters, and the widows and 'orphans' of the men killed were left with little effective support. Crucially, the Northumberland and Durham Miners' Permanent Relief Fund drew upon an older tradition of 'smart money' paid by employers to injured workers in the North-East coalfield and instituted a system of 'disablement' benefits in 1863 by which miners incapacitated by accident were paid a sum of money while they were unable to work.[39] Henry Baker was the first claimant on the permanent disablement fund and received benefit from January 1863 until his death in March 1875.[40] Other miners' permanent provident funds also paid disablement benefits in the decades that followed.

By the 1890s disablement benefits paid by the different permanent relief funds varied from 5s. to 10s. a week.[41] Northumberland and Durham paid 5s. a week to members disabled from working for periods under twenty-six weeks, the payments increasing to 7s. after the worker had been off for more than twenty-six weeks. This increase stands in contrast to the practice of friendly societies, where the level of payments decreased over time.[42] In contrast, Monmouthshire and South Wales Miners' Permanent Provident Society paid 8s. a week in disablement cases and did so indefinitely, without any reduction over time, but this was reduced to 6s. in 1902.[43] Benson has found, through analysis of the records of the permanent relief funds for Lancashire and Cheshire and for the West Riding of Yorkshire, that miners in receipt of disablement benefit in the late nineteenth century were off work for an average of around six weeks.[44]

The payment of these disablement benefits was one of the greatest challenges faced by the management boards of the funds, as many found that the payments accounted for a significant and growing proportion of their expenditure in the late nineteenth century. This, in turn, caused tension between workmen's representatives and those individuals more closely aligned with the interests of employers as pressure came to be exerted on claimants as a means to control expenditure.[45] This varied in extent from coalfield to coalfield as accident and disablement rates varied.

The board of the south Wales society noted the large number of disablement cases in 1885, for example, when it was observed that while there had been seventy-five deaths in the year up to March 1885, there were 6,207 disablement cases.[46] As a result, all disablement cases of more than twenty-six weeks' standing were investigated and, while very little 'malingering' was found, payments were reduced in many cases, seemingly on financial grounds alone.[47]

Table 1 Disablement cases and rates for certain miners' permanent provident funds, 1885–90

		Northumberland and Durham	Lancashire and Cheshire	South Wales
1885	Cases	14,924	7,054	7,805
	Rate per 100 members	17.2	18.5	20.8
1886	Cases	11,544	7,348	9,795
	Rate per 100 members	?	18.1	23.8
1887	Cases	14,409	7,409	10,801
	Rate per 100 members	15.7	17.9	25.6
1888	Cases	15,700	7,870	9,020
	Rate per 100 members	16.5	18.5	22.9
1889	Cases	16,000	7,921	10,985
	Rate per 100 members	16.0	17.7	23.9
1890	Cases	16,000	7,524	10,164
	Rate per 100 members	14.8	15.2	19.2

Source: Campbell, *Miners' Thrift and Employers' Liability*, Appendix A, Table H.

The fears of ever-increasing disablement payments often led to a similar policing of impaired claimants as that seen in the friendly societies. The 1899 rules of the Northumberland and Durham Miners' Permanent Relief Fund offered a 'fixed lump sum' for impairment, but this was subject to several conditions: applications had to be made within thirty-five days of the accident, a medical certificate had to be provided, there were visits by the Visitation Committee and the applicant had to be 'desirous of making an effort to help himself'. Added to this, claimants must not be 'trying work' after an accident.[48] The committee minutes demonstrate that these rules were regularly enforced, clearly with an eye on saving money on the costs of payment for impairment. One miner's benefits were suspended in 1906 'until he puts himself in order with the rules and makes a new application'.[49] The south Wales fund had similar policies, and in 1884 asked for the 'vigilance of the local officers' to make sure accidents 'have actually happened in connection with colliery working, and that they are duly vouched for by surgeons'.[50]

The relief funds were a crucial source of income for many impaired miners. The large numbers of miners who joined the societies demonstrate the worth that miners perceived in the societies' activities, while the significant numbers who received disablement benefits show the wisdom of that perception. Nevertheless, the permanent provident societies varied in the extent to which they enlisted miners in their coalfields in membership, with degrees of coverage varying from roughly 90 per cent in the 1890s in the north-east of England to between 5 and 10 per cent in south Wales in the Edwardian period, and so they varied also in the degree to which they met the needs of disabled miners in the respective coalfields.[51] In addition, Benson is correct to stress the collaboration that existed at the heart of the societies, but the quality and extent of that collaboration varied from coalfield to coalfield. The fund in the more consensual north-east of England continued as a viable concern into the 1930s and beyond, while its counterpart in the more combustible south Wales coalfield lost almost two-thirds of its members in the wake of the 1897 Workmen's Compensation Act and was largely defunct by 1906.[52] As such, the permanent provident society movement was never more than a partial solution to the financial problems caused by miners' impairments. Given the impossibiliy of family or community meeting the needs of impaired miners, and as the myriad of organisations and bodies in the voluntary sphere failed to prevent the considerable poverty that existed, many miners were forced to look to other sources of relief. Increasingly during the late nineteenth and early twentieth centuries this often meant the state and, in particular, the Poor Law, a flawed and stigmatising system that was despised by miners as much as by other workers.

Public provision for disabled miners: the Poor Law

From 1880 until its eventual disappearance in the twentieth century, the Poor Law played a complex role in the provision of assistance to disabled people in mining communities. Many viewed it as an option of last resort and it was often used only in times of crisis or destitution. For miners, similar to the population more generally, the Poor Law was one among a number of welfare providers and was drawn upon to supplement other forms of relief and benefit. The Poor Law is crucial to the history of disability in the nineteenth and early twentieth centuries. It set out the ideals and limitations which defined poverty and disability, and created a discourse of who was 'deserving' of welfare. The Poor Law Amendment Act of 1834 introduced the principle of 'less eligibility', which aimed to make relief as undesirable as possible and made the imposing and oppressive workhouse as much of a deterrent to the supposed problem of dependency as possible. The situation of the pauper, wrote the Commissioners of 1834, 'shall not be made really or apparently so eligible as the situation of the independent labourer of the lowest class'.[53] The 1834 Amendment Act's configuration of poverty as an individual and moral concern, many historians have argued, was a key ideological tenet throughout the Poor Law's life.[54] This served to create a statutory distinction between the 'deserving' and 'undeserving' poor, with disability often playing a key role in who was considered deserving of relief.

Deborah Stone's work contends that the New Poor Law was a powerful and influential factor in the conception of disability in the nineteenth century, and points out that the categories of pauper outlined in the 1834 Poor Law Amendment Act form part of modern conceptions and lexicons of disability: the 'sick', 'insane', 'defectives' and the 'aged and infirm' were positioned as separate categories with different levels of eligibility for relief or potential for fraud.[55] Stone describes their position within the Poor Laws as a supposed economic 'distributive dilemma' facing Poor Law administrators, in which welfare could be offered to deserving applicants so as to 'reconcile the distributive principles of work and need without undermining the productive side of the economy'.[56] Historians have seen these modes of categorisation as creating a long-lasting effect of pauperisation on disabled people. Anne Borsay describes the Poor Law, regardless of its initial intentions, as 'delivered through a system designed to stigmatize applicants without work and exclude them from the community'.[57] Furthermore, David Turner argues that the 1834 Act – along with contemporary media and other discourses – helped to propagate the long-running narrative of the 'fraudulent' disabled claimant of welfare, which continues to this day.[58] The Poor Law is commonly criticised in literature, which nevertheless adopts the discourse of the deserving poor, forced into penury through no fault of their own via disability and the failings of Poor Law. In *The Black Diamond* (1880), a miner's widow, who has been doing needlework to get by, loses her income through arthritis:

> How pitiable it is that the paralysis of one right hand will reduce, in the midst of our Christian society, a family from comfort and respectability, to beggary and misery. There is a great work yet to be done by some Christian philanthropist – a work that will supersede our clumsy inhuman Poor Law, with it prison-like workhouse, and police-like officials – which will not treat the widow and the orphan as criminals, but will provide for their necessities and take their part.[59]

The author was a Primitive Methodist Minister, which perhaps explains this vision of welfare in terms of Christian paternalism rather than state intervention. Elsewhere within coalfields literature the Poor Law, or parish relief, is used as a device to explore the politics of poverty, unemployment and industrial action. In 1929, Durham miner Harold Heslop argued that the cultural significance of receiving the 'mean charity'[60] of the Poor Law was changing in an age of industrial action (particularly the 1926 General Strike and lockout):

> Instead of the debt to the Guardians being regarded as a mark of shame, as in the old days, it was now a token of having suffered. Poor Law Relief, in these days

of clashing forces, assumed the aspect of sanctity. The relieving officers became the new historians, writing the histories of the workers, not in the books of a trade union, but in the ledgers bound in leather, with the quills of calm charity.[61]

The change in perception is how the applicant feels about receiving relief, rather than any change to the way the money is administered or Boards of Guardians treat applicants. In this way, coalfields literature illustrates both the unease felt about drawing upon poor relief – in large part because of the way that applicants were treated – and that stigmatisation was mitigated during times of industrial action because of an underlying political purpose that justified a period of worklessness and financial hardship.

The Poor Law undoubtedly carried a social stigma and was likely regarded by most as an emergency of last resort when one met with injury or disease: 'To be a pauper was the great danger to be avoided, and hell itself held no terrors greater than that for the bulk of them,' wrote Scottish miner, novelist and Labour MP James Welsh in 1924.[62] Reliance on the Poor Law in old age was particularly dreaded. Another Scottish miner, Tom Hanlin, who became a writer while convalescing from a mining injury, portrays a miner's widow with consumption fading away from the toil of widowhood, including 'telling your life story to a hard face in a parish office'.[63] These negative connotations are confirmed in the memoirs of the Welsh labour activist Elizabeth Andrews, who recalled that 'Many sickness clubs were formed in those days in the mining areas … There was a real dread of being buried by the Poor Law in a pauper's grave.'[64] Andrews' words, reinforced in coalfields fiction, illustrate the need for miners to utilise multiple forms of welfare so as to avoid the destitution that threatened to come with sickness or disability.

Despite its continued presence in the literature of the time, the period 1880–1948 saw the gradual decline of the Poor Law as the state increasingly recognised the need for other, wider forms of assistance and began to attribute poverty to environmental and structural causes rather than moral and individual failings. In particular, the reforms carried out by the Liberal government between 1906 and 1911 saw the architects of welfare policy acknowledging the need for a shift away from the individualism of the nineteenth century and towards a more collective provision for certain groups within the population. As a result, several changes occurred during the first half of the twentieth century that weakened the influence of the Poor Law: the Ministry of Health was created in 1919 and assumed responsibility for the Poor Law, with the original Boards of Guardians still overseeing local administration.[65] More significantly, the 1929 Local Government Act abolished the Boards of Guardians, to some protest by their members, and transferred the Poor Law administration to the Public

Assistance Committees of individual counties and county boroughs.[66] This signalled the final decline of the Poor Law until its functions were taken over entirely by the welfare state in 1948. Thus, any disabled miners who claimed poor relief in the period from 1880 to 1948 did so within a changing administrative and policy context, and one in which regional variations in practice and generosity determined the character of their experiences.[67]

Having exhausted any familial, community, self-help or mutualist sources of support that might have been available, disabled miners made application to relieving officers for assistance under the Poor Law to relieve the effects of poverty caused by impairment. The vast majority of such miners would have been relieved outside the walls of the workhouse and were made cash payments, or else were granted other forms of assistance in their homes. The proportions of relief given in indoor or outdoor forms varied from one Poor Law union to another and from region to region, but it is clear that the workhouse was not the experience of most paupers (disabled or not) in the late nineteenth century. A return for 1887–88 found that 70 per cent of all relief distributed in Durham was given in the form of out-relief, or 'domiciliary' relief, while the corresponding figure for 'South Wales' was 83 per cent; the average for England and Wales at the time was 59 per cent.[68] The figure was greater again in Scotland as a result of the lower level of institutional provision under its separate Poor Law system, partly determined by the poverty of the country's communities.[69] By the mid-1930s the proportion for England and Wales stood at 87 per cent, while that for Scotland was as high as 94 per cent.[70] Thus, disabled miners tended to receive domiciliary relief rather than to be relieved in the workhouse.

The 'mean charity'[71] of the Poor Law, it is clear, could provide an important resource for miners in their attempts to deal with disability. Lists of applications for relief presented by Carluke miners in the late nineteenth century featured several individuals claiming relief for rheumatism, bronchitis and broken or diseased legs, and there were a variety of outcomes. In the case of Andrew McAllister, a twenty-seven-year-old miner from Douglas, Lanarkshire, 6s. a week was granted in 1885 due to his incapacity to work following the amputation of a foot. John Gardiner, a twenty-six-year-old miner from the same parish with a wife and four dependent children, was similarly granted 6s. a week after being confined to his bed by an injury for ten months.[72] In neither case would 6s. have been enough to sustain their families, and the men would have had to seek additional assistance if their injuries were not to cause dire poverty for themselves and their families. These records demonstrate that miners used the Poor Law as a source of relief in conjunction with other agencies: in Govan parish in 1896 one collier was listed as 'wholly disabled' for two weeks from a bruised knee, and was granted outdoor relief alongside his relief from Dickson's Society and the Works Society.[73]

These cases from Carluke demonstrate the tendency for miners with disabling injuries to seek relief from the Poor Law authorities, but it is evident that occupational disease was also the cause of a great deal of poor relief granted to miners: again, records relating to the Poor Law in Carluke, Lanarkshire in the 1890s demonstrate a large number of miners relieved as a result of 'miners' asthma' or 'congestion of the lungs'.[74] Decades later, impaired miners continued to turn to the Poor Law for assistance. In a particularly revealing case from Bedwellty Union, south Wales, in 1924 that highlights the difficulty of negotiating the compensation system and how it could force miners to turn to the Poor Law, the relieving officer strongly urged the Board of Guardians to relieve a thirty-one-year-old miner with a wife and eleven dependent children who had previously been in receipt of 35s. a week in compensation payments as a result of nystagmus. The miner had resumed 'light employment' at Markham Colliery some time after his compensation award but the Tredegar Iron and Coal Company then suspended his compensation and he now suffered 'insufficient means'; the relieving officer described him as a 'very deserving case'.[75] Apart from such dole payments, Poor Law authorities also provided relief in kind to impaired miners: blankets, bedclothes, boots, clothing and foodstuffs were just some of the forms of relief granted to miners and their families.[76]

While out-relief was the most common form of assistance to disabled miners, some nevertheless tended to end up within the walls of the hated workhouse. It is evident that the workhouse test was applied in some cases to measure a disabled applicant's eligibility for relief.[77] In the case of Pontypool workhouse in south Wales in the 1880s, miners there listed as 'able-bodied' were often admitted with conditions such as facial paralysis, disease or 'dropsy' and appeared to use the workhouse's medical facilities to recover. Colliers listed as 'old/infirm' tended to be in their fifties or sixties and were listed with conditions such as asthma, rheumatism or, in one case, blindness. Many were 'discharged at [their] own request', suggesting that the workhouse was treated as a last resort in times of personal financial trouble or sickness.[78] Disabled miners used the workhouse when necessary, but were not necessarily bound there permanently.

While sick and disabled individuals were classed as deserving under the Poor Law system and were granted relief more readily than the 'able-bodied' poor, still there was concern that the potential existed for false claims and 'malingering'. Inspectors regularly exhibited a sense of distrust and reluctance when administering Poor Law relief to disabled people, and extensive documentation was often required before relief was granted. In 1910 the Easington Union Committee in Durham noted that a miner had a 'personal application made by his wife' that he was suffering from rheumatism. Though he successfully received weekly relief, he was 'requested to produce a medical certificate before any relief was paid and over [sic] and also a medical certificate each week', signed by the doctor of the local colliery. In this case it was reported that the man 'came to [the Committee member's] farm to beg and on questioning him had admitted that there had never been, nor was there at the present time, anything the matter with him'.[79] This sceptical attitude was not uncommon elsewhere. The *Glasgow Herald* in December 1911 reported that a man was charged of 'falsely representing that he had sustained an accident at Dechmont Colliery ... and was unable to work and required temporary ailment [sic – aliment] for himself and his family'.[80] Many suspicious individual cases were reported and dissected in the media, contributing to a climate of fear about potential fraud.

In addition, Poor Law officials were careful to ensure that the support received by miners from friendly societies or other welfare programmes was taken into consideration when granting relief. Assessments of need by relieving officers meant that all sources of income were accounted for before the decision to relieve was made. John Benson has studied the extent to which different Boards of Guardians considered friendly society benefits in their assessments of need and has noted that they were able to disregard friendly society payments of up to 5s. a week from 1894 onwards. The difficult circumstances of the lockout in 1926, with pressure from the central Poor Law authorities to exercise caution in the granting of relief, meant that Poor Law Unions varied in their inclusion of friendly society benefits in assessments but did nevertheless lessen relief payments according to any additional income from that source.[81] Such assessments of additional sources of income carried on into the 1930s. In 1935 the Northumberland Public Assistance Committee discussed whether the Miners' Permanent Relief Fund counted as a friendly society within the Poor Law, and amended the county's outdoor relief regulations to assert that,

> In granting outdoor relief to a member of a Friendly Society or to a person entitled to receive any benefit under the National Health Insurance Acts, the Guardians Committee shall not take into consideration any sum received from a Friendly Society as sick pay or any benefit under the National Health Insurance Acts, except so far as such sick pay or benefits exceeds 7s 6d per week.[82]

Thus, the Poor Law had a role, albeit a limited one, in a mixed economy of welfare for miners, most of whom saw it as a temporary measure. For some time before 1880, the Poor Law was the only available form of state welfare in this mix, but, beginning with the Employers' Liability Act of 1880, the state intervened to a greater extent to facilitate compensation for disabled miners.

State intervention: the Employers' Liability Act 1880 and the Workmen's Compensation Act 1897

The Employers' Liability Act of 1880 and the Workmen's Compensation Act of 1897 were to redefine the role of the state in the lives of disabled miners. They represented a growing awareness of the need for the state to intervene to ensure the payment of compensation and placed the onus of responsibility onto employers. The Acts made industrial injuries and disease compensation available to miners, but also brought with them all the difficulties of an adversarial legal system in which the extent or provenance of disability was disputed by employers who had a financial incentive to deny or lessen liability.

The Employers' Liability Act was passed in 1880 after a series of bills and Trade Union Congress petitions in the late 1870s, and the question of the liability of employers for accidents emerged as an issue in the 1879 general election.[83] The Act enshrined in law for the first time the principle that workmen injured by a fault at their workplace – defects in conditions of machinery, the negligence of employers or superintendents – had a right to compensation. However, some employers were able to 'contract out' of the Act by making 'joint' provision with their workmen through the establishment of permanent provident funds that offered death and disablement benefits in place of any compensation that might have been secured through the legislation.[84] Contracting out limited the scope of the Act to some degree, but it was other flaws that were most to blame for its rather toothless nature. This has led the leading historian of the legislation to describe it as 'a minor adjustment to, rather than a revolution in, liability law'.[85]

Such was the flawed nature of the 1880 Act that a great many efforts were made through the 1880s and 1890s to amend it. Different interests advocated a series of changes to the legislation, including variously the abolition or retention of contracting out, and a number of different bills were presented in Parliament. Ultimately, Joseph Chamberlain passed the Workmen's Compensation Act of 1897, which superseded the Employers' Liability legislation, and the measure made employers liable to pay compensation for any personal injury 'arising out of and [which] in the course of the employment is caused to a workman'. According to Bartrip, injured workers were now established as 'an elite group, analogous to war pensioners, eligible for special benefits denied to other, perhaps similarly injured, members of society'.[86]

Contracting out continued to be a possibility under the new legislation and helps to explain the significant differences in practice and experience in the various coalfields. The Northumberland and Durham Miners' Permanent Relief Fund continued as a viable concern into the mid-twentieth century and continued to tailor its activities to the changing compensation landscape: in 1938 it changed its rules to allow claimants with diseases such as nystagmus, compensatable under the Workmen's Compensation Act, to claim.[87] Contracting out continued in south Wales but was far more controversial and came to be challenged increasingly by the labour movement. Keir Hardie, the Scottish miners' leader and subsequently MP for Merthyr Tydfil, castigated the coalowners in south Wales for the arrangement by which they paid 25 per cent of the workers' contributions: 'The outcome is a death and disablement rate which entitles Wales to be regarded as the slaughterhouse of the coalfields of the kingdom.' He continued, 'In their haste to be rich mineowners seem to regard human life as the cheapest of all commodities.'[88] The result of this politicisation was that, in contrast to the north-east of England, miners abandoned the Permanent Provident Society after the 1897 Act was passed: membership more than halved from 1897 to 1898 and was dealt a further blow with changes to the legislation in 1906, such that there were fewer than 1,000 members by 1907.[89]

The workmen's compensation system underwent further revision in the years that followed, largely as a result of the changing nature of medical and scientific knowledge, but also as a result of trade union pressure. Many of these changes were devoted to scheduling miners' diseases and conditions as compensatable under the Act, including silicosis, nystagmus, pneumoconiosis and beat knee and elbow. Others changes were responses to major events and the changing economic situation, such as the 1917 and 1919 Workmen's Compensation (War Addition) Acts, which increased compensation for 'total disablement' and responded to the increased costs of living brought on by the war and the impact of this on disabled people.[90] Workmen's compensation was eventually criticised for its separate administration from other forms of welfare in William Beveridge's *Social Insurance and Allied Services*, and the final 1945 Royal Commission on Workmen's Compensation failed to report, signalling its replacement by the post-war welfare state.[91] The system was again radically overhauled in the 1940s with the passage of the Industrial Injuries Act in 1946, which socialised the costs of industrial injury, thus making the injured miner a cost on the state rather than one to be borne by private enterprise.

The Employers' Liability Act of 1880 and the Workmen's Compensation Act of 1897 brought employers and workers into dialogue with each other in relation to disability as never before, but also created new sources of contention and conflict. Although the right to compensation was guaranteed in both the

Employers' Liability Act and the workmen's compensation legislation, the process of making a claim and securing compensation was beset by delays, difficulties and anxiety for disabled miners. When meeting with accident or illness, miners were required to notify their employer of the issue. This would usually result in a medical examination of the miner by a doctor appointed by the colliery company. If the doctor attested to the presence and extent of the impairment, a sum of compensation would be paid to the miner, either in the form of a weekly payment or else as a lump sum. Where the colliery company disputed the causation or extent of the impairment, a miner had recourse to take his case through the court system, where, in an adversarial context, medical experts could be called, evidence presented by either side and a case made for compensation to be paid. Legal representation and medical testimony needed to be paid for, of course, and this was extremely difficult for any miner who did not have access to trade union resources.[92]

The extent to which this legal system was adversarial varied from one coalfield to another, depending on the nature of labour relations in those places. Labour relations were more combustible in south Wales and Scotland, with greater militancy on the part of trade unions and employers, and this was reflected in a great number of contested cases than in Durham, where a joint Arbitration Committee involved union and employer representatives in discussions over medical assessments and decisions on compensation payments.[93] The miners' union there routinely started each meeting of the Committee by nominating the same coalowner to chair the meetings, such was the trust felt in him by both sides.[94] Any decisions made by the Arbitration Committee were to be considered as binding on both parties as any decision given by a county court. It was stated in 1916 that such was this 'friendly arrangement between the representatives of the Durham Coal Owners and Miners in regard to the administration of the Workmen's Compensation Act' that 'costs are never asked for or paid, and verbal notice of an accident to a mine official is under certain circumstances accepted as sufficient by the Owner'.[95] Between 1898 and 1922 the Arbitration Committee dealt with over 5,000 cases.[96]

Despite such cooperation, compensation continued to be a source of contention in the Durham coalfield and the miners' union reacted with anger at what they perceived to be efforts by the employers to harass disabled miners and minimise their compensation liabilities. In particular, the Durham Miners' Association found in the 1920s that employers were allowed by the terms of the legislation to end compensation payments whenever they wished and require disabled miners and their union to take the case before a medical referee, the Arbitration Committee or the county court. Even where a medical referee decided in favour of the disabled miner, the employers could again stop payment almost immediately and require the miners to undergo a further examination, all the time saving on the payments that would otherwise be made to the miner. In contrast, a decision against the miner by the medical referee allowed little recourse to appeal and left the miner without any payment whatsoever.[97] 'When the Owners proclaim a desire for better and more harmonious relationships between themselves and the miner', the Miners' Association stated, 'we could better appreciate their desire if they made it more manifest by their better treatment towards the injured.'[98]

Joanna Bourke has noted that 'in the compensation court, the injured worker was customarily treated as though he were "on trial"' and the 'insurance doctors tended to be hostile to workers'.[99] Depictions of hostility between the doctor and compensation claimant are common in coalfields literature, where the encounter is often representative of wider class interests; the class allegiance of the doctor was seen to align with the interests of the coalowners and managers.[100] In T. Rowland Hughes's novel *William Jones*, Crad, who has worked in both quarries and coal mines, has silicosis but does not get compensation:

> 'Mi apeliais am un. Mi es i lawr at y *specialist* yng Nghaerdydd ac wedyn o flaen y *Board*, ond 'doedd dim digon o lwch ar fy mrest i imi gal compo. Glywist ti'r fath lol yn dy fywyd? 'Taswn i'n medru mynd dan ddaer am ryw flwyddyn arall i gal tipyn chwanag o lwch tu mewn imi, mi gawn i *gompensation* – a charreg fedd!'[101]

> 'I appealed for it. I went down to the specialist in Cardiff and before the Board after that, but there wasn't enough dust on my chest for me to get compo. Did you ever hear such nonsense in your life? If I had been able to go down below for a few more years to get a bit more dust inside me I would get compensation – and a gravestone!'[102]

Coalfields literature very often focused on compensation for silicosis, in part because lung disease was very common, but receiving the diagnosis of silicosis, rather than bronchitis or tuberculosis, was also crucial to gaining compensation.[103]

The author's class allegiance clearly influenced the depiction of the medical gatekeeping of compensation, particularly as it related to the perception of malingering. A. J. Cronin, who had worked as a colliery doctor in south Wales and Medical Inspector of Mines,[104] notes his personal suspicions of compensation claimants in his autobiography: 'my real invalids were numerous, but I had also to deal with the other sort ... many of the old time miners affected the symptoms of nystagmus and beat-knee, occupational diseases which entitled them to a pension.'[105] These suspicions influence a scene in *The Citadel* (1937), in which workers and the doctor clash over the denial of a compensation certificate to a long-time claimant. Ben Chenkin is claiming for nystagmus, but is portrayed as a malingerer: 'a great lump of a man, rolling in fat, who smelled strongly of beer and looked as if he had never done a full day's work in his life'.[106] The other 'compo cases'[107] draw ranks against Dr Manson, withdrawing their cards and refusing to be treated by him. Within the novel this is portrayed as working-class stubbornness against their own best interest, in contrast to the scientifically sound and therefore objective judgement of the middle-class doctor.

The basic trajectory of a compensation claim was further complicated by other factors that caused problems for the disabled miner in his attempts to secure financial recompense. When a workman made a claim for compensation, the wait for any form of payment presented an immediate issue. The Employers' Liability Act of 1880 ensured that proceedings for compensation should be started within six months of injury, while the Workmen's Compensation Act of 1897 stipulated that injuries must 'disable the workman for a period of at least two weeks from earning full wages at the work at which he was employed'.[108] However, the actual experience of waiting for compensation could be much longer than this. This was the experience of the Welsh miner Bert Coombes, who wrote, 'I think I waited nearly a month before they started to pay anything ... They cannot seem to realise that most of us are living on our next week's wages, and that even a day out of that means that someone must go short.'[109]

Those that did have to 'go short' while they were waiting for the administrative process of compensation had to make their own provision. Here, different steps existed in the different coalfields. In the more consensual atmosphere of the north-east of England, the practice of 'smart money' continued, partly as a recognition that disabled miners needed some form of income before compensation was paid. After the passing of the Workmen's Compensation Act in 1897, the Northumberland Coal Owners' Mutual Protection Association issued instructions to members stating that smart money 'is to be paid to the same classes of men as hitherto, but it is to continue for not more than two weeks. If the disability lasts more than that period then the compensation provided by the Act takes the place of smart money.'[110] The practice of paying 'smart money' continued well into the twentieth century: as late as 1935, the Durham Coal Owners' Mutual Protection Agency insisted that smart money was paid for the first four weeks of disablement prior to the commencement of compensation.[111] However, smart money was not paid as of right and could be withdrawn or rejected in any individual case. It was also very much confined to the North-East; the experience of Coombes confirms that many miners disabled from work had to resort to any combination of the mixed economy of welfare, including the Poor Law.

Compensation payments were never intended to replace lost income, and so they inevitably entailed a significant decrease in the income of the injured or sick miner. The Employers' Liability Act limited any compensation payments to the estimated earnings of three years of 'someone in similar employment'.[112] Weekly compensation payments for 'total or partial incapacity for work' under the Workmen's Compensation Act were based on earnings and calculated according to what claimants would have earned before the accident, but were to be 'not exceeding fifty per cent of his average weekly earnings during the previous twelve months', or one pound if the workman had been with the employer for less than one year.[113] Unsurprisingly, it was found that compensation needed to be supplemented with support from other agencies; as was stated in a House of Commons debate in 1940, 'thousands of men have to seek public assistance to eke out a miserable existence'.[114] Thus, not only did such a system entail a lower level of living after the development of an impairment but it also treated disability solely in terms of lost income and completely neglected the social, cultural and emotional impacts on the disabled miner through its failure to recompense him for the loss of a limb or an impairment of body function.

Impaired miners were faced with yet further difficulties and hardships as a result of the adversarial nature of the compensation system, which pitted them against their employers and gave such employers a financial incentive to contest the extent of disability. Weekly payments were not set in stone and could be reduced or terminated as a result of employer pressure. This was because the extent to which the impairment disabled a miner from working could change over time as the miner's condition changed or, more usually, because the coal company disputed the disabling effect of the impairment and sought revised medical opinions that could be used to reduce or end compensation payments. This was exacerbated by the close relationship that existed between the doctor and the colliery company, which meant that disabled miners were dependent on the medical testimony of their own doctors, who themselves owed their positions to the coal companies and therefore tended to provide expert views that did little to counter the medical testimony provided on behalf of the owners.[115] In other instances, the disabling impact of impairment could worsen as a miner's condition deteriorated and he would then be forced to seek higher compensation payments from a reluctant employer. In each scenario, the compensation system threw up all manner of obstacles in the way of the miner's securing adequate financial assistance to allow him to cope with his impairment.

Such complexities are best illustrated through individual cases, such as that of Robert Laird, a 'conveyor' in a colliery owned by the Fife Coal Company, who, in 1928, received weekly compensation when a septic wound in his injured hand made him 'totally incapacitated'. He was paid full compensation until a medical certificate stated that he was 'fit for any job he could do chiefly with his right hand rendering some assistance from his left'. He 'refused to accept the reduced compensation' and, once returning to work, applied for compensation 'on the footing of total incapacity' based on his hand's being in the same condition, which was refused. Laird's case displays an economic conceptualisation of disability – though one hand was 'incapacitated', the fact that he was able to perform work meant that he was denied full compensation. Though they were unsuccessful, Laird's efforts to receive full compensation highlight the importance that receiving payment meant to those injured.[116]

More complex again was the case of Wittrace Cope, a timber drawer at Houghton Colliery, Durham. Cope's situation also demonstrates the particular difficulties that could arise within the particular arrangements in place in Durham. He suffered a serious accident in 1903 in which he injured his back and hip. He was awarded full compensation at 17s. 8d. a week, but payments were ended in 1905 when he was adjudged fit for light work. Cope, it seems, struggled on in his light work despite continued difficulties as a result of his injuries until, in 1918, he brought forward evidence to state that he was unable to work due to the injuries he had received back in 1903 and insisted that he had been declared fit incorrectly. He was awarded compensation again, but only on the condition that he would not try to claim back pay to 1905. This was regretted by the officers of the Durham Miners' Association, however, and they looked to reopen the case within the Arbitration Committee, despite this not being allowed by the terms of the committee.[117] Significantly, James Robson, Miners' Agent, set out what he perceived as the injustice meted out too often to disabled miners such as Cope by the compensation system and, in doing so, articulated something of the experience of miners who did not succeed in obtaining compensation for their injuries:

> If ever a man suffered a gross injustice at the hands of fellow mortal, Cope has. He has been deprived of his compensation for 13 years, and he has had to bring up his family practically on the Parish. The effect upon a man's general health in having to live under such a great injustice must have been enormous, but to witness his family living under straitened circumstances as compared to what might have been for them under normal circumstances, and to be further deprived of any little assistance he was legally entitled to must have robbed him of any little pleasure he might obtain in life.[118]

Due to the nature of the disease, and the tendency for symptoms to improve as miners were removed from underground work, nystagmus cases were particularly subject to pressures exerted by employers to lessen liability. A number of nystagmus cases that came before the Durham Miners' Association's

Compensation Committee in 1914, for example, were found to have had their compensation payments reduced after the coal company alleged that the incapacity was at least partially due to causes other than the nystagmus, such as cataracts, detached retinas and other types of 'eye disease'.[119]

Coalfields literature picked up on the bitterness that was engendered by the compensation system and offers a scathing view of its inadequacies. Gwyn Thomas is typically sarcastic about the low rates of compensation, describing 'houses where there were to be found voters suffering greatly through the system, from bad lungs or legs, and getting so little compensation one would have thought their lungs and legs had actually improved as a result of being made bad.'[120] Indeed the system – work, pay and conditions – are presented as so poor that miner-characters repeatedly wish for their own deaths in order that their wives might benefit from the larger compensation payout:

> NED: Sandy, I'm tired ... I'm no' fit to be workin' doon here, but I've got to do it to keep my wife and weans respectable. *(Hopelessly)*. Ach! there's whiles I wish the roof would come doon on top o' me, and end it ... Mary would get compensation, and her worries would be a' by ...[121]

Another feature of the compensation system that further disadvantaged impaired miners was the practice of lump-sum payments. An amending Workmen's Compensation Act passed in 1906 allowed workers in receipt of compensation the option of receiving lump sums after at least six months of weekly payments, and it was believed that this was an attractive option for some miners. In his 1909 study *Accidental Injuries to Workmen*, published in reaction to the changes introduced in 1906, the surgeon Henry Norman Barnett maintained that a lump sum was potentially attractive, as 'the workman may be cognisant of his diseased condition and wish to make the most out of his accident to procure a lump sum in order that he may make provision for himself or his family should the disease prevent him from working'.[122]

Reasons for wanting a lump sum are explored in fiction, whereby a miner might have a chance of a new life. Sid Chaplin refers, perhaps rosily, to 'a dozen or so little shops which had been started by miners on compensation payments' in a short story in 1946.[123] The prospects for 'poor Mervyn' in Rhys Davies's *Jubilee Blues* (1938) include the unconvincing suggestion that 'perhaps he could study to be a chemist',[124] but he ultimately leaves the area with his family as part of a government work relocation scheme.

The amount of lump sum paid was very often tied explicitly to the circumstances of a miner's impairment. This is visible in the records of the Scottish Coal Workers' Compensation Scheme, which awarded a number of lump sums based on the consideration of how impairment affected work. The case of Michael Mooney v the Fife Coal Co., for example, concerned a man whose thumb and forefinger had been amputated. After a medical examination Mooney was found to be 'practically a one-armed man, whose damaged hand will only act as a guiding agent'. It was these considerations based on the impairment that led the case to settle for up to £200.[125] Others received lower amounts for reasons related to work and incapacity: Matthew Rutherford, who was 'very anaemic and ill nourished' and had 'poor sight', was found to have 'prospects of life … below normal, though his other organs appear sound', and thus received £75.[126] Thus, opinions on the extent of miners' impairments – almost always connected to the perceived ability to work – dictated levels of compensation.

At the same time, employers attempted to move disabled miners off weekly payments and onto lump-sum payments because it meant a reduction in the amounts paid overall, and trade unions were keen to advise their members not to commute their claims. As Arnold Wilson MP and Hermann Levy stated bluntly in their 1939 study *Workmen's Compensation*, 'A drowning man clutches at a straw; to an injured workman burdened with debt … a lump sum, however small, is "popular" only because it offers a temporary respite at the expense of the future.'[127] For his part, James Griffiths, MP for Llanelli in south Wales and later Minister for National Insurance responsible for the passage of the Industrial Injuries Act of 1946, remembered

> the tragedy of the 'compo' man of the south Wales valleys, the agents of commercial insurance companies who persuaded injured miners to settle for inadequate sums rather than risk taking employers to court: 'In my village … there are pathetic cases of industrial casualties left to limp their way through life'.[128]

Whatever the method of claiming or the complexities involved in securing compensation, the very act of collecting compensation could be a demoralising experience. Indeed, it could be made a demoralising experience. Discussing a new Workmen's Compensation Bill in 1933, Mr Tinker, the MP for Leith, told the House of Commons,

> When a miner is injured and has established his claim, he has to go to the colliery for his weekly compensation. It is not a pleasant job for the workman. He has to go to the colliery office and sometimes the pay clerk pays it to him, while at other times he has to go and see the manager. That is treating the workman almost as though he were begging something from the employer.[129]

As well as illustrating a manifestation of the power relations between employer and employee, Tinker's comments show the uncertainty and subservience that could go hand in hand with receiving compensation. Indeed, several MPs including Tinker suggested claiming through the Post Office in the same way as pensions were paid, so as to avoid 'the distasteful feeling that he is getting something to which he is not entitled', but this was not successful.[130]

Inscribed throughout the compensation system was the fear that workers might be faking injury or disablement in order to receive payments that they did not deserve. Such a fear undoubtedly existed in the minds of employers and doctors but it could also be used for rhetorical and practical effect to minimise compensation payments. Bert Coombes describes a demeaning effect which this culture of suspicion had upon recipients of compensation:

> I was paid compensation, but the amount and the method of paying it did not help me to get better. They gave the impression that I was trying to get something for nothing out of them. This compensation was handled by an insurance company, and all the injured were treated as if they had crippled themselves deliberately.[131]

Yet the discourse which divided the injured and disabled into the deserving and undeserving could be adopted by writers generally sympathetic to the workers' cause as a way of representing character. An ex-miner, Joe Corrie, contrasts two claimants in his novel, *Black Earth*, to show their integrity, or lack of it: 'So while an injury in the pit can mean hell for a man like Jack Smith it could mean Heaven for a man like Ted Jackson.'[132] Ted Jackson is a bookie, 'a pale-faced little man who walked with a limp', who is genuinely injured in the mine and undergoes surgery, but he exaggerates his injury for a larger compensation pay-out. The morning after the award, 'Ted was able to walk down to the pub without his crutches. A miracle had happened through the night.'[133]

Another group of miners, however, had no recourse to the compensation system and were left with few options for support. Some miners found that the toll of working in the industry caused a general deterioration in health and an accumulation of impairments that could not be attributed to any particular accident or compensatable condition and so did not have access to compensation. Richard Augustine Studdert Redmayne, the resident manager of Seaton Delaval Collieries in Northumberland and a former miner, told the Sankey Commission in 1919:

> If a miner is disabled through accident or ill-health occasioned in the mine and proved to have been so occasioned, then he receives compensation under the Compensation Act; but short of that, if a miner, through a breakdown of health, quite apart from that, short of his being on a permanent relief fund or some other fund, of course there is no means of compensating him.[134]

Miners' trade unions were clear in their view that the compensation system failed large sections of the disabled mining population and advocated new forms of welfare which shifted from a narrow, individualistic and legalistic view of industrial disability to a broader, fairer system of welfare that considered health and disability in a more holistic fashion.

The Workmen's Compensation Act remained active throughout most of the first half of the twentieth century, but the expansion of national state welfare under the post-war Labour government saw it brought to an end. 'The coming of a national scheme for health insurance and, in particular, the passing of the Industrial Injuries Act', wrote the *Colliery Guardian* in 1948, 'has made the Workmen's Compensation Act, from not a few standpoints, something of a back number.'[135] William Beveridge's 1942 report *Social Insurance and Allied Services* – the landmark document of the conception of the welfare state – had highlighted the shortfalls of the existing compensation system, which was 'below subsistence level for anyone who had family responsibilities or whose earnings in work were less than twice the amount needed for subsistence'.[136] The Workmen's Compensation Act was finally replaced by the National Insurance (Industrial Injuries) Act of 1946, passed by the former miners' leader, Jim Griffiths. It provided the first insurance-based compensation system for injured workers, taken from a fund contributed to by workers, employers and the state, and instituted more generous compensation payments than workers had received previously.[137] It was a recognition of the decades of support given to the Labour Party by the miners' trade unions and the importance of compensation to union politics and the lives of miners.

Conclusion

The period after 1880 saw the first legislation which recognised the principles of employers' liability and workers' rights to compensation, in a direct reaction to an economy of welfare which made it extremely difficult for disabled miners to attain any sense of financial security, even though they were supposedly statutorily entitled to it. The Employers' Liability Act and the Workmen's Compensation Act both contributed to a shift in attitudes towards the responsibility of employers and the disabled miner's right to compensation, but the actual process of claiming compensation was long and flawed, and rarely ended in a desirable amount being awarded. Disabled miners in the late nineteenth century and the first half of the twentieth – even those receiving compensation – had to rely on multiple sources of welfare from an unco-ordinated tapestry of voluntary and state organisations.

Furthermore, even though the principle of collective compulsory welfare was emerging, the principles of routine surveillance, unsteady payment and implied moral responsibility for impairment were visible in almost all of these welfare sources. Friendly societies and permanent relief funds, though declining, remained active, and the waning Poor Law was still turned to, largely as a last resort in cases of emergency. Likewise, existing domestic support networks based around family and community were crucial to miners who could not survive by relying solely on organisations. Literary representations of welfare and compensation tended to be influenced by the class alliances of the author. The interwar fiction by working-class writers focuses on the injustices and humiliations of unfair systems in contrast to the willingness of communities to help out injured miners with 'lifts', yet some also expressed anxieties about malingering. Undoubtedly, this period saw disease and injury in mining communities being reframed away from an individualised tragedy which could be addressed only through self-help or the stigmatised Poor Law, and towards an interpretation of disability as something that could be the fault of the employer and thus compensated. However, the need to rely on multiple forms of welfare and subsistence continued long after this change in the conceptualisation of disability came about, and dependency came to form the main experience of impaired miners.

Notes

1 For overviews, see Derek Fraser, *The Evolution of the British Welfare State: A History of Social Policy since the Industrial Revolution*, 3rd edn (Basingstoke: Palgrave Macmillan, 2003); David Gladstone, *The Twentieth-Century Welfare State*, British History in Perspective (Basingstoke: Macmillan, 1999); Alan J. Kidd, *State, Society and the Poor in Nineteenth-Century England*, Social History in Perspective (Basingstoke: Macmillan, 1999); Bernard Harris, *The Origins of the British Welfare State: Society, State and Social Welfare in England and Wales, 1800–1945* (Basingstoke: Palgrave Macmillan, 2004).

2 The changing portrayal of welfare was further reflected in the class and political affiliation of the writer, as working-class writers (many former miners, often with strong political ties to trade unions or to the International Labour Party/Labour Party) sought to show various ways in which the systemic inequality of wealth and power kept working-class people in constant risk of poverty and exposed to an unacceptably high probability of ill-health or injury.

3 Jose Harris, cited in Fraser, *The Evolution of the British Welfare State*, p. 13.

4 Laura E. Marshak, Milton Seligman and Fran Prezant, *Disability and the Family Life Cycle* (New York: Basic Books, 1999), pp. 9–10; Jane Lewis, 'Family Provision of Health and Welfare in the Mixed Economy of Care in the Late Nineteenth and Twentieth Centuries', *Social History of Medicine*, 8:1 (1995), pp. 1–16.

5 Glamorgan Archives (hereafter GA), D/D Vau 20, 'A Friend in Need is a Friend Indeed'; *Tarian y Gweithiwr*, 25 May 1899, p. 1.

6 T. Rowland Hughes (1903–49) was born in Llanberis, Caernarvonshire, the son of a quarryman, and worked as a university lecturer, and producer of Welsh feature programmes for the BBC. He was diagnosed with multiple sclerosis in 1937 and

during this period was a successful Welsh-language poet (twice winning the Chair of the National Eisteddfod, in 1937 and 1940) and novelist, producing a novel a year from 1943 to 1947.
7   T. Rowland Hughes, *William Jones* (Llandysul: Gwasg Gomer, 1991), p. 356.
8   T. Rowland Huges, trans. Richard Ruck, *William Jones* (Aberystwyth: Gwasg Aberystwyth, 1953), p. 288.
9   James Welsh, *The Underworld* (London: Herbert Jenkins, 1920), p. 19.
10 Welsh, *The Underworld*, p. 20.
11 Durham County Record Office (hereafter DCRO), CC/X 140, Minutes for Lord Mayor of London's Mining Distress Fund (later the Coalfields Distress Funds), Northern Coalfields Committee, 14 February 1929.
12 West Glamorgan Archives Service, D/D SHF/1, Swansea Hospital Ladies' Samaritan Fund Minute Book, Monthly Meeting, 12 September 1913.
13 National Archives of Scotland (hereafter NAS), Scottish Coal Workers' Compensation Scheme, Director's Minute Books, 1912–1914, F 148/12, John Black v. The Fife Coal Co Ltd.
14 DCRO, D/DMA (Acc: 1004(D)) 167, Durham Miners' Association Compensation Department Monthly Reports, 1918–1919, p. 16.
15 Lewis, 'Family Provision of Health and Welfare in the Mixed Economy of Care'.
16 Mike Mantin, 'Philanthropy and Deafness in Wales, 1847–1914', *Welsh History Review*, 27:2 (2014), p. 289.
17 Blind Persons Act (1920); GA, DBLI/RH/1, Minute Book, Management Committee Meeting, 9 September 1920.
18 GA, DBLI/RH/2, Minute Book, Special General Committee Meeting, 22 April 1925. The 'Conditions of Service' document was attached to the minutes, and thus was written before the meeting took place.
19 For examples, see Mary Wilson Carpenter, *Health, Medicine, and Society in Victorian England* (Santa Barbara: Praeger, 2010); Colin Lees and Sue Ralph, 'Charitable Provision for Blind People and Deaf People in Late Nineteenth Century London', *Journal of Research in Special Educational Needs*, 4:3 (2004), pp. 148–60.
20 GA, DBLI/RH/15, Minute Book, Management Committee Meeting, 8 September 1947.
21 GA, DBLI/RH/1, Minute Book, Management Committee Meeting, 9 September 1920; GA, DBLI/RH/5, Minute Book, Management Committee Meeting, 30 November 1931.
22 GA, DBLI/RH/2, Minute Book, Management Committee Meeting, 16 May 1927.
23 See David M. Turner and Daniel Blackie, *Disability in the Industrial Revolution: Physical Impairment in British Coalmining, 1780–1880* (Manchester: Manchester University Press, 2018).
24 DCRO, D/EBF 92/13, Rules of the Durham County Enginemen's, Boiler Minders' and Firemen's Mutual Aid Association and National Insurance Approved Society, 1913.

25 DCRO, D/X, 411/110, Revised Rules of the Tradesmen's Annual Friendly Society, 1885.
26 P. H. J. H. Gosden, *The Friendly Societies in England 1815–1875* (London: Batsford, 1973), pp. 82–4.
27 The National Archives, London (hereafter TNA), FS 15/842, Aberaman Colliery Friendly Society, Rules of the Aberaman Colliery Friendly Society, 1892.
28 For example, members of the Durham County Colliery Enginemen's Mutual Protection Association were fined up to £1 for being 'detected imposing in this way'. TNA, FS 28/6, Durham Colliery County Enginemen's Mutual Protection Association, Rules, 1883.
29 TNA, FS 15/847, Llanbradach Colliery Sick Benefit Society, 1895–1915, Rules of the Llanbradach Colliery Sick Benefit Society, 1905.
30 Swansea University, South Wales Coalfield Collection, MNA/NUM/I/34/165, Rules of the Glais Benefit Society, 1871.
31 DCRO, D/EBF 92/13, Rules of the Durham County Enginemen's, Boiler Minders' and Firemen's Mutual Aid Association and National Insurance Approved Society, 1913.
32 DCRO, D/IOR 57, North Eastern Counties Friendly Societies Convalescent Home, Rules of the North Eastern Counties Friendly Societies' Convalescent Home, 1893.
33 Harry Lindsay, *Rhoda Roberts: A Welsh mining story* (London: Chatto & Windus, 1895), p. 112.
34 John Benson, 'Coalminers, Coalowners and Collaboration: The Miners' Permanent Relief Fund Movement in England, 1860–1895', *Labour History Review*, 68:2 (2003), pp. 181–94.
35 George L. Campbell, *Miners' Thrift and Employers' Liability* (Wigan: Strowger and Son, 1891), pp. 6–7.
36 George L. Campbell, *Miners' Insurance Funds: Their Origin and Extent* (London: Waterlow & Sons, 1880), pp. 9–11.
37 Harold Heslop, *The Earth Beneath* (London: T. V. Boardman & Company Ltd., 1946), p. 161.
38 Campbell, *Miners' Insurance Fund*, pp. 6–7.
39 DCRO, NCBI/RS/1469, Draft of the Rules of the Miners' Provident Association, 1859; Tyne and Wear Archives Service (hereafter TWAS), CH.MPR/14/1 (MF2196), Miners' Disablement Fund (1863–1891); Turner and Blackie, *Disability in the Industrial Revolution*, pp. 99–100.
40 TWAS, CH.MPR/14/1 (MF2196), Miners' Disablement Fund (1863–1891).
41 Campbell, *Miners' Thrift and Employers' Liability*, p. 11.
42 TWAS, CH/MPR/10/1, Northumberland and Durham Miners Permanent Relief Fund, Rules, 1899, Rules 36 and 37; TWA, CH/MPR/10/5, Northumberland and Durham Miners' Permanent Relief Fund, Rules, 1923, Rules 37 and 38.
43 Cardiff Central Library, Monmouthshire and South Wales Miners' Permanent Provident Society, Report of Proceedings at the 2nd Annual General Meeting, 27

March 1883, p. 13; Report of Proceedings at the 21st Annual General Meeting, 25 March 1902, p. 18.
44 John Benson 'Non-Fatal Coalmining Accidents', *Bulletin of the Society for the Study of Labour History*, 32 (1976), p. 22.
45 Benson, 'Coalminers, Coalowners and Collaboration', p. 186.
46 Monmouthshire and South Wales Miners' Permanent Relief Society, *Report of the Fourth Annual Meeting, March 31st, 1885*, pp. 6–7.
47 Monmouthshire and South Wales Miners' Permanent Relief Society, 'Report of the Board of Management', Report of the Fifth Annual Meeting, March 30th, 1886, p. 17.
48 TWAS, CH/MPR/10/1, Northumberland and Durham Miners' Permanent Relief Fund, Rules, 1899.
49 TWAS, CH/MPR/1/7, Northumberland and Durham Miners' Permanent Relief Fund, Committee Minutes, Minutes of the General Committee Meeting, 22 September 1906.
50 Cardiff Central Library, Monmouthshire and South Wales Permanent Provident Society, Annual Reports, 1881–1893, Report of proceedings at the 3rd Annual General Meeting, 23 June 1884.
51 Benson, 'Colaminers, Coalowners and Collaboration', p. 18; Royal Commission on the Poor Laws and Relief of Distress, Appendix volume V, Minutes of Evidence (90th to 94th days) with Appendix, Cd. 4888, 1909, xli, p. 203.
52 Royal Commission on the Poor Laws and Relief of Distress, Appendix volume V, Minutes of Evidence (90th to 94th days) with Appendix, Cd. 4888, 1909, xli, p. 203.
53 Poor Law Amendment Act 1834, cited in Kenneth Morgan, *The Birth of Industrial Britain: Social Change 1750–1850* (Harlow: Pearson, 2004), p. 134. While the principle of 'less eligibility' was not enshrined in the Poor Law Amendment (Scotland) Act of 1845, Poor Law authorities north of the border introduced a poorhouse test into practice as a means to distinguish between deserving and underserving claimants for relief; see Stephanie Blackden, 'The Board of Supervision and the Scottish Parochial Medical Service, 1845–95', *Medical History*, 30:2 (1986), p. 147. See also Audrey Paterson, 'The Poor Law in Nineteenth-Century Scotland', in Derek Fraser (ed.), *The New Poor Law in the Nineteenth Century* (London: Macmillan, 1976), pp. 171–93.
54 See, for example, David Gladstone, *The Twentieth-Century Welfare State* (Basingstoke: Macmillan, 1999), p. 12; Lauren M. E. Goodlad, '"Make the Working Man Like Me": Charity, Pastorship and Middle-Class Identity in Nineteenth-Century Britain: Thomas Chalmers and Dr James Phillips Kay', *Victorian Studies*, 43:4 (2001), p. 592.
55 Deborah Stone, *The Disabled State* (Basingstoke: Macmillan, 1985), p. 40.
56 Stone, *Disabled State*, p. 51.
57 Anne Borsay, *Disability and Social Policy: A History of Exclusion* (Basingstoke: Palgrave Macmillan, 2005), p. 152.

58 David M. Turner, '"Fraudulent" Disability in Historical Perspective', *History and Policy* (2012), http://www.historyandpolicy.org/papers/policy-paper-130.html, accessed 5 January 2013.
59 Hugh Gilmore, *The Black Diamond* (London: Thomas Mitchell Primitive Methodist Publishing House, 1880), pp. 19–20.
60 Harold Heslop, *The Gate of a Strange Field* (New York: D. Appleton & Company, 1929), p. 135.
61 Heslop, *The Gate of a Strange Field*, p. 147.
62 James Welsh, *The Morlocks* (London: Herbert Jenkins Ltd, 1924), p. 45.
63 Tom Hanlin, *Once in Every Lifetime* (New York: The Viking Press, 1945), p. 173.
64 Elizabeth Andrews, *A Woman's Work Is Never Done: Being the Recollections of a Childhood and Upbringing amongst the South Wales Miners and a Lifetime of Service to the Labour Movement in Wales* (Rhondda: Cymric Democrat Publishing Society, 1957), p. 12.
65 Ministry of Health Act (1919).
66 Local Government Act (1929); Harris, *The Origins of the British Welfare State*, p. 203.
67 Generally, the Poor Law in Scotland tended to be less generous than that in England and Wales, and divergence in practice widened as the nineteenth century progressed; see M. A. Crowther, 'Poverty, Health and Welfare', in W. Hamish Fraser and R. J. Morris (eds), *People and Society in Scotland: Volume II, 1830–1914* (Edinburgh: John Donald Publishers Ltd, 1990), pp. 268–9.
68 Local Government Board, *Eighteenth Annual Report of the Local Government Board*, C. 5813, 1889, pp. xxxv, lxxvi–lxxvii.
69 Blackden, 'The Board of Supervision and the Scottish Parochial Medical Service', pp. 148, 161, 163–6; see also Crowther, 'Poverty, Health and Welfare', p. 275.
70 *Seventeenth Annual Report of the Ministry of Health, 1935–36*, Cmd. 5287, 1935–36, x, p. 121; *Seventh Annual Report of the Department of Health for Scotland, 1935*, Cmd. 5123, 1935–36, xi, p. 140.
71 Heslop, *The Gate of a Strange Field*, p. 135.
72 Mitchell Library, Glasgow City Archives (hereafter ML), C01 39/53, Douglas Parochial Board Record of Applications, 24 September 1885.
73 ML, D-HEW 17/297/1, Applications for Relief, Govan Parish, 25 August 1896.
74 ML, CO1 27/92, Applications for relief, Carluke, 1878–83; ML, CO1 27/93, Applications for relief, Carluke, 1884–93.
75 Gwent Archives, CSWBGB/C/29, Bedwellty Union Out Relief Advisory Committee Papers, 18 February 1924.
76 Gwent Archives, CSWBGB/C/29, Bedwellty Union Out Relief Advisory Committee Papers, 18 February 1924; see also Blackden, 'The Board of Supervision and the Scottish Parochial Medical Service', p. 161.
77 NAS, GD 176/1959, Circular letter as to the use of the Poorhouse as a test, Board of Supervision, Edinburgh, 26th July, 1883; for an example, see Gwent Archives, CSWBGB/C/29, Bedwellty Union Out Relief Advisory Committee Minutes, 3 July 1929.

78 Gwent Archives, CSW/BGP/I/222–230, Pontypool Union Workhouse Admissions and Discharges, 1858–1935.
79 DCRO, U/EA 24, Easington Union Relief Committee Minutes, 30 November 1898–7 February 1912, 6 April 1910.
80 *Glasgow Herald*, 11 December 1911.
81 John Benson, 'Poor Law Guardians, Coalminers, and Friendly Societies in Northern England, 1860–1894: Statutory Provision, Local Autonomy, and Individual Responsibility', *Northern History*, 44:2 (2007), p. 160.
82 Northumberland Archives (hereafter NA), CC/CM/PA/1, County of Northumberland Public Assistance Committee Minutes, 2 December 1929–2 January 1935, 11 June 1930.
83 P. W. J. Bartrip, *Wounded Soldiers of Industry: Industrial Compensation Policy 1833–1897* (Oxford: Clarendon Press, 1983).
84 Employers' Liability Act (1880).
85 P. W. J. Bartrip, *Workmen's Compensation in Twentieth Century Britain: Law, History and Social Policy* (Aldershot: Gower, 1987).
86 Peter Bartrip, 'The Rise and Decline of Workmen's Compensation', in Paul Weindling (ed.), *The Social History of Occupational Health* (London: Croom Helm, 1985), pp. 157–79.
87 TWAS, CH/MPR/10/8, Northumberland and Durham Miners' Permanent Relief Fund, Rules, 1938.
88 *Labour Leader*, 20 August 1898.
89 Cardiff Library, Monmouthshire and South Wales Permanent Provident Society, Annual Reports 1906–1920, Report of proceedings at the 28th Annual General Meeting, 30 March 1909; Monmouthshire and South Wales Miners' Permanent Provident Society, Annual Report, 1920, p. 15.
90 Workmen's Compensation (War Addition) Act, 1917; Workmen's Compensation (War Addition) Act, 1919; *Colliery Guardian*, 2 January 1920; Bartrip, *Workmen's Compensation in Twentieth Century Britain*.
91 William Beveridge, *Social Insurance and Allied Services*, Cmd. 6404 (1942); *Report of the Royal Commission on Workmen's Compensation*, Cmd. 6588 (London: HMSO, 1945).
92 Angela Turner and Arthur McIvor, '"Bottom Dog Men": Disability, Social Welfare and Advocacy in the Scottish Coalfields in the Interwar Years, 1918–1939', *Scottish Historical Review*, 96:2 (2017), p. 209.
93 On the differences in industrial relations in the different coalfields, see Stefan Berger, Andy Croll and Norman LaPorte (eds), *Towards a Comparative History of Coalfield Societies* (Aldershot: Ashgate, 2005); Alan Campbell, Nina Fishman and David Howell (eds), *Miners, Unions and Politics, 1910–47* (Aldershot: Ashgate, 1996); John McIlroy, Alan Campbell and Keith Gildart (eds), *Industrial Politics and the 1926 Mining Lockout: The Struggle for Dignity* (Cardiff: University of Wales Press, 2004); on the Arbitration Committee, see W. R. Garside, *The Durham Miners 1919–1960* (London: George Allen & Unwin Ltd, 1971), pp. 308–10.

94 Departmental Committee on Workmen's Compensation, *Minutes of Evidence, Volume1*, [Cmd. 908], 1920, xxvi, p. 242, para.5952.
95 North East Mining Archive and Research Centre (hereafter NEEMARC), NUMDA/6/1/1/1, DMA Reports of the Compensation Department, Volume I, Arbitration Committee, 3 March 1919.
96 DCRO, D/DMA Acc 1004 D 169, Durham Miners' Association, Review of the Work of the Compensation Department for the year 1922, p. 355.
97 DCRO, D/DMA Acc 1004 D 169, Durham Miners' Association, Review of the Work of the Compensation Department for the year 1922, p. 358; see also, DCRO, D/DMA Acc 1004 D 169, Durham Miners' Association, Review of the Work of the Compensation Department during the year 1925, p. 488.
98 DCRO, D/DMA Acc 1004 D 169, Durham Miners' Association, Review of the Work of the Compensation Department during the year 1925, p. 488.
99 Joanna Bourke. *Dismembering the Male: Men's Bodies, Britain and the Great War* (London: Reaktion, 1999), p. 48.
100 There was a similar suspicion towards the judiciary about enquiries into accidental deaths in mining. See B. L. Coombes, *These Poor Hands: The Autobiography of a Miner Working in South Wales, with an Introduction by Bill Jones and Chris Williams* (Cardiff: University of Wales Press, 2002) or Lewis Jones's *Cwmardy* in Lewis Jones, *Cwmardy and We Live* (Cardigan: Parthian, 2006).
101 Hughes, *William Jones*, p. 139.
102 Hughes, trans. Ruck, *William Jones*, p. 93.
103 For example, Rhys Davies's short story, 'The Pits Are on the Top', in Rhys Davies, *Collected Stories: Volume I*, edited by Meic Stephens (Llandysul: Gomer Press, 1996) pp. 261–6, involves a miner who had just died from lung disease, but had not received compensation because he was diagnosed with bronchitis.
104 Discussed further in Chapter 6.
105 A. J. Cronin, *Adventures in Two Worlds* (London: Victor Gollancz, 1952), pp. 159–60.
106 A. J. Cronin, *The Citadel* (London: Vista, 1996), p. 117.
107 Cronin, *The Citadel*, p. 119.
108 Employers' Liability Act, 1880; Workmen's Compensation Act, 1897.
109 Coombes, *These Poor Hands*, p. 63.
110 NA, NRO 00263/C/1/2/1, Northumberland Coal Owners' Mutual Protections Association, Minute Book, Workmen's Compensation Act, 1897, Instructions to Members.
111 DCRO, D/DCOMPA 208, Durham Coal Owners' Mutual Protection Association, Workmen's compensation Acts: Instructions to Members, May 1935.
112 Employers' Liability Act, 1880.
113 Workmen's Compensation Act, 1897.
114 Hansard, 30 January 1940.
115 DCRO, D/DMA Acc 1004 D 169, Durham Miners' Association, Review of the Work of the Compensation Department during the year 1924, pp. 869–70.

116 NAS, SC21/12A/1928/18, Robert Laird v The Fife Coal Company, Dunfermline Sherriff Court, 18 September 1928 and 8 November 1928.
117 DCRO, D/DMA 167, Durham Miners' Association, Compensation Department Monthly Reports, September 1918–December 1919.
118 DCRO, D/DMA 167, Durham Miners Association, Compensation Department Monthly Reports, Report for October 1918, p. 21.
119 NEEMARC, NUMDA/1/6/39, Durham Miners' Association Compensation Committee Minutes, 1914.
120 Gwyn Thomas, *The Dark Philosophers* (Cardigan: Parthian, 2006 [1946]), p. 206.
121 Joe Corrie, 'Hewers o' Coal', in Joe Corrie, *Plays Poems & Theatre Writings*, Linda MacKenney (ed.) (Edinburgh: 7:84 Publications, 1985), p. 109. See also John Swan's *The Mad Miner* (London: The Houghton Publishing Company, 1933), p. 151 and Gwyn Thomas, "Oscar", in *Where Did I Put My Pity?* (London: Progress Publishing Company, 1946), p. 34.
122 Henry Norman Barnett, *Accidental Injuries to Workmen: With Reference to Workmen's Compensation Act, 1906. With Article on Injuries to the Organs of Special Sense* (London: Rebman, 1909), p. 114.
123 Sid Chaplin, 'Half Moon Street', in Geoffrey Halson (ed.), *The Leaping Lad and other stories* (Harlow: Longman Group Ltd., 1970 [1946]), p. 19.
124 Rhys Davies, *Jubilee Blues* (London: Heinemann, 1938), p. 213.
125 NAS, Scottish Coal Workers' Compensation Scheme, Director's Minute Books, 1912–1914, F3235/14, Michael Mooney v The Fife Coal Co. Ltd.
126 NAS, Scottish Coal Workers' Compensation Scheme, Director's Minute Books, 1912–1914, F287/13, Rutherford v The Fife Coal Co. Ltd.
127 Arnold Talbot Wilson and Hermann Levy, *Workmen's Compensation* (London: Oxford University Press, 1939), p. 134.
128 James Griffiths, *Pages from Memory* (London: J. M. Dent & Sons Ltd., 1969), p. 82.
129 Hansard, 10 February 1933.
130 Hansard, 10 February 1933.
131 Coombes, *These Poor Hands*, p. 63.
132 Joe Corrie, *Black Earth* (London: Routledge, 1939), p. 233.
133 Corrie, *Black Earth*, p. 232.
134 Coal Industry Commission, *Vol. II: Reports and Minutes of Evidence on the First Stage of the Inquiry*, Cmd. 360 (London: HMSO 1919), p. 1163.
135 *Colliery Guardian*, 11 June 1948.
136 Beveridge, *Social Insurance and Allied Services*, p. 7.
137 Bartrip, *Workmen's Compensation in Twentieth Century Britain*; McIvor and Johnston, *Miners' Lung*, p. 203.

4

THE SOCIAL RELATIONS OF DISABILITY

While disabled people in mining communities worked, sought medical care and received welfare, they also existed in a complex web of social relations. Such social relations were varied and complex, were determined by a broad array of social, cultural and other factors and had profound consequences for experiences and understandings of disability. But just as existing social relations helped influence the experiences of disabled people, so disability brought about new social relations between individuals, groups and agencies. Thus, disability was both reflective and constitutive of social relations, and the question arises whether the varied social relations between different coalfields, themselves the product of a range of disparate factors, led to different social relations of disability in the case-study coalfields.

This chapter considers everyday social relations within coalfield society, and does so from a spatial perspective.[1] It considers a range of 'public', 'private', interstitial and liminal spaces in which disabled people lived their lives and came into contact with others. The home is, of course, a crucially important location for the production and reproduction of social relations, but disabled people also spent a great deal of their time in the broader community, from public places such as parks, squares and the street to community institutions such as places of worship, sports grounds, cinemas, clubs and pubs, social centres and so on. In adopting this perspective, the chapter draws upon Brendan Gleeson's socio-spatial approach to disability. Railing against the paucity of historical and spatial approaches to disability, Gleeson set out to analyse the 'social space of disability' by exploring the spatial dimensions of everyday life for disabled people in the city.[2] Convinced of the 'irreducibly spatial character of social relations', he set out to do this through a focus on the home and institutions as significant social spaces for the social construction of disability, in addition to 'interstitial' spaces such as the street or the informal economy.[3] Through consideration of these various spaces, a 'landscape of disability' can be mapped and used to better understand the experiences and understandings of disability in coalfield society.

This attention to spatial perspectives as a means to consider the everyday realities of disabled people's experiences also serves to emphasise the importance of movement – from one place to another, or through spaces – and thereby also gives a better sense of the everyday lives of disabled people in mining communities and the particular circumstances in which social relations were produced. In this sense, space becomes more than mere location or a tangible, physical environment, and more a 'lived space' in which bodily experiences – in addition to cultural norms, political views and other emotions – help to inscribe it with meaning and significance. The spatial approach also serves to prioritise the aspects of life that were important to historical actors themselves, rather than the more intangible, abstract social, cultural and political contexts that are traditionally given greater prominence by academic perspectives.[4]

While the social relations of disability were reflected and constituted in the workplace, as demonstrated in the first chapter, they were also manifest in the two other important spheres of life: home and community. This study has regarded the home as a workplace (mainly of unpaid women servicing industrial workers), while coal historiography since the late 1990s has brought into focus the importance of home and community as spaces in the constitution of social relations in coalfield communities.[5] The home, in particular, with its gendered divisions of labour and family roles, is a key location in which to address the intersection of male disability and gender. It is also the space most likely to be inhabited – and affected – by disabled women in the coalfields.

Work in disability studies since the 1990s has illustrated how the construction of disability is itself informed by class, gender, race, ethnicity, religion and age, in addition to marital status and family composition. An early feminist disability study, *Pride Against Prejudice* (1991) by Jenny Morris, was a groundbreaking challenge to the generalisations of social model theory for their failure to adequately include disabled women. She argued that 'a feminist perspective can help to redress [the lack of disabled people's voices], and in doing so give voice to the experience of both disabled men and disabled women'.[6] Other work has seen an intensified effort to address the lack of women's perspectives in disability studies and to integrate feminist theory into an intersectional disability studies.[7] Likewise, the interplay between disability and masculinity is an important and emerging question. Like Morris, Tom Shakespeare argues that the structural focus of the social model has obscured personal experiences of oppression: 'Masculinity and femininity are in a process of transitional change in western societies, which makes it difficult to generalise about the strategies of individual disabled men and women.'[8]

Disability and the home

While the focus in the labour history of mining communities was once on trade unions, strikes and industrial relations, the broadening of the historiography in the 1970s and 1980s led to attention being given to other aspects of the social history of such communities. These included the home, in terms of both the provision and quality of the physical structure and, more importantly, the social institution in which people resided and formed social relations. The best work in this field emphasised the interdependence of the home, the community and the workplace in the production and reproduction of social relations, and the extent to which the home was as crucial a location, in the creation of the mining community, as the colliery.[9] As a space, the form of miners' housing had consequences for the lives of their disabled inhabitants that helped to condition social relations.

Miners' houses varied in character and quality from one coalfield to the next, but certain common characteristics were evident. They tended to be small, crowded and frequently lacking adequate sanitation, creating multiple health risks in addition to the threat of smoke pollution from both pit and domestic chimneys.[10] Nevertheless, differences are discernible across different coalfields and would have had a material influence on the experiences of disabled people and their families. In the Scottish coalfields, single-roomed cottages, many dating from earlier in the nineteenth century but others still being built as late as the early twentieth century, constituted almost 20 per cent of the housing stock in some districts by that time. More numerous were the two-roomed houses consisting of a kitchen and a smaller additional room.[11] In the north-east of England, small, single-storey houses of two rooms – a kitchen and another room – were also common, but both here and in the Scottish coalfields later developments were a little more commodious as houses with two or three bedrooms were built in larger numbers by the end of the nineteenth century.[12] Houses in mining communities in south Wales, usually built in the late nineteenth and early twentieth centuries, when bye-laws governed the physical character of the buildings, tended to be of this higher quality, with kitchens, bathrooms and two or three bedrooms.[13] According to the census of 1911, overcrowding (by the census measure) stood at 5.6 per cent of the population in the Rhondda valley and 5.9 per cent in nearby Aberdare, in south Wales, whereas the level was as high as 34.2 per cent in Stanley, 32.2 per cent in Brandon and Byshottles and 41 per cent in Annfield Plain, all in the north-east of England.[14] If levels of overcrowding varied from coalfield to coalfield, the consequences of living with a disability or convalescing in a single room shared with six or seven other people could be severe.[15] As Carr observes, the houses in the north-east were 'no fit places for the care and rehabilitation of the sick'. The lack of space, the frequent absence of fireplaces or windows that opened, and the poor sanitary state of the housing were inimical to good health, convalescence and everyday life with an impairment. Severely ill or disabled people were required in these conditions to lie on a sofa or bed, or were propped up in an armchair, perhaps in the one living room of the household, where ordinary domestic routines continued.[16]

Homes that were ill-equipped to serve as spaces for disabled people could potentially cause fear and anxiety to families. A Mass Observation report in 1942 aimed to investigate this issue. It recounted the views of a Medical Officer of Health who complained that:

> It's all the worse because people here have always taken a great pride in their houses. They are self-respecting people. I had a letter from a woman only the other day. Her son's been invalided out of the Army with tuberculosis. He's got to come back to a house that's running with damp. The letter was most pathetic. But there's nowhere else they can go.[17]

Thus the report revealed the difficulty in reconfiguring houses to accommodate disabled family members in the available domestic space.

The physical form of the miner's house had some influence on social relations, but it was the home, as an idea and as an institution, that was more important in the experience and production of social relations. The relationship between husband and wife in the mining household has long been stereotyped as the breadwinner-worker and the equally hard-working but dependent wife in a clear sexual hierarchy. Gender historians have qualified this generalisation and have challenged one-dimensional or overly broad stereotypes to offer more nuanced portrayals in which love and affection are as evident as any pragmatic utilitarianism and in which wives are not necessarily powerless victims of male authority.[18]

The most obvious way in which disability reflected and was constitutive of social relations was in the context of care giving. In her history of women in pit communities, and also drawing on her family's experiences in a mining village in north-east England in the early twentieth century, Griselda Carr describes women's care for both disabled and temporarily sick husbands: they 'nursed them with tender care, feeding them, helping them to wash and removing the slops. They dosed them with medicines, bandaged and poulticed them, all the while attempting to maintain in a small and often crowded living room as much peace and quiet as they could.'[19] The grandmother of Carr's husband,

Bill, for example, 'shouldered' the care for two sons, 'one who was born with a short crippled leg and another who was a Down's Syndrome child'.[20]

While women's working lives in particular could be transformed by the arrival of a child with a congenital disability, they could also be turned upside down by the sudden permanent disablement of their husbands or sons in industrial accidents. Social relations between previously able-bodied adults in the context of severe head injury, loss of a limb or paralysis could change considerably. Such injuries and conditions were common in mining communities and, given the particular gender relations in these communities, often meant a significant burden of care giving placed on women's shoulders in addition to their usual domestic responsibilities. While such injuries could heal to a greater or lesser extent, even a temporary disablement would have an impact on income and require care giving. The disability of the male worker generated a great deal of additional work for the miner's wife, including taking on domestic tasks usually carried out by the man. One miner from south Wales remembered, for example, how his wife was forced to assume his usual responsibility of carrying in the coal delivered to the front of the house to the coal shelter in the back yard as his strength failed as a result of pneumoconiosis.[21]

Daughters were also required to assume greater responsibilities and assist their mothers in care giving and domestic tasks, even to the extent of giving up their hopes of continuing with their education.[22] Examples can also be found of parents, sons, daughters, siblings, aunts and other relations who were the sole support of disabled miners, and this serves to remind us of the variation in family and household composition in the past and the complexities of care giving and support for disabled miners.[23] Slightly differently, it was common for families with sick or disabled members to employ a 'girl' from the neighbourhood to assist with everyday domestic tasks, whether the wife of the miner was present in the household or not.[24]

Interestingly, the miners' union in south Wales used the experiences of miners' wives as care givers in their recruitment campaigns in the interwar period, and in their attempts in the 1930s and 1940s to convince their members of the importance of rehabilitation. This material communicates the considerable physical and emotional labour that faced women when a miner was carried home injured from the pit.[25] In an article published in the union magazine *The Miner* in 1946 a miner's wife wrote:

> With the means at my disposal, along with the kind assistance of neighbours, I nursed and cared for my husband for eleven months in ... crowded conditions. It was a hard and trying time as I had at this time five young children, the eldest of whom was nine years of age and the amount of compensation I received for this period was 24/- per week.

She noted how she was forced to do the work required in the garden that year because of her husband's incapacity and was again required to look after him, later on in life, in the eight years before he died, when he was confined to home due to pneumoconiosis.[26] Given the added demands placed on women by the injuries and illnesses of their male relations within a context of little external support, it is unsurprising that one study from the 1930s found that it was the wives rather than the miners who 'remembered occasions and details of illnesses and death minutely, no doubt on account of their close association with the sickness'.[27]

The caring or supporting role expected of men was markedly limited by gender. Men provided or were given money for their families, but were not, on the whole, expected to provide hands-on care. In some instances the lack of practical caring may have been due to competing duties in paid employment. Ramsay Guthrie's historical novel *Black Dyke* (1904), set in pre-union days, depicts a miner with an invalid wife who has been 'badly', 'On an' off this five yeers',[28] who cannot 'bide at home' with her, despite his desire to do so: 'His heart was sore in the thought of leaving his wife in her suffering. He was angered at the tyranny which compelled him to do so. A fine of half a crown was the penalty of absence unless a doctor's certificate of personal illness could be produced.'[29] Other examples of men depicted in care-giving roles can be found in literature, even while care continues to be considered 'women's work'. The paralysed miner in the Scottish novel *Black Earth* is mainly cared for by his wife, but a male collier friend visits to shave him – a specific caring task perhaps considered more suitable for a man because shaving is part of male grooming and associated with barbershop work.[30] Women are also depicted receiving care from male family members,[31] such as Ann, a miner's wife in Jack Jones's novel *Bidden to the Feast* and whose husband becomes one of her main carers after she suffers a paralysing stroke, as his daughter Megan comments: 'Dad'll look to mam. He'd rather, an' she's better with him than with [her daughter] Moriah –. or anybody for that matter.'[32]

Such emotional engagement with illness and care giving on the part of working-class men was perhaps more easily articulated through imaginative literature than in the macho world of mining communities, but recollections of the time nevertheless suggest that working-class men could transcend their traditional gender roles while away from the judgemental gaze of neighbours and friends, within the privacy of the home. Male care giving is described in Jones's autobiography, *Unfinished Journey*, when he helps with the care of his collier father, sick with pleurisy. Jones has been working his father's shift in the pit, but realises that, without relief, his mother will also become ill from strain and then 'it would be domino on all of us'.[33] Coalfields literature thus depicts a mixed picture of caring relationships between family members. Despite the presumption of female care, and the view that care is 'women's work', male family and friends may also contribute when the primary carer herself is incapacitated or overwhelmed.

Existing gender relations in mining communities clearly influenced this pattern of care giving: apart from the more general, widespread belief in the 'natural' abilities of women as carers, the low levels of economic participation by women in coalmining communities confined them to the home in greater numbers than those women in other urban or industrial contexts. But it is also clear that such care giving brought about new gender relations as the usual roles of men and women, particularly the former, changed. Disability within mining culture, with clearly prescribed gender roles, had profound consequences for men and their sense of themselves.

It is extremely difficult to get a clear sense of the psychological impact of disabling injury and impairment on men and their sense of masculinity in this particular context. Documentary evidence, is scarce since social relations in this context were unremarkable, everyday aspects of home life and did not, therefore, give much cause for comment or discussion, especially where they might have involved feelings of shame and inadequacy. In addition, large numbers of disabled workers, particularly those who suffered paralysis, would have suffered social isolation in the home as a result of their inability to join in the usual social activities of mining communities and the absence of any contact with other people. Nevertheless, careful scrutiny of a range of historical, autobiographical and literary sources can help to sketch some of the main aspects of the impact on masculinity and some sense of the social isolation experienced by many disabled people.

What we can infer from the historical sources and literary depictions is that the strength of the breadwinner model and ideals of masculinity in mining communities meant that physical impairment that prevented work and social interaction was disabling in social terms. Miners prided themselves on their physical strength, skill and capacity for hard work and these conferred status and prestige within the occupational and broader community. The loss of income and status contingent on disabling injury, on top of the impact on a man's ability to perform his role as head of the household and an active member of the community, would have had a considerable impact. In addition, impairment and a period of convalescence at home removed the man from his 'masculine' public sphere of work and, possibly, from community social life and confined him to the 'feminine' private sphere of home, though, as we shall see the separation between these spheres was not as binary as the division suggests. Nevertheless, a disabled worker's usual means of performing his masculinity were removed from him and he was he was left without the main aspects of his life by which he defined himself.

Durham miner-writer Harold Heslop's *The Earth Beneath* (1946) portrays the impact of permanent disability following a mining accident in the character of Butch, a typical 'big hewer' figure whose 'biceps almost burst his shirt sleeves at times'.[34] Butch is injured in a roof fall, fracturing both legs and his back; his left leg is permanently shortened and even with the aid of two sticks '[h]e hobbled painfully ... [w]henever he jarred his back the pain almost made him faint'.[35] Butch remarks to a fellow miner: 'It's rotten lying waiting for the bones to knit, George. And it's very painful, hinny. Ye're so helpless, if ye ken my meaning. ... I'm done, laddie ... A man knows when he's done, George.'[36] It is both the physical pain and his changed role in the family that causes him distress; he is 'done' and 'helpless' because he 'had been forced to lay aside the task of bread-winner'.[37] Heslop portrays Butch's response as typical for a miner:

> To the miners it was a tragedy that the power within the muscles of a comrade should be sapped and wasted before its time. A man never retired from labour in their sphere. He stepped from the mine into the grave, his work done. And the sexton covered up his shame. To be cut off as Butch Rowlands had been cut off was a gaping tragedy.[38]

In spite of the severity of this statement, Heslop describes how Butch and his wife get by, in part through the support of the community. They have a collection of money from the colliers to start with, occasional donations of a shilling, tobacco or a fish from their friend George, and Butch's wife also works harvesting fields, making mats and selling nettle beer. Butch is still active in the community through participation in chapel life.[39] He was a lay preacher before his injury; now, with physical support from George, he attends chapel weekly, passing comment on visiting preachers: 'for Butch, if he could not preach, could mount guard on God's word'.[40] So, although Butch is 'cut off' from performing the masculine role of 'bread-winner', though he cannot walk unaided and is prone to fainting (a condition gendered as feminine), Heslop's novel ensures that this 'gaping tragedy' is mitigated by the support of comrades such as George and a network of community support, particularly the chapel in this case.

In addition to the individual strains faced by miner and wife under the changed circumstances of a serious injury or impairment, the relationship between husband and wife inevitably evolved. Few historical sources address this emotional cost on miners' wives, but writers took up the issue in their work. In Joe Corrie's *Black Earth*, Jack's paralysing injury from a roof fall portrays the emotional strains of his disablement and its toll on his wife, Maggie:

> It seemed that he was terrified she should go out of his sight lest something should happen to him. He couldn't bear to have her out of his sight. ... Maggie had to do everything. Twice a week Tom Marshall came in to shave him. Even that obligement wasn't appreciated, for he hated the process. But Tom persisted. ... Jack was either silent or abusive. Tom knew only too well that Jack couldn't help it and would curse himself at times for thinking that he might show more patience and reasonableness lying there. But he saw how Maggie was breaking down under the strain. Day after day the same, never sitting down for a minute but he wanted something. It was more than any woman could stand. A pity that he hadn't been killed that day.[41]

This passage, including its shocking final thought, utilises many of the 'burden' and dependency tropes of disability in literature and culture. Yet its portrayal of frustration and anxiety from both the injured miner, family and friends in the weeks and months after a life-changing injury was, for many mining families, very real.

Disablement of the main breadwinner, whether temporary or permanent, also brought about a reconfiguration of social relations between fathers and their children. The contemporary definition of masculinity cast the man as a father with responsibilities to his children as much as a husband to his wife, and disability had consequences for this part of the man's identity and social relations also. In the first instance, disability, and particularly the reduced income brought about by its effects on earning capacity, led some families to limit family size and have fewer children, and this was especially the case during the interwar economic depression. More to the point here, existing children were often forced to start work earlier than they might have done otherwise, rather than continue in education, or else assist with the domestic tasks in the home.[42] Sons, especially, were expected to take on the responsibility as primary earner. In a 1973 interview the Welsh miner Dai Daniel Rees discussed the need to step up when his father 'failed' from pneumoconiosis: 'I was the eldest and I had to keep working. That is how I started a bit sooner like see.'[43] Similarly, John Paterson remembered having to leave school and start work at fourteen as his father's health failed as a result of pneumoconiosis in the Lanarkshire community of Benhar.[44] This entailed an immediate change in the financial responsibilities within the family and, depending on the particular personal relations, possibly the status and authority of the different individuals within the family.

The sense of duty and responsibility on the part of sons for their old, infirm or impaired parents was given official force by practices within state welfare policies, especially the Poor Law.[45] For example, the *Aberdare Times* reported in October 1894 on two brothers summoned to court 'to show cause why they should not maintain their father', who was described as '75 years of age and a cripple'. The brothers' own family situations were examined: one was a 50-year-old widower, the other had a more complicated scenario – 'when his wife was ill he wanted him [the father] to try and get a place with his sister Mary. John said he was willing to pay ... and wanted the old man to be kept in the Union.' The ruling found that both brothers should continue to pay for 'the old man'.[46] Poor Law officials in Scotland in the late nineteenth century bemoaned the lack of commitment to the welfare of parents on the part of some children and were keen to compel sons and daughters to acknowledge their responsibilities and contribute to the upkeep of their parents.[47]

In other instances, the disability of the male breadwinner meant that his children were not able to enter the world of employment and were required to assist in the home, and this was especially the case for daughters. A Poor Law Relieving Officer noted the case of a miner in Blaina, south Wales in 1926 who had been out of work since 1921 as a result of a fractured spine. He had a wife and three dependent children, and his sixteen-year-old daughter was 'unable to take up domestic service. Needed at home to assist to nurse her father.'[48] It seems unlikely that such a change in the relations between this man and his daughter transformed the authority that he held over her as her father, but subtle changes in their relationship, on an emotional as well as a practical level, would seem to be entirely likely. It was a common practice for daughters to leave school at age fourteen to help mothers with domestic tasks, and this would seem even more likely in the event of the impairment of the father in the family.[49] David Meek, a collier from Bothwellhaugh, Lanarkshire remembered how, when his mother developed multiple sclerosis, his fifteen-year-old sister would rise at five o'clock in the morning to prepare breakfast for his brothers and their father; the work became too much for her, since she was also responsible for looking after the younger children in the home, and he, his brothers and his father simply made their own breakfasts from that point onwards.[50] Significantly, though, the added burdens assumed by girls in these situations not only affected their position in the family but also had consequences for their own well-being and future pospects.

While some historians quite correctly emphasise the extent to which state welfare policies classified men as providers and women as dependents, and ensured that the traditional gender relations were upheld, it is nevertheless possible to discern some cases in mining communities where daughters became the primary supporters of their impaired parents. For instance, the records of the Bedwellty Poor Law Union during the 1926 miners' lockout frequently demonstrate the extent to which daughters were made financially responsible to make up for the loss of income brought about by the illnesses and impairments of their fathers. One head of a mining household in Abertillery, for example, was listed as having gastroptisis with an income of 'self', National Health Insurance, and '4 daughters working at the laundry earning 19/-'. Two sons were listed as unemployed.[51] This was an extreme case, in the particular circumstances of 1926 when any adult sons would have been out of work, but it reflects the necessity of children in mining families, including daughters, contributing to the household income in the event of impairment, or even being the main support for their fathers.

At the same time, it would be simplistic to argue that disability led to emasculation and the complete reordering of gender relations in the home. The period of convalescence did not constitute merely the absence of work and its replacement with the 'female' aspects of the domestic environment. Various adjustments were necessary that marked this out as an unusual period in the life of the family in which the usual gender norms did not, perhaps, operate. For example, working-class families adjusted their living arrangements to meet the impaired mobility of the injured miner, often through setting up a convalescent bed in the front parlour or 'living room' on the ground floor.[52] This reorganisation of the normal domestic arrangements marked this out as a period in which the usual norms did not apply, and so might have mitigated any emasculation to some degree.

Other aspects of the experiences of disabled and convalescent miners undermine any tendency to offer easy generalisations of emasculation. Some miners took up hobbies or interests that, on first sight, had traditionally feminine connotations, but adopted them on their own terms and according to a more complex sense of masculinity. Janet Chapman remembered that her father, who worked at the Kinneil Colliery in the Midlothian coalfield, took up baking 'and he wis a lovely baker, he wis. And he wis great. He wis gettin' on great tae he took ill and he wis moved tae the Deaconess.'[53] This is of course, only one example but it hints at a home life and identity beyond that of 'injured miner', via activities that traditionally did not fit stereotypes of masculinity.[54] Perhaps the best illustrative example of the complexity of experiences from the effects of disability on masculinity can be seen in the case of George Preece (Figure 4). He lost both his legs following an accident undergound at Abercynon in 1909 and went to live with his niece and her children, where he developed an interest in crocheting. One piece of Preece's crocheting work that has survived consists of an image of a battleship (Figure 5).[55]

Even in the absence of waged work or any interest in masculine hobbies and activities, it was still possible for wholly isolated disabled ex-miners to maintain some semblance of their masculine identity and their position as the source of the family's well-being. The continued performance of traditionally masculine duties by disabled miners, and its role in the avoidance of complete emasculation,

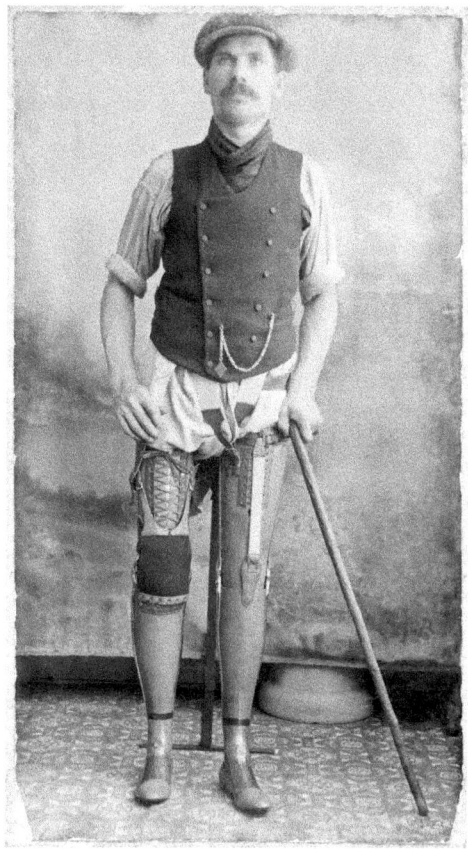

4 Disabled miner George Preece, c.1909

was made possible as a result of the welfare provision that a worker made before becoming impaired. Trade unions, friendly societies, medical schemes, commercial insurance companies and other self-help and mutualist agencies appealed to the masculine identities of workers and their responsibilities to their dependent wives and children. In a leaflet published in 1936, for example, the South Wales Miners' Federation listed some compensation cases that it had won on behalf of local miners and urged miners at Bedwas to support the union. It told them 'Let your Wife and other Dependents see how you are stripped of all protection by being outside the Federation. Let them see how you are cruelly risking all their interests, and robbing them of all help and guidance should anything happen to you. Their protection and yours is the Miners' Federation.'[56] In return

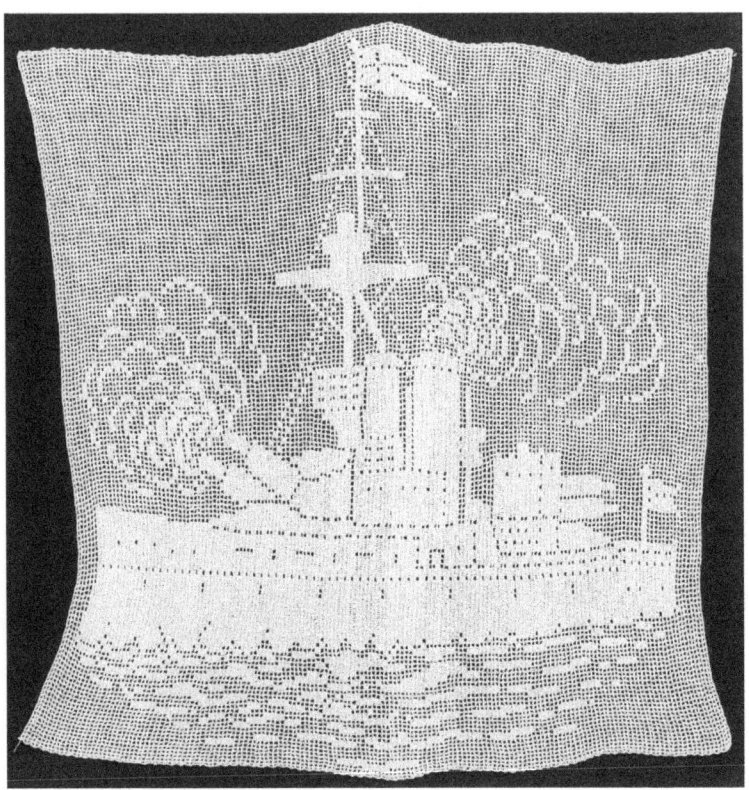

5 Crochet panel depicting a naval gunship made by George Preece during his re-habilitation after a mining accident at Abercynon Colliery in 1909

for membership of the union the miner would gain eligibility for union assistance to pursue compensation claims and for the support of his dependent family members; the friendly societies offered sickness benefits to assist the family during times of illness and incapacity. In these ways, through the payment of compensation or sickness benefits, an injured miner could feel that he was continuing to play the breadwinner's role even in the absence of waged work and was encouraged to think that he was doing his duty as a man.

This insistence on the male breadwinner model as the basis for gender relations, and its encouragement whatever the circumstances, was further strengthened in the cases of disabled miners who were still cast as providers with responsibilities for 'dependents', despite a reduced income as a result of their impairments. An 1887 court case in south Wales reported by *The Cambrian* newspaper demonstrates what happened when this contract was broken, when a disabled miner, 'a lame man', appeared in court 'for not complying with an order of 4s. per week made upon him towards the support of his wife'. The miner was ordered to pay £1 of the money owed to his wife within a fortnight or spend a month in prison.[57] Thus, just as the welfare and legal systems compelled children to take responsibility for their impaired fathers, they also ensured in other cases that disabled miners, where possible, continued to play their role as 'independent' men with responsibilities to dependents.

More than any other factor, however, it was perhaps the sheer power and customary character of male dominance that reduced the possibility of complete emasculation and ensured that the man's position as head of the household endured. Jim Bullock, a miner and later mine manager in west Yorkshire, remembered that his father finished work in 1903 at the age of fifty-three as a result of rheumatism, and that, while he now became dependent on adult sons who earned enough underground to support him and the rest of the family, he remained the 'king in his own home'.[58] This was surely replicated in a great many other cases: members of a miner's family were long accustomed to his authority and status as the head of the household, and neither impairment nor disability, whether temporary or permanent, was likely to erode these things completely.

Not all miners who became disabled were married, and not all disability in coalfields communities was the result of industrial accident. The consequences of disability on marriage prospects, particularly where young disabled people were not economically active, are not well documented, but it is likely that they faced difficulty in forming relationships. Few sources exist which address this directly, but the 1997 testimony of Janet Chapman offers some insight. Chapman was a 'pithead lassie' who lived with her father (born in 1893 and died in 1947), a despatch clerk described as 'hunchback' who worked at Kinneil Colliery in Scotland. An interview with Janet hints at the emotional bonds created by the family structures, and also the prejudice and hostility faced by disabled members of the community when they intended to marry:

> Mother wis Bo'ness wumin. Ma father wis in a wheelchair when ma mother met him. She married him when he wis in the wheelchair. That she did. Ah know that.
> [Interviewer: That took courage, that took courage, aye?]
> It did. It did, aye. That's why the folk used tae say tae her that she wis bein' stupid, you know ... And bein' honest, ma gran, Rintoul, ma father's mother, didnae want ma father tae get married tae ma mother. She didnae want him to get married at all because he wis ... wi' him bein' in the wheelchair and that, she jist did not want it to happen. But ma father wanted tae marry ma mother, and that wis it.[59]

Chapman's testimony hints at a desexualisation of miners and prejudicial barriers to their relationship and marital possibilities, but it is also evidence of at least some people being able to see beyond disability as 'disqualification'.[60]

Sexual and marital relations are explored in coalfields literature, most notably in depictions of miners who become paralysed as a result of a mining injury.[61] The changed relationship between husband and wife, Jack and Maggie, is a central focus of crisis in Scottish miner Joe Corrie's *Black Earth*. Jack worries that, without his ability to provide for Maggie, either as 'breadwinner' or as a marital partner, she will want to seek out a new sexual partner: 'she had no more use for him. Standing there, the healthy animal that she was, thinking, no doubt, that she should have another man. Ay, that's what was wrong with her, the greedy vixen.'[62] Jack's changed personality, being cold and angry towards his wife, is related to his feelings of fear and powerlessness: 'It wasn't people he hated so much as life, ay, that's what it was, and life to him meant the long days in that bed, and Maggie, full-breasted, in perfect health, for ever in his sight. And yet when he thought of death he would tear at the bedclothes in fear. He was a coward, yes, he was a coward.'[63] Jack feels taunted by the sight of his wife, particularly because he cannot be a sexual partner in the traditional phallocentric sense. A medicalised focus on male sexual function is highlighted by Tom Shakespeare as 'particularly oppressive and undermining of disabled men.'[64] Jack here focuses on the physical aspect of his marriage; as for Maggie, she is particularly hurt by losing his emotional support: 'never once had he asked how she was managing to carry on ... it was indifference to them all that hurt her.'[65] The qualities she misses are related as much to his personality as to his physical ability; she prays for him to return to 'the man who had no selfishness in him, the man who could laugh, the lover of the early days and the father of the latter days, the man who could take a drink, who could sing a song, who could look forward and see peace and happiness at the end of things.'[66] Disability has disrupted the marital relationship in both physical sexual and emotional terms; it is a crisis which has been gendered by the husband focusing more on their sexual relationship and the wife focusing more on their emotional relationship. Jack is not despicted as asexual; rather, his crisis stems from frustration that he cannot act on his continued feelings of sexual desire, and he feels that this brings his masculinity into question.

Thus disability had various, complex and conflicting consequences for a man's masculinity and his affective, sexual and social relations with members of his family (and his ability to form a new family), but it also altered the position of women and their relations in the home. Unsurprisingly, the assumption of care and emotional work by miners' wives had the potential to render women's own disabilities invisible. As Carr states, 'Although they were the linchpins of their families' survival, most of the women almost totally neglected their own health.'[67] A sense of sacrifice for the sake of the rest of the household was assumed here, with less rest, poor diets and rare doctor appointments creating ill health and disability. Thus, the physical and emotional labour involved in mining women's care for disabled family members exacerbated the strains that their bodies experienced and made their own chances of debilitating conditions or permanent disability that much more likely.[68] At times the strain was too much, and instances can be found of miners' wives petitioning the Poor Law authorities to admit their disabled husbands into the workhouse; one miner's wife at Easington, County Durham nursed her husband for two years after he fractured his spine but felt compelled to have him admitted to the workhouse after she was diagnosed with stomach cancer.[69]

The home was clearly a significant space for the production and reproduction of the social relations of disability – or, in Gleeson's terms, an important 'social space of disability' – but it also acted as an important liminal space. Providing as it did the space in which injured, impaired or sick miners convalesced, the home can be considered as a transitional space between impairment and able-bodiedness (or, at least, a space in which a worker transitioned to a state of reduced impairment) in addition to a threshold between the private world of family and the public world of neighbourhood. Indeed, such a conceptualisation of the home collapses the public–private binary and emphasises the interpenetration of these two spheres of everyday life.

The home as a liminal space: neighbours and community

As we have seen, mining communities' systems of welfare and support were not limited to the formal, organised societies, unions and clubs. Women provided a massive amount of unpaid care-giving and emotional labour in the home, but they did not do so alone or in isolation. Many historians of working-class life have emphasised the close relationships between neighbours within a locality and the interdependence that facilitated survival in the face of poverty and hardship.[70] Oral history accounts place emphasis on the everyday interactions with neighbours as a crucial form of support and care for disabled members of the community. This is seen in Bruley's oral history of women in the south Wales coalfield:

> If a misfortune occured, neighbours would close in, usually bringing cawl (broth) or Welsh cakes. They would take home washing, look after children and take turns to nurse the sick or injured. Oral history respondents were keen to tell me how strong the bonds of community were.[71]

Disability, then, is included as part of 'misfortune', with an unspoken but assumed bond between neighbours and friends to help when it occurred. The automatic division of nursing and care labour seen here shows how common it was, and how communities helped each other.

This was not specific to south Wales. Carr, in a discussion of neighbours in the north-east of England coalfield, noted the many different people involved in care for men's long-term sickness: along with 'panel' National Health Insurance doctors and district nurses, miners got 'support from relatives and neighbours as well as from the older women "healers" of the village'. Carr's concession, though, that 'mostly they [i.e. miners' wives] shouldered their responsibilities with a sturdy independence', hints at the limitations of neighbourly care.[72]

Even in the absence of active involvement of friends and neighbours in care giving, the social isolation of disabled workers in the home was broken down in other ways, and these again stress the interpenetration of home and neighbourhood, marking the house as a liminal social space of disability. The experiences of the Welsh writer Edward Young offer an instructive example of the interconnectedness of the 'private' sphere of the convalescent's sick-room, on the one hand, and the 'public' sphere of work, politics and community matters on the other, and the falsity of any hard and fast divide between the two. Young worked in the local tinplate industry in Pontardawe in the Swansea valley, south Wales before becoming a collier and, under his bardic name Eos Wyn, achieved some local fame as a poet from the 1860s onwards. Following a bout of smallpox in his early twenties, however, Eos Wyn gave up work in the colliery and was confined to his bed by complications that left him in considerable pain and dependent on laudanum for the rest of his life. Nevertheless, he continued to compete in eisteddfodau (cultural festivals) and to publish poems in local newspapers. More importantly, he started to author a regular column entitled 'Ystafell y Cystuddiedig' ('The Convalescent's Room') in a local newspaper until his death in 1892.[73] The authorship of this column, which focused on a range of issues including the state of local trade and industries, the struggles between Anglicanism and nonconformity, local and national politics, and other social and cultural issues, was itself an involvement in, and contribution to, the public sphere of ideas, discourse and discussion.

Not every convalescent miner could enter the public world through journalism or publication, of course, but Eos Wyn's column suggests another way in which the boundary between public and private worlds, male and female spheres, could be traversed or even made insignificant. Some of the earliest editions of his column were written in the form of a conversation between a convalescent patient and a group of acquaintances and former work colleagues upon their visit to see him in his sick-room. The conversations included discussion of his condition and his attitude towards his impairment, but also ranged widely over such topics as the international situation, school boards, chapel and church rivalries, political reform, the local fair and a range of other issues.[74] Eos Wyn would often comment in his column on the visits he received from well-wishers; in this way, through such visits to a convalescent acquaintance, the outside world of work, politics and other masculine issues was brought directly into the private sphere of the sick-room, which itself came to form a liminal space between the home and the broader, public community.

In addition, this intersection of public and private spheres was also achieved through more formal and communal visits to Eos Wyn's home. Local columnists, writing a form of local travel writing in which the literary personalities of any locality warranted a visit as much as any waterfall or mountain vista, urged other poets and litterateurs to call by Eos Wyn's home if they happened to be travelling through the area.[75] Similarly, his columns often noted the passers-by he encountered while sitting at his front door during spells of good weather.[76] More interestingly, a Sunday school treat at which 600 children and old people were provided a banquet of food in May 1872 ended with a procession that called at Eos Wyn's house and performed one of his compositions 'Y Gwanwyn' ('The Spring') outside his home and within his hearing.[77] A little later, in 1874, a procession of two local lodges of the Oddfellows stopped at his house and the accompanying brass band played a tune while he listened from his chair at the front door.[78] His brothers in the Oddfellows also bought him a carriage that could be pulled by a donkey, enabling him to leave his home and gain some mobility in the community. In these ways a prominent member of the community, best known for his literary and other cultural activities, was not isolated in his home by his disability and continued to be considered a valuable member of his community.

Such activities were not replicated in the cases of most disabled miners, but visiting sick or impaired friends and work colleagues must have been common in these close-knit communities. Indeed, the practice of moving a convalescent worker, and even sick parents, wives and children, downstairs helped to facilitate such interactions and counter some of the negative, isolating effects of impairment, and this comes through strongly in coalfields literature.[79] A young new pastor in a 1934 novel notices the difference between visiting 'the loving ones in the kitchen' (loving because they are welcoming to him as a guest) who are 'the sick and very aged, some seated or lying on the couch in the kitchen', and the experience of visiting those with 'senile decay, consumption, cancer, spinal trouble, all sorts of diseases, "upstairs out of the way"'.[80] To be 'upstairs out of the way' is isolating and implies that illness and disability is being hidden from the more public, downstairs areas of the home, where family (and often visitors or neighbours) come and go freely. In this way, to be downstairs was practical, but was also shown to serve an important secondary function in keeping the family member involved in day-to-day family life and facilitating visits from other individuals.

Furthermore, any injured or sick miner in receipt of sick pay from a friendly society was visited by one or more of his brothers in the society, partly as a means to guard against malingering but also as a practical manifestation of the fraternity that stood at the heart of these mutual organisations. Thus, impaired miners, whether temporarily or permanently confined to a sick-bed, were not necessarily isolated completely from their communities and continued to remain part of the social relations that characterised their occupational and community groups.

Nevertheless, care needs to be taken not to overstate this form of interaction or to under-estimate the considerable social isolation faced by many impaired miners. James Hanley noted the case of a miner paralysed in his work who had lain in his bed for eleven years, 'a permanent cripple, without any hope', 'shut off from all activities, intercourse and seeing the life about him', but he used this case as an explicit analogy of the south Wales economy in the interwar depression, and so the accurate portrayal of lived experience seems less of a priority here.[81] Willie McGill, a miner who worked at Sanquhar, Dumfriesshire, remembered that the pit was a dusty one and that a great many of the workers contracted pneumoconiosis. He noticed that as old men they were soon confined to the home after they finished work in the industry: 'See, whenever they retired, whenever they retired, ee maybe seen them for six month, and ee never seen them again, ken.'[82] Such perspectives would seem to coincide with Gleeson's characterisation of the home as a space that isolated disabled people, but other evidence presented here suggests that in working-class, mining communities the home could function as a liminal space in which friends, neighbours and members of the extended family visited, socialised and assisted impaired individuals.

The street: disability in interstitial spaces

Following a period of convalescence in the liminal space of the home, most impaired individuals, excluding paraplegics perhaps, were able to enter other spaces and come into contact with other individuals with whom they entered into social relations. In the first place, such impaired people entered what Brendan Gleeson has described as 'interstitial' spaces, such as the street, the informal economy and other places in the public sphere.[83] Indeed, for Gleeson, the street, at least in terms of industrial communities, is the space in which disabled people were most visible, in contrast to the home and institutions that isolated them from the community at large and confined them out of sight.[84]

The ubiquity and visibility of impairment in coalmining communities, of streets 'thronged with the maimed and the mutilated', is a striking feature of the writings of a number of observers, especially of those writers from outside these mining communities who observed the extent of impairment for the first time.[85] Touring south Wales in 1887, for example, two socialist missionaries noted the 'plentiful crop of cripples' whom they observed in Dowlais.[86] In a later period the Polish sociologist Ferdynand Zweig interviewed a miner for his 1948 study *Men in the Pits*, who told him: 'Can't you see for yourself the number of disabled men with amputated legs or arms or fingers, or even blind, or with twisted spines or necks, or otherwise laid on their backs?' For his part, Zweig agreed with this impression: 'Nowhere else can you see the same relative numbers of disabled men as in a colliery village.'[87]

Such comments clearly testify to the visbility of impairment in mining communities, but they also pose intriguing questions. Did such visibility and ubiquity lead to greater acceptance of disabled people in mining communities? Did their presence in such large numbers on the streets make impairment an unremarkable and everyday reality of life? Or did their impairment mark them as different in an ableist society and lead to isolation? One clue, perhaps, is offered by Ernst Dückershoff, a German miner who worked in a Northumbrian pit at the turn of the century. In his study of *How the English Workman Lives*, Dückershoff noted the presence of 'cripples' begging in the street because 'they [had] long since spent the money they received as compensation and can make no further claim'.[88] Dückershoff, writing with the more comprehensive social insurance system in Germany in mind, saw such begging as a failure of welfare provision in British mining communties, and it is possible, given the importance of respectability in working-class communities and the strength of the breadwinner model, that begging in this manner involved a significant degree of social marginalisation for disabled miners.

The 'cripples' whom Dückershoff witnessed begging in the street were not only located in an interstitial space, between the home and the institutions of the public sphere, but were also located in the interstices of the economy, forced to resort to begging to obtain some sort of income. Another example of such a combination are the disabled ballad singers who performed in the street to earn an income, many of them in coalfield districts and some of them former miners.[89] Ballad culture was strongest in pre-literate communities, before the advent of mass education and mass communications, but could still be observed in late nineteenth- and early twentieth-century Britain. Ballad singers would sing their songs or sell their ballad sheets on the street corner, in the market or at local fairs in order to raise money, often for themselves but also for other causes in the community such as other disabled individuals, the widows and 'orphans' of colliery disasters, or striking miners. Some of the most famous ballad singers in nineteenth-century Wales used bardic names that testified to their impairments (Richard Williams was Dic Dywyll (Blind Dick), Levi Gibbon was Y Dryw Dall (The Blind Wren) and Lewys y Goes Bren (Lewis with the Wooden Leg)), which were a major factor in their entry into ballad singing. Similarly, in the north-east of England, Tommy Armstrong, the 'Pitman's Poet', gained fame and a modest income from his songs after giving up work in the pit as a result of the impairments caused by childhood rickets and a serious accident underground.[90]

More intriguingly, some ballads gave first-hand accounts of the experiences of these disabled singers and might be considered the type of 'vernacular' and 'experiential' – as opposed to 'institutional' – sources that Elizabeth Bredburg praised as essential to disability history.[91] Not only do they testify to the precarious financial position of disabled people in the period, but they also comment to some degree on the social relations that existed between impaired ballad singers and others in the community. In 'Mwnwr Tlawd' ('Poor Miner') for example, the singer recounts his experience underground when a fall damaged his spine, while in 'Cwyn y Cloff' ('The Lame Man's Lament') the balladeer explains how he migrated from rural west Wales to work in the mines of Glamorgan but lost his leg to an accident.[92] The financial imperatives that drove these 'singers of the penny songs' onto the roads were highlighted in the ballads.[93] William Bowen, a ballad-singer who lost his sight after an accident in Penycae, Ebbw Vale, sang:

Gwraig a phlant a ymddibyna	A wife and children depend on me
Am eu bara yn ddiball,	For their bread without fail,
Ac edrychant am gynhaliaeth	And look for sustenance
Trwy ymdrechion cantwr dall;	Through the efforts of a blind singer;
Myned i bob ffair a marchnad,	Going to every fair and market,
Teithio'r hollwlad raid yn siwr,	Travelling the whole country surely,
Dyma dynged William Bowen,	This is the fate of William Bowen
O! tosturiwch wrth y gwr.	O! Pity the man.[94]

Thus the ballad singer occupied an interstitial space – the street – in an interstitial part of the economy (i.e. informal, insecure, low paid), and it might also be argued, following Rosemary Garland Thomson, that ballads were perhaps more than a mere niche in the economy and means of subsistence, and can be conceived as a means to handle disability and negotiate interactions and social relations with non-disabled people. She argues that in their encounters with non-disabled people individuals with impairments must learn to manage relationships from the beginning and 'use charm, intimidation, ardour, deference, humour, or entertainment to relieve nondisabled people of their discomfort'. 'Those of us with disabilities are supplicants and minstrels,' she argues, 'striving to create valued representations of ourselves in our relations with the nondisabled majority.'[95] If successful, these strategies neutralise the stigma of disability and create the context in which more meaningful relationships can be formed between disabled and non-disabled people, and the personhood of disabled individuals is allowed to develop more fully.[96]

While impaired miners were visible on the streets of mining communities, they could also be seen in other interstitial spaces. Many writers on working-class life in the late nineteenth and early twentieth centuries have commented on the close proximity of housing in working-class districts and the resultant lack of privacy. Campbell, for example, notes how the 'physical constraints of household space ... fostered a communal street culture in the areas immediately surrounding houses'.[97] This is most evident in mining communities, and especially in the case of terraced housing with little available space around the house, in the practice of inhabitants of the houses sitting out on the front door-step or the pavement on a stool when the weather allowed. And this was exactly the practice of injured and sick miners during the late nineteenth and early twentieth centuries, where they were able to greet passing neighbours and friends, engage in conversations and renew their relations with members of the community. In the novel *The Back-to-Backs*, the author describes a sunny day in the community of Haggar, where elderly people and men impaired by their work in the colliery are brought out of their homes to enjoy the good weather. 'Every form of mutilation was exhibited on the pavement,' Grant wrote. 'Every cottage seemed to have at least one hopelessly mutilated inhabitant.'[98] In a not dissimilar situation, the social function of this practice in the creation of affective ties in the community was emphasised in Bert Coombes' account of a Whit Sunday procession of the chapels in his community in the Neath valley in south Wales. Coombes wrote that it was not so much a procession as a 'saunter', since older and infirm members of the community took their place in the ranks of the marchers. More than that:

> the many cripples, or the helplessly old who manage in some way to get to the front doors, must have their greetings, too. No old friend must be passed, and by the time an old man has forsaken the lead to totter across and shake hands with some old crippled friend, and returned to his place for the walk to be resumed, quite a time has passed.[99]

Some such men, including Gwilym, a pneumoconiotic miner, Coombes noted, were not able to get to leave their beds and watch the passing procession. Nevertheless, the front door-step, and the pavement immediately beyond it, was an interstitial space occasionally inhabited by impaired miners, and one in which social relations could be made and renewed.

Other spaces in the community became important locations for disabled miners to congregate and, interestingly perhaps, form some sort of community among themselves. The pneumoconiosis catastrophe of the 1930s and 1940s in south Wales focused attention on the sufferers of this particular occupational disease and their everyday lives and social position in mining communities. In her study of pneumoconiotic miners in south Wales in the early 1930s, Enid Williams commented on the old and infirm miners who gathered in Aberdare public park each day: 'Anyone would notice that the majority of these men had aged before their time and that they were very short of breath and frequently coughed.'[100] Similarly, the miner-writer Bert Coombes wrote that 'Practically every fine day I see a group of about a dozen men around the war memorial in the village near here. To use a local phrase which applies to them "their chests have gone."'[101] At Ammanford, another community in the anthracite district, 'silicosis' was said to be claiming 'victim after victim'; 'frequently sufferers are to be seen in the streets of the town gasping for breath', it was reported.[102]

Such instances confirm Gleeson's observation of physically impaired individuals in the industrial city that 'their frequently-restricted ambulance conditioned a different type of participation in streetlife, usually the fixed occuaption of a key node, such as a street corner'. Gleeson was referring to physically disabled people with limb, spine or nervous system impairments, but the point is also true of these pneumoconiotic miners whose impaired lung capacity made walking through these spaces difficult.[103] The observations by Williams and Coombes perhaps also suggest some sort of comradeship of disability among impaired former miners, an identity of interest perhaps and co-dependency, but they also emphasise the altered reality for these men who found themselves denied their former roles as workers and were now required to exist in an interstitial limbo between the spheres of work and home. However much sympathy and practical support their former work colleagues offered to disabled miners no longer able to work, their apartness was emphasised on a daily basis and it is no surpise that one of these victims of pneumoconiosis described himself and others who suffered the disease as the 'forgotten men' of the coalfields, the 'living dead of the mining industry', 'sentenced to a hopeless, destitute and empty future'.[104] Ferdynand Zweig similarly suggested some sense of this social isolation when he described sufferers of pneumoconiosis as 'a great number of men walking idly with grim, sullen faces and with a genuine grievance' through mining communities.[105] The rhetorical aspects of these sources colour the portrayals here, but there is a strong sense in which impairment and disability were clearly and visibly marked.

Public spaces: leisure and religion

Apart from these interstitial spaces, mining communities were characterised by a range of particular public institutions, in addition to locations for the pursuit and consumption of leisure, that helped to create a sense of community. These institutions were just as crucial to the production and reproduction of social relations as the home and the workplace, and disabled miners found themselves enmeshed in a complex network of relations here too. Similar to the home and the workplace, these spaces were heavily gendered and were constructed according to clear and powerful ideas about the norms that should govern the daily lives of men and women.

In his study of the 'Little Moscows' of interwar Britain, Stuart Macintyre set out the most important social spaces of men in Maerdy in the Rhondda Fach valley and Lumphinnans in the Fife coalfield, and noted the pub, the cinema, the football match, the institute and the library as the main locations of male sociability and community formation. In contrast, the women of mining communities had fewer opportunities for social interaction, but shopping, the cinema and religion offered some scope for female sociability, even if such activities 'lacked the rich diversity, systematic character and purpose of intercourse among working men'. Macintyre also notes that the physical configuration and proximity of houses in the Maerdy terraces and the Lumphinnans rows encouraged female interaction, while the communal laundries and the 'greens' where washing was dried frequently brought women together in Lumphinnan's case.[106] Similarly gendered spaces for men and women were observed in the north-east of England by Ernst Dückershoff.[107]

Such spaces changed over time and, in many cases, became more numerous as social facilities in mining communities were developed. Whether funded by employer paternalism, middle-class philanthropy or the miners' own efforts, the numbers of institutes, halls, cinemas and sporting spaces increased in the first half of the twentieth century and provided more opportunities for social interaction, though to a greater degree for men than women.[108] This increase in community facilities was further encouraged by the formation of the Miners' Welfare Fund. The Mining Industry Act of 1920 introduced a tax of 1d. on each ton of coal raised in Britain for the accumulation of a fund to invest in miners' welfare through medical, educational and lesiure facilities; the building or maintenance of miners' institutes and sporting facilities was one of the most popular forms of provision made by the Fund, providing recreation and education to miners and their families.[109]

And yet the accessibility of these spaces to disabled people is uncertain. Those with mobility needs would have faced trouble getting into these new leisure spaces. As one disabled miner commented, 'a man's life is not confined to his work. He has a social life, and the consequence of an accident like the loss of a leg or an arm or an eye, was with him, when he was trying to enjoy some social life and domestic life, and not simply that he couldn't work. We're not simply cogs in a wheel.'[110] This was certainly the experience of Will Devereux, a pneumoconiotic miner from Glynneath in the Neath Valley. Such was his impairment that he was unable to walk the short distance from his home to the Miners' Welfare Hall, the 'centre of village life', unless he received some help to get there. 'So there is little he can do', it was commented, 'but sit at home, while his wife goes out to factory work.'[111]

In some instances, former work colleagues and other members of the community were important in breaking down the social isolation of former miners with impairments who might otherwise have had little opportunity to pursue their former leisure interests. Dick Cook, a blind miner, remembered the impact of his disability on his social life and the reaction of his friends:

> If I wasn't seeing I was listening and that is the biggest thing I think of is loneliness when you are blind or deaf, things like that, loneliness. You can be lonely in a crowd unless you are spoken to, you can be in big crowds[.] I was many times and I remember your Dad used to take me to rugger matches ... [Y]our Dad [the interviewer's father] used to always put his arm under mine and tell me what was going on.[112]

Cook's interview shows the importance of relationshps within the community and with colleagues in gaining access to otherwise impossible spaces.

Physical access to these public spaces was an important means by which disabled miners came together, but it was also important as a means to access the support that the neighbourhood might extend to them in their poverty. Bert Coombes offers an instructive insight into the importance of the public house in this context of communal solidarity. After noticing a gravely ill friend sitting in the corner, Coombes learns that he has come to the pub to sell tickets to raffle his gramophone to raise money for his family in order to make ends meet. Coombes and his mate immediately buy more tickets than they can comfortably afford and another group of miners buy tickets without hesitation, while, interestingly, two railwaymen are initially reluctant before eventually agreeing to do so. Coombes commented: 'you will never see a miner refuse help to another who is sick or injured, for it may be his own turn next; but the others who make up the mining communities may live with them for years and yet not take any interest in the problems of those who create the industry on which they live.'[113]

Apart from the means by which to access the communitarian spirit within mining communities, public houses also form a place of leisure. In the fiction of the coalfields, the pub and social club are shown as accessible, and regularly frequented by people with a range of disabilities (though not severe mobility impairments). Jack Jones's *Black Parade* (1935), a novel which depicts the fortunes of a Merthyr mining family from the 1880s to the early 1930s, portrays the various ways in which families could support disabled members, socially as well as materially. This is most frequently through the agency of the central character and mother, Saran, but male bonding around alcohol and the pub is also important. Ossie, a man blinded during the Great War, goes out drinking with his father- and brother-in-law, his 'hand on [Sam's] right shoulder'. He is carrying a half-crown given to him by another disabled man, his brother-in-law, Lewis, who has turned bookie after having a hip shattered in the war who is also planning 'to go out for the night and part of next morning.'[114] The pub is presented as an exclusively male space in this and other novels (when a young Saran enters a public house to find Glyn when the two are courting, he is mortified).

The male spaces of working-men's clubs offer another leisure space for men. 'What is a social club for but to sit about with your friends and talk?' asks the narrator of Rhys Davies's *Jubilee Blues* (1938).[115] The aged and disabled are part of this social world – in person and as a topic of conversation. Significantly, the discussion of impairment is bound up with both industrial action and another typically male interest, sport. The 'older club members' sit talking 'of the old days' of 'strikes … and limb-losses'. Among them is 'Ieuan Mold, ex-boxer, ex-collier, ex-married-man, ex-fighter in agitations of long ago, and saviour of two lives in a pit flood, whose battered face no one liked to look on for long in daylight, so misshapen it was.'[116] In one embodied figure is inscribed the cultural and 'misshapen' industrial history of the region. Ieuan's sporting days are behind him by the time he sits among the old men reminiscing, but disability did not automatically preclude men from engaging in the less formal forms of 'sport' which took place – at least not in the world of coalfields novels. The unregulated outdoor boxing matches depicted in *Black Parade* spill over into street fighting in which Harry, the former bare-fist boxing champion, continues to 'compete', despite having had a leg amputated after a mine accident: 'fighting with his back 'gainst the wall and his peg drove into the ground.'[117]

While sport and leisure were important areas of male sociability that might or might not be accessed, depending on the severity of impairment and the quality of relations with others in the community, perhaps the most important community space for many inhabitants of mining communities was the church or chapel. The three regions were distinctive in their religious traditions. Broadly, the dominant institutions were the Presbyterian Church in Scotland, Primitive Methodism in the colliery districts of the north-east of England and Calvinistic Methodism and a handful of other nonconformist denominations, including the Congregationalists, in south Wales, where the chapels were often at the heart of Welsh-speaking communities. In all three regions Catholicism was regarded with some suspicion as connected with the poverty and purportedly lax morality of Irish immigrants.[118]

In the north-east of England, Robert Colls has argued: 'the heroic relationship of Methodism and Mining in the industrial revolution, a legend even today [1977], was a cliché by 1907'.[119] Coalfields novels, many of them written by ministers and published by religious presses, contributed to this picture. A prominent feature of many of the late nineteenth- to early twentieth-century novels is the role of mining accidents in religious conversion. The routine accidents of the pit, rather than the major disasters, are a way of calling a man's attention to his bodily frailty. The spiritual salvation which results makes injury and even permanent disability welcome. *The Black Diamond* (1880), by Hugh Gilmore, portrays the conversion of the wild Ralph Lowton following a serious crush injury which renders him a temporary 'invalid' and puts him on the path to spiritual and social betterment.[120] One pious collier remarks: 'Who knoweth but this young man may have to say like the psalmist, "It was a good thing for me that I was afflicted?"[121] Amen. May the Lord use his bodily affliction to the recovery of his soul.'[122] It is a sentiment repeated in Harry Lindsay's *Rhoda Roberts* (1895) when a miner claims, 'what we sometimes call accidents are merciful dispensations of an All-wise Providence'.[123] This view is immediately contested, as another miner takes issue with the idea that mass death and injury is the will of God. Thus, while physical injury may be connected to *individual* salvation, large-scale disaster should not be seen as divine punishment of a community.[124] In general, injury or disability leading to religious conversion focuses on the individual, an emphasis which is rooted in Methodist interest in personal revelation: 'some sort of personal experience of salvation was, at the beginning of the period [1870–1926], almost an essential requirement for becoming a Methodist'.[125]

Although religion was on the wane in the twentieth century, it remained a significant community presence. Despite the prominence of religion in coalfields literature, however, there are few historical records which shed light on the particular relationship of chapels and churches to disabled people or the experience of disabled members of different congregations in the Sunday service or in other social activities arranged by and within places of worship. The very architecture of places of worship could of course exclude people with impaired mobility, as Nancy Eiesland points out in *The Disabled God*, noting her own experience of being denied eucharist as a consequence.[126] Nevertheless, some church community support groups, such as the St James United Reformed Church Newcastle Women's Guild, founded in 1930 to provide services, including taking patients to and from hospitals and visiting people in their homes, certainly demonstrated a concern for the well-being of disabled people and offered different forms of support.[127] Ernst Dückershoff was impressed by the activities of chapels and churches in mining communities in the north-east of England on behalf of families in need.[128] Such welfare activities on behalf of injured and sick miners and their families indicate perhaps some measure of concern and engagement that might have lessened any feelings of social isolation, but arguably also made disabled people the objects of charity, with all that that implied.[129]

By the interwar period, with a predominance of literary texts written by working-class authors with strong political convictions, disability becomes part of the emerging struggle between socialism and nonconformity. The chapel tends to be seen no longer as a radical friend of the labouring poor and working classes, but as a place that excludes the poor (who are dirty and ragged and therefore not godly) and, in some cases, disabled people.[130] Ellis Lloyd's *Scarlet Nest* (1919) includes a disabled collier boy, Dafydd, who has been severely burned, paralysed and brain damaged in a colliery explosion. The socialist Owen John, a fellow collier, helps Dafydd by paying for him to go on all the 'treats' put on by chapels. But this is strongly resisted by the inflexible deacon Hezekiah. Thus Owen John, the supposed atheist, embodies Christian love and fellowship by supporting Dafydd out of a sense of solidarity, while the chapels are exposed as self-serving 'strongholds of the modern Pharisees and the Capitalists'.[131]

Following the 1926 General Strike, tensions only increased as the oppositional stance of the established Presbyterian church in Scotland and some nonconformist denominations meant many miners 'ever after regarded the mainstream Christian churches as agents of capital'.[132] This divide between chapel and worker is a recurring theme, often involving disability. In 'The Benefit Concert' (1946), as mentioned in Chapter 2, Rhys Davies subverts the tradition of chapel-led charity. The concert of the title is to provide funds for a prosthetic leg for a miner, Jenkin. The money raised is significantly in excess of that required for the leg (given as £100, of which £1 was spent on the leg), and Jenkin wants to use the extra to set up a tobacco shop, thus securing an independent livelihood. Rather than support the disabled man, the chapel deacons (described as 'business men') announce 'on the glory of Horeb the extra money will be spent'.[133] The material prosperity of the chapels, set against the abject poverty of the colliery districts during the Depression, was also the focus of scathing attack by the satirist Gwyn Thomas, who regularly used disability and black humour to ram home his point. His novel *Sorrow for Thy Sons* (c.1936) includes diatribes against the grasping materialism of the chapel which directly leads to disablement.[134] One member, Charlie, has been starving his children in favour of paying handsomely for chapel membership, to the despair of political activist Howells:

> Rickets, Charlie, it's rickets. It hasn't got anything to do with heaven or hell, sin or goodness, except that those people who allow kids to develop rickets are committing a sin for which the punishment should be some form of hell on earth. Rickets come from lack of food. Your kids lack food more than they ought to, because you go handing three or four bob a week over to the Apostolic pastor, so that he can eat enough on earth to avoid rickets in the life after, or that somebody can decorate the walls of that tin shanty you call your church with some new season blooms.[135]

This tirade calls out the hypocrisy of expecting the wages of the working classes to fund bourgeois frivolities such as 'new season blooms', and to enable a relatively luxurious lifestyle for the middle-class pastor, humorously suggesting that he can overeat to the extent that he is well nourished in the afterlife. As well as attacking the sanctimonious ideology that welcomes suffering as mortification of the spirit – roundly condemned in much coalfields literature – the novel draws the reader's attention to the wider casualties of industrial society in this period of mass unemployment. The people marked, or disqualified, by 'diseases' of poverty are excluded from the dogmatic and hypocritical values of certain strains of chapel religion that ascribe moral value to a clean, healthy, middle-class appearance. As a consequence, 'God's image will become more and more the exclusive property of the middle and upper classes ... the unemployed masses [will] see that godliness is only another form of that joblessness which is denied them.'[136] In writers such as Thomas we can see challenges to the stigmatising, exclusionary and disempowering narratives and structures found in some aspects of religious culture, discussed further in Chapter 6. Thomas is drawing on an alternative moral view based on socialism, challenging the Christian alignment of bodily perfection and moral purity for disenfranchising the working classes, whose bodies were made imperfect by working conditions, unemployment or deprivation. While the limited historical sources suggest that organised religion did try to provide some charity directly targeted at disabled members, many working-class coalfields writers cast doubt on the social role of chapels within a capitalist system and on the workings of charity itself.

While sources exist to suggest the ways in which impaired men accessed and experienced social and community spaces, it is far more difficult to ascertain the experiences of disabled women. Few sources suggest how women experienced these spaces, but, at the same time, women had little access to public houses, sporting venues or other spaces in the community. Bill Williamson, writing about the Northumberland pit community of Throckley in the early twentieth century emphasises the narrowness of women's lives and the extent to which they were focused on the domestic tasks of the home. Such was the time-consuming and arduous nature of those tasks that a woman had little time for leisure outside or far beyond the confines of the home and, instead, faced a 'kind of imprisonment, a grinding necessity' in which 'her work and her leisure were fused'.[137] This left the immediate neighbourhood as the place in which women's social lives were lived and experienced in mining communities, and Williamson emphasises the importance of the social networks that were built and maintained in these spaces:

> Maintaining the links of neighbourliness and friendship was a central theme in her working life, part of the business being a pitman's wife. Thinking about these things, being concerned about them was another essential part of being a house-wife; without those contacts her life would have been considerably impoverished and insecure.[138]

Valerie Gordon Hall notes the increase in leisure opportunities for young women in mining communities in the interwar period, and the importance of the church and chapel for women's social lives, but sources offering any perspective on the experience of disability in such contexts are lacking.[139] This is, in itself, indicative of the invisibility of female impairment in mining communities.

Conclusion

It is no easy task to study the social relations of disabled miners. They were made and remade in the numerous mundane, quotidian encounters in face-to-face situations that nobody would have thought to record at the time. Only through autobiographical accounts such as oral history interviews or through portrayals of mining communities, whether by insiders such as Bert Coombes or outsiders such as Ernst Dückershoff or Ferdynand Zweig, can we piece together something of these relations. More importantly, such social relations were extremely complex, dependent on so many different factors and intersections, and dependent on personal dynamics, so that relations between different individuals were all unique in their own particular ways. Significantly, however, a greater challenge is posed by the fact that it was interactions in the past that generated comment or some trace in the sources, whereas the absence of such contact has failed to leave any mark: social isolation leaves only silences in the sources.

Nevertheless, even in the face of imperfect source material, it is possible to glimpse the social relations into which disabled people in coalfield communities entered. As individuals, they sat at the heart of a complex web of social relations that reached from the home into the neighbourhood, and beyond into the wider community. Disabled people in mining regions faced undoubted social isolation, but it was not as complete in this particular context as some works on disability studies have insisted, nor did they necessarily suffer the totality of 'socio-spatial exclusion' that Gleeson discerns in other contexts.[140] Gleeson might have discerned the 'disabling city' in nineteenth-century Manchester and Melbourne, but, with this more empirical approach to mining communities, it is more difficult to discern 'disabling coalfields' to quite the same degree, and the complexities and varieties of disabled people's experiences need to be recognised.[141]

Notes

1 On the 'spatial turn', see Fiona Williamson, 'The Spatial Turn of Social and Cultural History: A Review of the Current Field', *European History Quarterly*, 44:4 (2014), pp. 703–17; Ralph Kingston, 'Mind Over Matter? History and the Spatial Turn', *Cultural and Social History*, 7:1 (2010), pp. 111–21; Leif Jerram, 'Space: A Useless Category for Historical Analysis?', *History and Theory*, 52:3 (2013), pp. 400–19.
2 Brendan Gleeson, 'Domestic Space and Disability in Nineteenth-Century Melbourne, Australia', *Journal of Historical Geography*, 27:2 (2001), pp. 223–40; see also his 'Recovering a "Subjugated History": Disability and the Institution in the Industrial City', *Australian Geographical Studies*, 37:2 (1999), pp. 114–29.
3 B. J. Gleeson, *Geographies of Disability* (London: Routledge, 2002), p. 27.
4 Jerram, 'Space: A Useless Category', p. 402.
5 For some examples of work that considers the home as integral to the creation of social relations in mining communities, see Valerie G. Hall, *Women at Work, 1860–1939: How Different Industries Shaped Women's Experiences* (Woodbridge: Boydell Press, 2013); Alan Campbell, *The Scottish Miners, 1874–1939. Volume One: Industry, Work and Community* (Aldershot: Ashgate, 1999).
6 Jenny Morris, *Pride against Prejudice: Transforming Attitudes to Disability: A Personal Politics of Disability*, reprint edition (London: The Women's Press Ltd, 1991), p. 10.
7 For two examples, see Kim Q. Hall (ed.), *Feminist Disability Studies* (Bloomington: Indiana University Press, 2011); Alison Piepmeier, Amber Cantrell and Ashley Maggio, 'Disability Is a Feminist Issue: Bringing Together Women's and Gender Studies and Disability Studies', *Disability Studies Quarterly*, 34:2 (2014), http://dsq-sds.org/article/view/4252, accessed 5 August 2016.
8 Tom Shakespeare, 'The Sexual Politics of Disabled Masculinity', *Sexuality and Disability*, 17:1 (1999), p. 55.
9 For an early example, see John Benson, *British Coalminers in the Nineteenth Century: A Social History* (Dublin: Gill and Macmillan, 1980). Also important is M. J.

Daunton, 'Miners' Houses: South Wales and the Great Northern Coalfield, 1880-1914', *International Review of Social History*, 25:2 (1980), pp. 143-75.
10 Griselda Carr, *Pit Women: Coal Communities in Northern England in the Early Twentieth Century* (London: Merlin, 2001), p. 69.
11 Campbell, *The Scottish Miners, 1874-1939. Volume One*, pp. 217-18.
12 Benson, *British Coalminers in the Nineteenth Century*, pp. 95-8.
13 Campbell, *The Scottish Miners, 1874-1939. Volume One*, pp. 219-20.
14 Daunton, 'Miners' Houses', p. 171.
15 Campbell, *The Scottish Miners, 1874-1939. Volume One*, p. 216.
16 Carr, *Pit Women*, pp. 65-6. Bert Coombes noted the sufferers of pneumoconiosis who were required to spend their nights sitting up in a chair to sleep because they would not be able to catch their breath lying down; B. L. Coombes, *Those Clouded Hills* (London: Cobbett Publishing Co. Ltd., 1944), p. 56.
17 Mass Observation Archive, SxMOA1/2/64/1/B/1, Typescript of report on Blaina and Nantyglo, October 1942.
18 Carol White and Sian Rhiannon Williams (eds), *Struggle or Starve: Women's Lives in the South Wales Valleys between the Two World Wars* (Dinas Powys: Honno, 1998), p. 10.
19 Carr, *Pit Women*, p. 68.
20 Carr, *Pit Women*, p. 71.
21 South Wales Miners' Library, Swansea University (hereafter SWML), AUD/164, John Morgan Evans oral history interview.
22 Gwent Archives, CSWBGB/C/32, Bedwellty Union Out Relief Advisory Committee Papers, 29 December 1926; see also, White and Williams, *Struggle or Starve*, pp. 161-74.
23 For examples, see Mitchell Library, Glasgow City Archives (hereafter ML), CO1 27 95, Applications for Poor Relief, Carluke, 1898-1902.
24 West Glamorgan Archives Service (hereafter WGAS), D/D SHF, Swansea Hospital Ladies' Samaritan Fund Minutes, 12 February 1926; 9 November 1928.
25 For a literary study on the topic of care work, disability and mining wives see Alexandra Jones, '"Her Body [was] Like a Hard-Worked Machine": Women's Work and Disability in Coalfields Literature, 1880-1950', *Disability Studies Quarterly*, 37:4 (2017).
26 *The Miner*, August 1946, pp. 6-7.
27 Enid M. Williams, *The Health of Old and Retired Miners in South Wales* (Cardiff: University of Wales Press Board, 1933), p. 22. See also the discussion of miners' health and care in relation to marches in Chapter 6.
28 Ramsay Guthrie, *Black Dyke* (London: Charles H. Kelly, 1904), p. 29.
29 Guthrie, *Black Dyke*, pp. 5-6.
30 Similarly, the paralysed miner in J. C. Grant's novel *The Back-to-Backs* (London: Chatto and Windus, 1930) receives care from both his sister and a male family friend.

31 See also Gwyn Jones's *Times Like These* (London: Victor Gollancz, 1979 [1936]), where Olive receives care from her unemployed collier husband.
32 Jack Jones, *Bidden to the Feast* (London: Corgi Books, 1968 [1938]), pp. 76–7.
33 Jack Jones, *Unfinished Journey* (London: Hamish Hamilton, 1938), p. 96.
34 Harold Heslop, *The Earth Beneath* (London: T. V. Boardman and Company Ltd., 1946), p. 83.
35 Heslop, *The Earth Beneath*, p. 290.
36 Heslop, *The Earth Beneath*, p. 290.
37 Heslop, *The Earth Beneath*, p. 291.
38 Heslop, *The Earth Beneath*, pp. 290–1.
39 Harold Heslop's father was a Methodist preacher; Methodism is treated in this novel as part of the history of political activism among the miners and a vital aspect of the formation of the first trade unions. Butch, for example, is an agitator for the Union as well as a lay preacher. On the topic of Methodism and politics in the Durham mining community, see Robert Moore, *Pit-men, Preachers and Politics: The Effects of Methodism in a Durham Mining Community* (Cambridge: Cambridge University Press, 1974.)
40 Heslop, *The Earth Beneath*, p. 292.
41 Joe Corrie, *Black Earth* (London: Routledge, 1939), p. 227.
42 E. L. Collis and Major Greenwood, *The Health of the Industrial Worker* (London: Churchill, 1921), p. 409.
43 SWML, AUD/238, Dai Daniel Rees interview.
44 Scottish Oral History Centre (hereafter SOHC), John Paterson interview, 1998. It is with such experiences in mind that some miners could characterise sons as 'capital for your old age'; too many daughters, on the other hand, was considered by some as 'the dark tragedy of the mining family'; Jim Bullock, *Bowers Row: Recollections of a Mining Village* (Wakefield: E. P. Publishing, 1976), pp. 65, 77.
45 Marjorie Levine Clark, 'The Gendered Economy of Family Liability: Intergenerational Relationships and Poor Law Relief in England's Black Country, 1871–1911', *Journal of British Studies*, 45:1 (2006), pp. 72–89; Clark discerns a more widespread use of the 'liable relatives clause' from the 1870s onwards as part of the 'crusade' against out-relief (p. 78).
46 *The Aberdare Times*, 13 October 1894.
47 For example, see *Thirty-Fifth Annual Report of the Board of Supervision for the Relief of the Poor and of Public Health of Scotland, 1879–80*, c. 2661, 1880, xxviii, 'Report by General Superintendant of the Poor, Southern (Highland) District, for the Half-Year ended 31st March 1880', p. 8.
48 Gwent Archives, Bedwellty Union Out Relief Advisory Committee papers, 18/20 October 1926.
49 Stuart Macintyre, *Little Moscows: Communism and Working-Class Militancy in Inter-War Britain* (London: Croom Helm, 1980), p. 137.
50 Campbell, *The Scottish Miners, 1874–1939. Volume One*, p. 236.

51 Gwent Archives, CSWBGB/C/30, Bedwellty Union Relief Advisory Committee Papers, 1925 and 1926.
52 For examples, see Carr, *Pit Women*, p. 52; SWML, AUD/164, John Morgan Evans oral history interview.
53 SOHC, Iain McDougall Coal Mining Oral History Project, interview with Janet Chapman, 1999.
54 This potentially complicates the contested place of arts and crafts in the history of disability as individually chosen rehabilitation and social readjustment rather than inherently patronising. See, for example, Carolyn Malone, 'A Job Fit for Heroes? Disabled Veterans, the Arts and Crafts Movement and Social Reconstruction in Post-World War I Britain', *First World War Studies*, 4:2 (2013), pp. 201–17.
55 Mike Mantin, '"From Pithead to Sickbed" Exhibition Blogs: George Preece, Disabled Miner', Disability and Industrial Society website, http://www.dis-ind-soc.org.uk/en/blog.htm?id=45, accessed 30 August 2018.
56 South Wales Miners' Federation, *To the Bedwas Workmen and Their Womenfolk* (Caerphilly: Owen Jones, 1936).
57 *The Cambrian*, 29 July 1887, p. 3.
58 Bullock, *Bowers Row*, pp. 18, 23.
59 SOHC, Iain McDougall Coal Mining Oral History Project, interview with Janet Chapman, 1999.
60 Several disability theorists discuss disability as a 'master trope of disqualification'; see, for instance, Toibin Siebers, *Disability Aesthetics* (Ann Arbor: University of Michigan Press, 2010), p. 27.
61 For further examples, see J. C. Grant's North-East English novel *The Back-to-Backs* (1930) and Scottish miner Tom Hanlin's romantic novel *Yesterday Will Return* (New York: The Viking Press, 1946). In *The Back-to-Backs* the paralysed miner, Tom, is frustrated by falling in love with his brother's wife, and focuses on feelings of sexual impotence. The plot of *Yesterday Will Return* is driven by the suspicious death of a paralysed miner, Matt, who broke his back a week after they were married and died falling from his bed; his wife, Mima, a *femme fatale* type of character, is suspected of murdering him for the lump-sum compensation.
62 Corrie, *Black Earth*, p. 224.
63 Corrie, *Black Earth*, p. 246.
64 Shakespeare, 'The Sexual Politics of Disabled Masculinity', p. 58.
65 Corrie, *Black Earth*, p. 182.
66 Corrie, *Black Earth*, p. 255.
67 Carr, *Pit Women*, p. 72.
68 On working-class women's health and disability, see M. Ll. Davies, *Life as We Have Known It* (London: J. and A. Churchill, 1931); M. Spring Rice, *Working-Class Wives: Their Health and Conditions* (Harmondsworth: Penguin Books, 1939).
69 Durham County Record Office, U/EA 12, Easington Union Board of Guardians' Minutes, 27 June 1912.

70 Joanna Bourke, *Working Class Cultures in Britain, 1890–1960: Gender, Class, and Ethnicity* (London: Routledge, 1994).
71 Sue Bruley, *The Women and Men of 1926: A Gender and Social History of the General Strike and Miners' Lockout in South Wales* (Cardiff: University of Wales Press, 2010), p. 21; see also Carr, *Pit Women*, p. 33.
72 Carr, *Pit Women*, p. 68.
73 For an obituary of Eos Wyn, see *Cwrs y Byd*, May, 1892, pp. 81–4. The title of his column suggests he was aware of, and influenced by, the writings of Harriet Martineau; see [Harriet Martineau], *Life in the Sick-Room. Essays by an Invalid* (London, 1844). See, also, Maria H. Frawley, *Invalidism and Identity in Nineteenth-Century Britain* (London: University of Chicago Press, 2004).
74 *Y Gwladgarwr*, 24 December 1870, p. 2; 31 December 1870, p. 3; 11 February 1871, pp. 2–3; 18 February 1871, p. 3; 4 March 1871, p. 2; 11 March 1871, p. 2.
75 *Y Gwladgarwr*, 13 January 1872, p. 2.
76 *Y Gwladgarwr*, 24 August 1872, p. 2.
77 *Y Gwladgarwr*, 1 June 1872, p. 5.
78 *Y Gwladgarwr*, 5 September 1874, p. 6.
79 See, for example, Jones, *Times Like These* and Richard Llewellyn, *How Green Was My Valley* (London: Penguin Books, 1991 [1939]).
80 Jack Jones, *Rhondda Roundabout* (London: Hamish Hamilton, 1949 [1934]), p. 98.
81 James Hanley, *Grey Children: A Study in Humbug and Misery in South Wales* (London: Methuen, 1937), p. 255.
82 SOHC, Iain McDougall Coal Mining Oral History Project, Willie McGill interview, 4 September 1999.
83 Gleeson, 'Domestic Space and Disability in Nineteenth-century Melbourne'. Similar to what we find in relation to coalfield communities, Gleeson noted that disabled people were a common sight on the streets of nineteenth-century Melbourne and that their bodily differences were often very evident.
84 Gleeson, *Geographies of Disability*, p. 99.
85 Jules Ginswick (ed.), *Labour and the Poor in England and Wales 1849–1851: The Letters to The Morning Chronicle. Vol. III The Mining and Manufacturing Districts of South Wales and North Wales* (London: F. Cass, 1983), p. 49.
86 'Socialist Campaign in South Wales', *Commonweal*, 27 August 1887, quoted in Ken John, 'Sam Mainwaring and the Autonomist Tradition', *Llafur*, 4:3 (1986), p. 65.
87 Ferdynand Zweig, *Men in the Pits* (London: Society of Friends, 1948), p. 5.
88 Ernst Dückershoff, *How the English Workman Lives* (London: P. S. King & Son, 1899), p. 93.
89 Gerald Porter, 'The English Ballad Singer and Hidden History', *Studia Musicologica*, 49:1/2 (2008), p. 141; Roy Palmer, *The Sound of History: Songs and Social Comment* (Oxford: Pimlico, 1988), pp. 92–7.

90 The Tommy Armstrong Society website, http://www.pitmanpoet.org.uk/Welcome/welcome.htm, accessed 14 August 2018. See also Palmer, *The Sound of History*, pp. 28–9, 96–7.
91 Elizabeth Bredburg, 'Writing Disability History: Problems, Perspectives and Sources', *Disability and Society*, 14:2 (1999), pp. 194–5.
92 David White, *Mwnwr tlawd, yr hwn a gafodd niwaid mawr dan y ddaear* (Caerfyrddin, n.d.); Anon., *Cwyn y cloff* (n.d.). Digital copies of both texts are held at Welsh Ballads Online: https://www.library.wales/discover/library-resources/ballads/. *Mwnwr tlawd*: http://hdl.handle.net/10107/1106801 and *Cwyn y cloff*: http://hdl.handle.net/10107/1101239 (accessed 24 September 2019).
93 *Y Goleuad*, 13 Hydref 1905, p. 10. Turning to literature to make a living was common across the coalfields. For instance, William Francis Barnard (1840–1903), a miner born at Red Row, Clackmannanshire, started selling poetry when his son, Andrew, was injured in the mine and he needed extra money because of lost income; D. Edwards, *Modern Scottish Poets v.10* (Brechin: D. H. Edwards, 1887), p. 292. Andrew Barnard (1860–?), slowly recovered from this accident, mastering a variety of crafts (knitting and lace-making, along with joinery, fretwork and tailoring), and became a poet himself. Perhaps inspired by the success of the two Barnards, a collier friend of Andrew's, James Ballantyne (1860–87), also turned to poetry following a mining accident which left him partially paralysed. James and Andrew 'often rhymed and talked together', suggesting that they influenced each other's work; D. Edwards, *Modern Scottish Poets v.13* (Brechin: D. H. Edwards, 1890), pp. 132–3.
94 *Y Cantwr Dall, neu amgylchiadau William Bowen, Y Cantwr* (Aberdare: Jones & Son, c.1873–87).
95 Rosemarie Garland Thomson, *Extraordinary Bodies: Figuring Physical Disability in American Culture and Literature* (New York: Columbia University Press, 1997), p. 13.
96 Thomson, *Extraordinary Bodies*, p. 13.
97 Campbell, *The Scottish Miners, 1874–1939. Volume One*, pp. 222–3.
98 Grant, *The Back-to-Backs*, p. 202.
99 B. L. Coombes, *Miners Day* (Harmondsworth: Penguin, 1945), p. 113.
100 Enid M. Williams, *The Account of an Investigation into the Health of Old and Retired Coalminers in South Wales* (Cardiff: University of Wales Press, 1933), p. 1; see also p. 40.
101 Coombes, *Those Clouded Hills*, p. 56.
102 *Amman Valley Chronicle*, 3 March 1938, p. 8.
103 Gleeson, 'Domestic Space and Disability in Nineteenth-Century Melbourne', p. 227.
104 *The Miner*, December 1944, p. 14.
105 Zweig, *Men in the Pits*, p. 103.
106 Macintyre, *Little Moscows*, p. 139.
107 Dückershoff, *How the English Workman Lives*, pp. 39, 55–75.

108 Robert James, *Popular Culture and Working-Class Taste in Britain, 1930–39: A Round of Cheap Diversions?* (Manchester: Manchester University Press, 2014); Peter Bailey, *Leisure and Class in Victorian England: Rational Recreation and the Contest for Control, 1830–1885* (London: Methuen, 1987); Daryl Leeworthy, *Fields of Play: Sporting Heritage of Wales* (Aberystwyth: Royal Commission on the Ancient & Historical Monuments of Wales, 2012).
109 Viscount Chelmsford, *The Miners' Welfare Fund* (London: HMSO, 1927); W. John Morgan, 'The Miners' Welfare Fund in Britain 1920–1952', *Social Policy & Administration*, 24:3 (1990), pp. 199–211
110 SWML, AUD/382, D. C. Davies oral history interview.
111 *Picture Post*, 27 January 1945, p. 18.
112 SWML, AUD/222, Dick Cook interview.
113 B. L. Coombes, *These Poor Hands: The Autobiography of a Miner Working in South Wales, with an Introduction by Bill Jones and Chris Williams* (Cardiff: University of Wales Press, 2002), p. 165.
114 Jack Jones, *Black Parade* (Cardigan: Parthian, 2009 [1935]), pp. 413, 342.
115 Rhys Davies, *Jubilee Blues* (London: Heinemann, 1938), p. 222.
116 Davies, *Jubilee Blues*, p. 222.
117 Jones, *Black Parade*, p. 412.
118 Key works of literature were produced by Catholic miners, including the ex-miner writers Joseph Keating in Wales and Tom Hanlin in Scotland.
119 Robert Colls, *The Collier's Rant: Song and Culture in the Industrial Village* (London: Croom Helm, 1977), p. 164.
120 Hugh Gilmore, *The Black Diamond: A Tale of Life in a Colliery Village* (London: Thomas Mitchell, Primitive Methodist Publishing House, 1880), p. 60. Gilmore (1842–91) was born in Glasgow. A homeless orphan, he trained briefly as a bottle-maker's apprentice in Liverpool before moving to Newcastle-upon-Tyne, where he converted to the Primitive Methodist church. He became a lay preacher, and later an itinerant preacher, travelling the northern circuits, including Weardale and Darlington. He was a well-known and popular speaker, as well as writing numerous articles under his initials 'H. G.' for Methodist magazines such as the *Christian Ambassador*.
121 The reference is to Psalm 119:71.
122 Gilmore, *The Black Diamond*, p. 49.
123 Harry Lindsay, *Rhoda Roberts: A Welsh Mining Story* (London: Chatto and Windus, 1895), p. 8. Henry Lindsay Hudson (1858–1926) was born in Belfast, educated in Liverpool, and worked as a teacher for a period in Wales. A lay preacher and Steward of the Weslyan Methodists, he also worked as a journalist.
124 For a helpful short overview of the ways in which disability is 'interpreted in various ways as a function and sign of [the] proximity' to 'the human life-world' of 'the divine and metaphysical orders' (p. 6) – from antiquity to the present – see Ato Quayson, *Aesthetic Nervousness: Disability and the Crisis of Representation* (New York: Columbia University Press, 2007), pp. 5–9.

125 Robert Moore, *Pit-men, Preachers and Politics: The Effects of Methodism in a Durham Mining Community* (Cambridge: Cambridge University Press, 1974), p. 23.
126 Nancy Eiesland, *The Disabled God: Toward a Liberatory Theology of Disability* (Nashville: Abingdon Press, 1994), p. 100.
127 Tyne and Wear Archives Service, C.NC7/1/18/1, St James' United Reformed Church, Northumberland Road, Newcastle, Women's Guild Minutes, 1930–3.
128 Dückershoff, *How the English Workman Lives*, pp. 84–7.
129 In this context, see A. J. Kidd, 'Philanthropy and the "Social History Paradigm"', *Social History*, 21:2 (1996), pp. 180–92.
130 Richard Llewellyn's *How Green Was My Valley* (1939) is a significant exception and the relationship between religion and literature is discussed in Chapter 6.
131 Ellis Lloyd, *Scarlet Nest* (London: Hodder and Stoughton, 1919), p. 189.
132 Callum G. Brown, *Religion and Society in Twentieth-Century Britain* (Harlow and New York: Pearson Longman, 2006), p. 157.
133 Rhys Davies, 'The Benefit Concert', in Rhys Davies and Meic Stephens (ed. and intro.), *Collected Stories: Volume II* (Llandysul: Gomer Press, 1996), pp. 17–25.
134 *Sorrow for Thy Sons* was published posthumously in 1986, but was written during the 1930s.
135 Gwyn Thomas, *Sorrow for Thy Sons* (London: Lawrence and Wishart, 1986), p. 234.
136 Thomas, *Sorrow for Thy Sons*, pp. 238–9.
137 Bill Williamson, *Class, Culture and Community: A Biograhical Study of Social Change in Mining* (London: Routledge & Kegan Paul, 1982), pp. 132, 131.
138 Williamson, *Class, Culture and Community*, pp. 130–1.
139 Gordon Hall, *Woman at Work*, pp. 61–4.
140 On the social isolation of disabled people in industrialisation, see Michael Oliver, *The Politics of Disablement* (London: Macmillan, 1990); Gleeson, 'Domestic Space and Disability in Nineteenth-Century Melbourne', esp. pp. 225–6.
141 Gleeson, *Geographies of Disability*, p. 106.

5

THE POLITICS AND POLITICISATION OF DISABILITY

Introduction

On 22 May 1922, Dai Watts Morgan, MP for the Rhondda valleys in south Wales, described the bitterness felt by permanently injured miners in his constituency to his honourable colleagues in the House of Commons. He outlined in uncomfortable detail their long struggle to receive a level of compensation that allowed a decent standard of living:

> In no case where [the miners] have been totally disabled for life have they received the maximum of £1 a week. Such men, when they meet us from day to day or from week to week, say: 'When are you going to do something to assist us and to put our cases upon a just level, and to give us the rights that we ought to receive?'[1]

Watts Morgan, a former miner himself, conveyed in his speech the level of anger and injustice about disability that was felt in the coalfields. It was an impassioned contribution to the politics of disability, bringing to light both the grievances of individual miners and the wider structures of injustice that faced disabled people in the coalfields. While disability is inevitably a political issue in every chronological and cultural context in which it is found, the precise character of the politics of disability varies in time and from place to place, and it is possible to see differences in the ways in which such politics played out in the different coalfields.[2] Such differences coincide with important issues within the historiography of comparative coalfield societies, which discerns different political trajectories and traditions in each of the coalfields. Differing degrees of conflict and consensus, on the one hand, and variations in change and continuity over time, on the other, meant that each coalfield in Britain possessed its own, distinct political context.[3] Such distinctions and differences are just as evident in the politics of disability. More than that, it might be argued that disability, while always political, underwent a process of further politicisation in the period under consideration. An adversarial compensation system, initiated in 1880 and brought into full existence in 1897, pitted workers – through their trade unions – against their employers in legal contest, and led to significant amounts of time, effort and resources being expended by both sides to influence and amend legislation passed in the House of Commons. This, of course, had profound implications for the experiences of impaired miners and their families and the power relations in which they found themselves enmeshed.

Literature and disability politics are also closely interrelated in this period. Several prominent writers were ex-miners and politicians, including Scottish miner James C. Welsh MP,[4] and Durham miners John Swan MP[5] and Jack Lawson MP.[6] Some contested as parliamentary candidates but were unsuccessful, such as Joseph Keating,[7] Harold Heslop[8] and Jack Jones.[9] Many writers were involved with the Communist Party (CP), such as Lewis Jones or Jack Jones,[10] or took active roles in the trade union, such as Harold Heslop or John Swan.[11] The experience of disability, often connected to unemployment, was the focus of many writers, while disability metaphors were prolific in representing political solidarity, in which the strength of the people united (including those with impaired bodies) represents an embodied political strength.[12]

This chapter outlines the many ways that disability informed the politics of coalmining in the period from 1880 to 1948 and the myriad ways in which disability issues figured in industrial relations within the industry during this period. It uses an approach which moves from the everyday politics of disabled people's lives to the campaigns conducted by the labour movement at regional, national and United Kingdom-wide levels, and on to the pressure exerted by 'miners' MPs' and others in Parliament to secure or influence legislation. It aims, like Watts Morgan, to bring the two together to illustrate how central disabled people were to the broader politics of the coalmining industry. Politics as expressed via the cultural life of the community, particularly the emergent body of coalfields writing in the 1930s, is also touched upon. In this literature, concerns for the body and health of the miner and his family were central to the political sentiments expressed. Crucially, it is important not to treat people with disabilities solely as the objects of all this campaigning activity, but to give attention to their agency and the extent to which they were able to bring their influence to bear on these political and industrial matters.

Industrial relations, coal-mining and disability

The politics of disability in mining communities and within the industry as a whole occurred within a distinctive context, and some understanding of the broader aspects of industrial relations in the coal industry is first necessary. In a British context, the industry was arguably characterised by some of the stormiest and bitterest industrial relations of the late nineteenth and early twentieth centuries. Despite the existence of various mechanisms of collective bargaining, conflict resolution and conciliation, still the industry was marked by a greater propensity to industrial action and strike activity than other areas of the economy.[13] Moreover, the troubled history of the industry had profound consequences for industrial relations in Britain more generally as the miners' 'triple alliance' with rail and transport workers led to a major dispute in 1921 and as trouble in the coal industry led to Britain's only general strike in 1926.[14]

The period from about 1880 onwards saw huge increases in trade union membership in Britain. The half-million union members in the mid-1870s had increased to four million by 1914, comprising nearly a quarter of the working population, a growth which James Hinton characterised as the formation of 'mass labour movements' and a shift in British working society.[15] Attempts to unionise coalminers had occurred on a fitful and partial basis through the nineteenth century but, on the whole, unions tended to be weak and short lived, and were rarely coordinated across more than one coalfield. As far as the comparators in this study are concerned, the earlier development of the coalfield in the north-east of England, and the relative maturity of the labour movement, are reflected in the establishment of county unions for Northumberland and Durham, respectively, in the 1860s and their ability to weather the trade depression of the 1870s more effectively than their counterparts in other coalfields.[16] More effective trade union organisation did not come to the Scottish coalfields or south Wales until later. Alan Campbell has outlined the 'painstaking, uneven and irregular' growth of trade unions in Scotland before the 1890s, where small, local and fragile miners' associations rose and fell in rapid succession.[17] More robust county unions were formed in the Scottish coalfields from about the mid-1890s, and trades unionism rapidly grew in strength as larger numbers and proportions of miners joined their respective unions in the last years of the century and the period before the First World War. Greater collaboration across the county unions was brought about by the formation of the Scottish Miners' Federation (later the National Union of Scottish Mineworkers) in 1894.[18] In south Wales, the small and disparate organisations, often based on individual valleys and acting not as proper trade unions but more as committees to administer the sliding-scale pay mechanism, were only united in a coalfield-wide organisation for the purpose of collective bargaining with the formation of the South Wales Miners' Federation in 1898.[19]

More generally, the 1890s witnessed a significant increase in union membership across the coalfields so that, by the turn of the century, something like two-thirds of all workers in the industry belonged to their respective trade unions and, as John Benson notes, it was from this point that the unions 'were able to exercise a really decisive influence on the life of the individual family'.[20]

Trade unionism in the coal industry was given further impetus with the formation of the MFGB, a union of miners' unions, in 1889, and this organisation was to become crucial for the miners' political strategies in relation to disability matters into and during the twentieth century.[21] With the foundation of this organisation, an attempt was made to unite miners across Great Britain in common cause and to exert pressure on employers in the industry – who were themselves cooperating across their different coalfields to an increasing extent – through the Mining Association of Great Britain, founded in 1854. Differences of opinion meant that it was some time before all coalfield unions were affiliated to the 'national' Federation. Some small Scottish unions affiliated upon the MFGB's inception, while the Scottish Miners' Federation also entered into formal affiliation on its creation in 1894.[22] The miners of south Wales affiliated to the MFGB later, in 1899, following the abandonment of their commitment to a sliding scale in the previous year, while Durham and Northumberland, opposed to the campaign for an eight-hour day, did not do so until as late as 1907. All district unions were affiliated to the Federation by 1913, by which time it represented the interests of 645,900 miners.[23]

The MFGB was crucial to the politicisation of disability in the twentieth century, since it was the main campaigning body that pursued legislation on disability issues on behalf of miners. Employers' liability and workmen's compensation legislation were matters of real concern to the MFGB right from its inception, as was the campaign for an eight-hour day. Success in the latter, with the passing of an Act of Parliament in 1908, convinced many of the importance of this campaigning, political strategy of the Federation, and subsequent years witnessed attempts to influence safety legislation, medical research, nationalisation of the coal industry and other issues relating to the industry.[24]

Thus, the political landscapes and labour movements of coalfield societies were by no means homogeneous. Unions arose at different times, varied in their strength and the extent of their militancy and entered into different forms of industrial relations with their respective groups of coal employers. Not all miners subscribed to class struggle or even solidarity, and differences according to party political affiliation, religion, ethnicity and nationality served to undermine unity, albeit to different degrees, in each coalfield. Added to that, of course, a large a proportion of miners were not members of their respective trade unions and this varied from coalfield to coalfield and in each coalfield over time. Such structural factors, characteristic of the labour movements in each coalfield, were the context in which disabled miners and their families experienced impairment and in which the politics of their disablement was played out.

Miners' trade unions were thus large organisations that were able to wield an increasingly powerful influence on behalf of their members. The organisations that set out to represent miners' wives, and the women of British coalfields more generally, were, in contrast, far smaller and were unable to exert anywhere near the same degree of power. Given the relative paucity of employment for women in coalfield communities, female trade unionism was unimportant and far more activism came through the Labour Party and the Women's Co-operative Guild. Women in the Labour Party were organised in the Women's Labour League, formed in 1906, but this was replaced by 'women's sections' affiliated to local branches with the revision of the Party's constitution in 1918.[25] As part of this change, the Labour Party also appointed Marion Phillips as its first Chief Woman Officer in 1918, and Elizabeth Andrews performed the same role in Wales from that date; both were tasked with organising Labour women and assisting them in their activities.[26] Another organisation that campaigned to improve the lives of women in mining communities, in addition to working-class women more generally, was the Women's Co-operative Guild, a women's auxiliary organisation within the Co-operative movement, founded in 1883.[27]

Both these organisations enrolled working-class women in relatively large numbers and looked to utilise their perspectives to help determine the welfare policies they advocated. By 1933, for example, the Labour Party in Wales had 11,207 male members and 9,160 female members (45 per cent of the total) and the south Wales coalfield was a particular stronghold: in 1929 there were ninety-five sections in the East Glamorgan area alone.[28] As far as the Women's Co-operative Guild is concerned, the historian of the Guild in Wales has identified over 100 branches in existence for at least some time in south Wales during the period between 1891 and 1939,[29] but, there were fewer than 2,000 members in the whole of Wales by 1933.[30] These various working-class women's organisations shared members in common and cooperated with each other on a regular basis. Such cooperation was also manifest in a more formal alliance from 1919 onwards as the Standing Joint Committee of Industrial Women's Organisations was established. This included representatives of the Labour women's sections and the Women's Co-operative Guild, in addition to female trade unions, and it worked throughout the interwar period and into the 1940s to further welfare issues that were intended to improve the lives of working-class women, including housing, maternity and child welfare, and pithead baths.[31]

Disability, advocacy and representation

Histories of industrial relations have usually focused on the high-level negotiations of the representative leaders of workers and employers that were held to discuss the industry as a whole, or else major sectors of those industries. They have tended to concern themselves with the broader matters that affected the particular trade or industry, and so it has tended to be collective bargaining mechanisms, wage agreements and industrial disputes that have occupied the attention of labour historians. Similarly, the historiography of trade unions has prioritised industrial struggles involving issues such as wages, hours of work and working conditions in rather abstract ways, rather than the meaning of such issues in the personal experiences of individual miners.[32] In none of this labour history is there much attention given to the material circumstances of life for individual miners and their families, or to the more mundane but crucially important work carried out by branch or lodge officials in defence of the individual worker with a grievance.[33] Perhaps ironically, considering the commitment to history from below, historians of trade unions have not studied labour politics from the viewpoint of individual union members and have failed to appreciate what trade unions did for, or meant to, individual members on a day-to-day basis. This perspective nevertheless suggests itself as a meaningful way in which to consider the politicised character of disability, since it forces us to consider the experiences and viewpoints of the disabled person.

The vast majority of disabled miners did not see their unions launch large-scale campaigns on their behalf, or at least not on their behalf alone, nor did they find MPs taking their particular cases up in the House of Commons or appealing them in the House of Lords. Rather, the most common experience for disabled miners, if they were indeed members of their respective trade union, was far more mundane: to meet the lodge secretary, to discuss the particular circumstances of their case and for the lodge secretary to seek an adjustment to working conditions or some form of compensation from the manager at the particular colliery. These local, personal relationships with a lodge undersecretary are represented in a novel by Jack Lawson (who would become MP for Chester-le-Street from 1919 to 1949) in *Under the Wheels* (1934). Jabez Sill, the secretary, is a paternal, even quasi-religious figure (referred to as 'the new prophet') who walks through the community checking on the people and dispensing advice to injured men about compensation and other work disputes.[34] This lower, micro level was no less political than the higher reaches of the British political establishment, however, since it constituted the play of power relations in the most real, intimate and significant level of people's actual lives.

While a perspective that focuses on the individual miner and his impairments is extremely important, miners' trade unions found that, despite each case having unique characteristics, in terms of the circumstances of the individual miner or the manner in which his impairment was caused or affected him, most cases also had a great many features in common. This was because employers, or their insurance companies, tended to take a systematic approach to compensation matters and utilised a set of strategies to limit liabilities across the board. What this meant in practice for trade unions is that while each impaired miner was a case, assisted through personal case work by the union staff, whether at lodge or at 'national' level, such cases also became part of broader union campaigning. For example, any individual miner called for examination by his employer's doctor to judge the severity of his impairment would not have found himself alone but would probably have been joined in the queue at the doctor's surgery by many of his workmates who also suffered impairment. Bert Coombes gives a vivid sense of the scale of routine compensation assessments:

> In the room on the left about twenty men are seated on plank forms waiting for the compensation doctors to come and examine them. The signs of injury are plain on most of them, for several have their arms slung, and four are on crutches. It resembles the dressing-station after a battle. Across the passage is another group waiting in a line for the clerk to pay them some compensation. He counts some money out, and calls each man forward to sign for his payment. They will receive not more than thirty shillings, usually less, for a week's compensation, but they are easier in their minds than those in the opposite room, because their claims have been admitted.[35]

Individual cases fed into union industrial strategies whereby broader issues were taken up by union districts or executive committees, or even by the MFGB or miners' MPs in negotiations with employers' representatives. An excellent illustrative example can be found in the case of a miner suffering nystagmus that was taken up by the South Wales Miners' Federation and that reached the House of Lords in 1936. The man had had his claim for compensation dismissed in the county court after returning to work without being certified as being recovered and thereby declaring himself fit to work. This decision was apparently in accordance with a decision taken in the Court of Appeal some years previously and reaffirmed when this particular case was referred to it. The case was considered of such importance that the Trades Union Congress (TUC) appealed the case in the House of Lords, which gave the decision in the miner's favour and established the principle that a return to work did not necessarily mean that an injured worker was fully recovered.[36] It is therefore difficult to draw a clear line between individual case work and the broader industrial strategies of the miners' trade unions. Inevitably, the one informed the other in a very direct fashion, and this is implicit in the discussion that follows.

In the first place, however, not all miners were members of their respective trade unions; at times, quite large proportions of the mining workforce stood outside union membership. To a degree, non-members have been neglected by a labour historiography that has prioritised institutional approaches, for which primary sources have survived and which place union activists and members rather than non-unionists in the foreground. Miners not in union membership have not left many sources to the historian, but they still warrant attention. In the context of disability, non-members might have found their dealings with employers more difficult than their counterparts who benefited from the advocacy available to them by virtue of their union membership. Certainly, trade union officials stressed that employers were more likely to deal favourably with compensation claims from individual miners if they knew the miner was a member of the trade union. There was undoubtedly a rhetorical intent to such assertions, clearly designed to bolster union membership, and no statistical material on the relative success of members and non-members exists to allow us to test the validity of such assertions. But, following union officials' logic, it seems reasonable to assume that employers, intent as they were on limiting liabilities in as many ways as possible, would have resisted claims from non-members quite as vehemently as they did, if not more so, in relation to union members and that the cases of non-union members, who lacked the negotiating skills or were unable to afford the legal representation that union officials could draw upon, could not be carried as far. A somewhat fatalistic assessment, in the case of a miner who fainted from overwork and lost his arm to the conveyor, that 'the Company was always exonerated' is made in Gwyn Jones's *Times Like These* (1936), reflecting a view that the balance of power was deeply unequal.[37]

Relative to their unionised counterparts, disabled miners not in union membership would have found themselves in a disadvantaged position in their dealings with their employers and would have had to rely on the generosity of the colliery company official with whom they dealt or any personal political capital on which they could draw.[38] Older miners who had served the particular company for an extended period of time might have been able to draw upon a moral economy – especially during the nineteenth century – that laid a certain level of responsibility for old and infirm miners on the companies in whose service the miner had expended his strength and fitness, while 'good' and 'loyal' workers could be favoured by employers who might have wished to stress values such as respectability, thrift and independence or to project a public profile of benevolence and altruism.[39] This moral economy was eroded by the workings of the workmen's compensation system, as such old and infirm men became a greater liability than other men, but, even by the 1920s, some sort of altruism continued to be shown to impaired workers, albeit in certain, particular circumstances.[40] In the correspondence between different managers of the Powell Duffryn Coal Company in south Wales, for example, can be seen estimations of the worth of particular individual miners who applied for tickets of admission to a convalescent home – applications from men considered by managers to be a 'decent chap' or 'a regular and fairly good workman' were granted.[41]

Nevertheless, miners who were not members of their trade union found themselves in a relatively powerless relationship. The moral claims that they could call upon or the personal political capital that they could utilise in their dealings with the colliery manager were slight, and very few such miners in this situation would have secured their aims in these instances. Whether they sought light employment or compensation payments, non-union members had few means at their disposal to compel employers to grant their demands. This is not to argue that impaired miners in union membership were in a powerful position, of course, and it is clear that employers were able to bring considerable pressure to bear and to utilise all manner of tactics to lessen their compensation liabilities.[42] But, as union officials were keen to point out, individual union members were supported in their cases with access to expert medical opinion and good-quality legal representation in order to fight their cases.[43] In their 'Non-Unionist Campaign' in the early 1930s, for example, the Ferndale and Tylorstown Joint Miners' Lodges in the Rhondda Fach valley drew attention to a case in which a miner had secured a compensation payment of £556 due to silicosis as a result of the Ferndale Lodge's efforts in a disputed case. It stated that 'To substantiate the claim, a Professor of Geology had to be engaged to certify the rock, chemists to analyse it, medical men to proceed with the usual tests, apart from those engaged with the legal aspect of the case'; 'what ordinary workman could hope to finance a case of this kind, which involves such considerable expense?' it asked. The campaign leaflet also noted that two men had died in an accident at Ferndale previously, one of whom was a member of the union and whose family received £300 and the other, not a member, whose family were granted £15.[44] Similarly, the Durham Miners' Association opined in the 1920s, in light of the harassment they alleged the employers directed at men on compensation, that 'Were it not for the Trade Union the position of the injured would be made helpless and hopeless.'[45]

Upon becoming injured, a legal responsibility was placed on the individual miner to report his accident and his injury to the colliery company. He would also have reported the injury or complaint to his lodge secretary or, a little later into the twentieth century, the dedicated compensation secretary on the lodge committee. From that point, he would have been represented in negotiations by that union official. Lodge officials took up large numbers of individual cases and this was clearly an important part of their everyday administrative activities as union officers. The Ebbw Vale District of the South Wales Miners' Federation, for example, recorded 247 individual general notices of claims for injury compensation in between July 1900 and March 1901.[46] Union officials insisted that their organisation was 'more than a trade union', rather a 'social institution' providing an 'all-round service of advice and assistance', with lodge officials who were 'acknowledged social leaders called upon to advise in all kinds of domestic and social problems' 'between the cradle and the grave'.[47] The lodge secretary in the Durham coalfield was referred to as the 'father of his people', and the centrality of the lodge officials to the community was echoed too in the autobiographical writings of miners' leaders. In his memoir, *A Man's Life*, Jack Lawson wrote: 'If an accident happens, the union looks after the compensation of the unfortunate. And there are men in every northern colliery who can expound the Compensation Law like a lawyer.'[48] Indeed, the individual on the lodge committee, whether the secretary or the compensation official, built up a great deal of experience in compensation matters and was assisted by guides to the legislation prepared by the union for its officials, and briefing sessions on new developments.[49] In many cases, lodges appointed men as compensation secretaries who had first-hand experience of the compensation system and its intricacies through their own cases; this served the twin purpose, perhaps, of drawing upon the skills and experiences of particular individuals to assist other members while benefiting the individual, ensuring them a role in the union bureaucracy when they were no longer able to work in the industry itself.[50]

The initiation of claims to changed work conditions or compensation payments for disabled miners was replicated across the British coalfields, yet there were subtle but important differences in the ways in which different unions pursued these cases. The coalfield in the north-east of England was developed much earlier than its Scottish and Welsh counterparts and, by the late nineteenth century, possessed a more robust union culture and more stable industrial relations. Writers of the north-east of England coalfield repeatedly express pride in the formation of the union, its strength and the special political character of the north-eastern miner. For example, in Harold Heslop's *Last Cage Down* (1935) the Darlstone (alias for Durham) miners 'have kept one hundred years of unbroken organization' and are political fighters, unlike the 'new type of miner, the modern, tranquil, mechanized miner, the unorganized and unhistorical miners of the Midlands'.[51] Methodism's place in the creation of this enduring political culture and a type of miner who is serious, focused and politically committed is emphasised.[52]

The greater industrial relations stability in the north-east of England was evident in the more consensual politics that surrounded the permanent provident fund movement in the region in the nineteenth century relative to, for example, south Wales, where suspicion and struggle were more characteristic.[53] Such cooperation was also evident in the new era of workmen's compensation as the 'friendly arrangement' between employers and unions on the Arbitration Committee ensured that fewer cases were contested in the courts.[54] In Durham a case would be passed on to the Arbitration Committee if the lodge secretary was unable to secure an agreement with the colliery company on the workman's behalf, and would go to court only if agreement could not be reached at that stage.[55] The result, predictably, was that fewer cases were taken to law: between 1898 and 1922, the Arbitration Committee dealt with over 5,000 cases.[56] The Durham Miners' Association opined that, even with the increase in contested cases taken to court following the amendment to workmen's compensation legislation in 1923, 'We have yet to be convinced that in the total, our injured would get a greater measure of justice and more compensation from County Court Judges than from the Arbitration Committee.'[57]

In south Wales and Scotland, where no such Arbitration Committee existed, the case would be dealt with at colliery level by the lodge official and, in the event of failure to effect an agreement, would then be passed up the union structures, usually to the miners' agent, before reaching the executive committees and subsequently being passed to the MFGB itself for action. These different levels of union structure took cases through the hierarchy of law courts, and legal representation, whether by solicitors or barristers, was secured as appropriate. Lodge officials tended to see cases through the local magistrates' courts, while agents tended to administer cases that had reached the county courts and the MFGB oversaw appeals at the Court of Appeal and the House of Lords.[58]

The advocacy work of lodge compensation secretaries on behalf of individual miners was clearly crucial to the men themselves and to their experience of disability, and this is illustrated most clearly in the constant war of attrition that employers waged on men on partial compensation. Indeed, the constant struggles between 'partial compensation men', also known as 'light employment men', and employers gives a clear insight into the particular power relations between disabled miners and their employers, and demonstrates the considerable disparities in power between the two sides, even when union support was forthcoming.[59] While problems with the way the Act of 1923 defined incapacity gave rise to a considerable amount of difficulty, at least part of the trouble faced by men on partial compensation payments was due to the character of their impairments.[60] Such men were not sufficiently impaired to be considered incapacitated ('total compensation men') and, instead, tended to have temporary impairments that might change, or indeed lessen, over time, or else permanent conditions where the degree of impairment could lead to disagreement among medical experts. In short, 'partial compensation men' faced impairments where the degree of incapacity was less certain and more open to challenge, interpretation and disagreement.

More generally, the coal industry was a particularly labour-intensive sector of the economy and the costs of labour made up a large proportion of the employers' outgoings. This resulted in constant tension between employers and unions over wages but, in light of the relatively dangerous nature of the coal industry and the comparatively high levels of compensation liabilities, also focused attention on how to reduce the 'burden' of payments to impaired miners.[61] Coal employers sought and found myriad ways in which to resist or frustrate compensation liabilities and relieve themselves of the financial burdens imposed upon them by the statutory system.

The particular approach to these matters of any coal company varied from place to place and over time. There are instances in which unions observed that the employers were happy to settle cases without recourse to legal action, but these are few and far between and the usual state of affairs was one of conflict and struggle.[62] At the same time, it is possible to see that there were certain periods in which the number of contested cases or manipulation of the situation by employers was greater. This is especially true of the 1920s, for example, as an amendment to the Workmen's Compensation Act in 1923 included clauses that allowed employers to seek new ways to minimise liabilities. The Durham Miners' Association was exercised by what it perceived as the deliberate harassment of injured miners by the employers through Section 14 of the Act. This gave greater rights to employers to require men in receipt of compensation payments to undergo further medical examinations by the employers' doctors. The subsequent reports invariably found either that the men were recovered or else that the disability had lessened, and the injured miner was given ten days' notice that their payments would lessen or end. To prevent this from happening, the miner was required to submit a counter medical report within those ten days, and this placed enormous pressure on the individual miner and, by extension, his trade union. With over 300 such cases in the last three months of 1925 alone, the Durham Miners' Association believed that the employers deliberately swamped them with more cases than they could manage.[63] They found that the individual miner, rather than be 'humbugged' by the employer and appear before the employer's doctor, merely restarted work, often before he was ready to do so. Either the miner continued work and did not come back onto the compensation lists or, if the miner failed his work subsequently, he found that it was a costly and time-consuming business to restate his case for compensation, without any guarantee that it would be established successfully. The summoning of such miners to repeated medical inspections, asserted the Miners' Association, heaped 'unnecessary humiliation and indignities' on the disabled individual: 'It is provocative', stated the Association, 'and conveys the impression that the injured person is a thief and getting money by false pretences, or that our people took a pride in getting mutilated.'[64] The Rhondda No. 1 District of the South Wales Miners' Federation similarly found that employers in its area were using the clauses of the new Compensation Act to dispute cases and that considerable pressure was placed on union financial resources by the large volume of work created for the union.[65]

Another common tactic utilised by employers to harass light employment men was to cut compensation payments when wage increases were implemented across the industry. This was possible because, for much of the period, the compensation payments of partially disabled miners were calculated with reference to the differences between their pre- and post-injury wages, and miners were awarded half of the difference (it was often referred to in negotiations as 'half difference compensation'). This meant, of course, that impaired miners, unable to earn at the same level as previously, found that their partial compensation payments were insufficient to take them up to their previous income levels, and so disability entailed a fall in living standards for the injured miner and his family. The miners' unions, and indeed the labour movement more generally, campaigned throughout the first half of the twentieth century for compensation payments that were equal to the full wages, but were not successful in this aim, even under the majority Labour government of 1945 that passed significant reforms in social welfare and workmen's compensation legislation.[66] Employers also took the opportunity to cut compensation payments to individual miners upon the granting of wage awards to miners generally. This was because a wage increase would take an impaired miner's wages closer to, or indeed equal to, the previous level of income and so closed or removed the gap between previous and current wages, with the effect that employers felt justified in cutting the partial compensation accordingly. This happened in response to the 'war bonus' during the First World War, the 'Sankey award' in the immediate post-war years, a wage agreement in 1937 and the 1939 'war bonus'.[67] Each time, miners' unions were forced to attempt to represent members on partial compensation through negotiation and legal action.[68]

The direct harassment and humiliation of impaired miners was exacerbated by what the disabled men and their trade unions perceived as a more mundane, petty unpleasantness that similarly made clear the precise character of the power relations that existed between men on compensation and their employers. For example, the Fife and Kinross Miners' Association lodged an official complaint with the coalowners' association in 1910 in relation to the rudeness and incivility of colliery officials to men who collected their payments at the colliery office each week.[69] Similarly, in 1917 the Caerau Lodge of the Miners' Federation in south Wales complained to the local coal company at the insensitivity of a representative of the company who had visited an injured man and informed him that he had broken his spine. His condition had been kept from him by his family and doctor, and the 'uncouth' way in which the colliery official had informed him of his condition had plunged him into depression. A report of the incident was passed on to the miners' agent and MP, Vernon Hartshorn, who was to seek to have the official censured.[70]

This particular lodge was required to take up a number of complaints about the rough treatment meted out to disabled members by representatives of the colliery company, particularly in the early 1920s as the company placed pressure on partial compensation men to sign away their rights to compensation in return for permanent jobs on the surface. A series of complaints against the company's doctor, Bentley, culminated in 1924 when the lodge made a stand 'to wipe out these grievances at the Caerau Colliery'. The final straw was a miner with nystagmus who was 'treated like a Dog by Doctor Bentley' in a medical examination. It was reported that 'He told him to stoop down. [The miner] put his hand on the table as he was stooping down. Doctor Bentley knocked his hand off the table and [the miner] asked him if he was just finished. Alright he said you can carry on for a few weeks.'[71] Colliery doctors often had a gruff and robust way about them, and complaints about their bedside manner were not uncommon, but the sense of grievance felt by miner patients and their supporters was that much greater in these cases involving impairment.[72] These instances also made clear, and indeed were intended to make clear, the particular power relations that disabled miners found themselves in relative to their employers.

While considerable advocacy work was carried out by unions in support of their disabled members, it is important to avoid any overly optimistic or celebratory account of the roles of trade unions. At times, in unfortunate situations and for a variety of reasons, union compensation officials simply failed their members or even refused to offer support. Such failures raise important questions about the power relations that disabled miners entered into with their trade unions, the bodies that were ostensibly intended to defend their interests and bring about an amelioration in their situation. In these instances, the particular power relations between the unions and the disabled miners were not what might have been assumed from the rhetoric utilised by trade unions that posited disabled members as an important responsibility for the labour movement and that placed the victims of industrial capitalism at the heart of union campaigning.[73] This is not to discount the considerable time, effort and resources that miners' unions devoted to the lives and well-being of their disabled members, but only to note that not all disabled miners would have held a favourable view of their respective trade unions.

In the first place, miners in arrears with their union dues were denied assistance in compensation cases; in another instance, a miner from Harthill in Lanarkshire was denied assistance because his injury was sustained while strike breaking during the lockout of 1926.[74] Union discipline and rules of eligibility needed to be maintained for the sake of industrial strength, and disabled members found themselves in a similar position to other members. At the same time, such rules were not always interpreted strictly: unions often allowed the cases of miners in arrears to progress if they cleared their debts to the union and, in one instance, the chairman of a lodge personally paid off the arrears of one member to allow his case to continue.[75] Rules were clearly relaxed in order to ensure unity and to offer assistance where it might have been denied.

More frequently, and intriguingly, lodge, district and executive committees were required to deal with complaints from members unhappy that union officials had not taken their cases beyond a certain point, or from miners who were dissatisfied with the quality of the assistance that they had been afforded by the respective union. In some ways, the former type of case was more straightforward and tended to arise through a lack of funds that prevented unions from taking more cases to law than they would have wished.[76] More frequently, union officials, instructed by their legal counsel, made estimations of the likelihood of success in taking cases to court. As the Fife and Kinross Miners' Association noted:

> if we cannot prove the accident, or if the medical evidence is very contradictory and unsatisfactory, then it behoves the Executive to carefully consider whether the case should be pressed, because no matter what our sympathy for the particular man may be, if the law has not provided for the case, or if we cannot legally prove it, then there is little use in pressing it to a litigation.[77]

It is perhaps the second type of case, however, where miners complained about the quality of assistance provided to them, that is most revealing of the power relations that existed between disabled miners and their trade unions, since they rarely resulted in the union admitting fault or making amends for it.[78] Such cases did not arise particularly often, or at least not as far as trade union minutes record, but it should come as no surprise that the considerable pressures and strains, and the importance of the matters at stake, resulted in dissatisfaction and disagreement. Of the small handful of cases that crop up in the records of the South Wales Miners' Federation, it is the case of Rowland Ellis, a 'disabled collier', before the Rhondda No. 1 District that is most instructive. Ellis contrasted the compensation payment of £90 secured for him by the Federation with the larger payment won for a widow and her children at the same time. Dai Watts Morgan, the Miners' Agent for the District, pointed out that the numbers of children had been taken into account, but also how Ellis had been in receipt of weekly compensation payments in the time before his lump-sum award. More interestingly, Watts Morgan had completely lost patience with Ellis and accused him of ingratitude. Watts Morgan stated: 'I know him. He is a person whose case we fought for right along from beginning to end, and who then went directly behind the backs of the officials, the solicitor, the District Committee and myself. He thought that we were doing him wrong.' In the event, the meeting passed a resolution that confirmed the District committee's action in the case.[79] Faced by the considerable power of the trade union, therefore, disabled miners dissatisfied with the quality of representation provided by it had very little recourse to restitution, and union officials possessed considerable authority that was difficult to challenge.

More generally, and apart from the provision or denial of assistance by the trade unions in compensation cases, disabled miners stood in a slightly ambivalent position relative to their trade unions. There were, for instance, a number of factors that lessened the ability of individuals to engage with union activities. Many impaired miners were often disabled from attending trade union meetings or other activities and were not able to make their feelings known. Lewis Jones's novel *Cwmardy* (1937), for example, describes entire valleys of people attending political meetings 'with the exception of the bedridden' (the effect here is to show how unanimous is the support, but the point is based on recognising incapacity), while Bert Coombes similarly observed that many former miners in the Neath Valley were so debilitated by chest disease that they were unable to leave their homes, except for a trip out of the house in the summer to see the annual chapels procession.[80] At the same time, however, applications for assistance from impaired miners were a routine matter of business at union lodge meetings, whether the miner was able to attend or not, as friends or family members, or indeed committee members, represented their interests to the meeting. Harold Heslop's novel *Last Cage Down* includes a scene of a union meeting at the Miners' Hall where, alongside the 'usual trite questions', there were several applications for relief from disabled miners, including 'the weekly applications for trusses and water-beds and loans of the wheel chairs held by the lodge for people suffering from diseases necessitating these things'; the minutes of lodge meetings also confirm this picture.[81] More significant still, perhaps, was the fact that some union lodges offered reduced benefit club membership fees to disabled miners in recognition of their lessened financial status.[82]

A more intriguing aspect of disabled miners' relations with their trade unions is provided by a consideration of industrial disputes, since it is clear that the disabled men on light work and in receipt of partial compensation possessed a different status to their fellow workers. The miners' unions were keen to ensure that employers admitted and observed their liabilities to disabled members, in terms of both compensation payments and the need to provide light employment to them. As such, they insisted that, in the event of the employers giving notice to the workmen of a termination in contracts (i.e. that the miners would be locked out of their work should they fail to accept new working conditions or wage rates offered by the employers), the men on partial compensation payments would retain their right to compensation. In this way, the unions argued that employers could not absolve themselves of their responsibilities to partial compensation men and that they continued to face a responsibility to offer light employment and to pay partial compensation, even in the event of a cessation of work. Lodges in the Rhondda No. 1 District of the South Wales Miners' Federation attempted to make this argument to employers in the District in the lockout in 1921, for example, despite the legal advice they received that they would be unlikely to win any case they took to court on this matter. The legal advice stated while the employers were liable for any loss of income arising from the impairment, it was unlikely that the disabled miner would be able to prove that they were unable to obtain work elsewhere because of their impairment, when it was disruption in the industry, such as happened during an industrial dispute or during a depression in trade, that was responsible for the loss of employment of a large number of men.[83] Nevertheless, the South Wales Miners' Federation advised all its members just prior to the commencement of the lockout that they should not attempt to go to work, with the exception of the light employment men.[84] The advice given by the Federation was thus intended to preserve the men's rights to partial compensation because it could not be claimed by the employers that they were not available to work, similar to their non-disabled colleagues, and used by them to deny payments to these men.

In light of the desire for unity in strike actions, and given the treatment meted out to strike breakers, this is a remarkable action on the part of the trade unions. The precious unity that was so sought after was sacrificed, at least to some small degree, by the exemption of partial compensation men on light employment. Breaking a strike was considered the ultimate sin in most mining communities, and yet the union placed the rights of disabled men to compensation and light employment above this cardinal rule of industrial unity. This was clearly a principle that was worth defending. Even this commitment to the needs of disabled members could not survive the heightened stakes of the 1926 dispute, however, as the unions called both partial employment men and safety workers – responsible for ensuring that the pits would still be workable after a dispute – out on strike. This was despite the demand from some employers that the partial compensation men should continue to work and was a clear sign of the determination to pursue the dispute to the utmost of the unions' power.[85] Most employers, however, were particularly hostile during the 1926 lockout. John Swan, the compensation secretary for the Durham Miners' Association, recalled that 'the owners saw to it that no truce existed. War was waged almost on every man in receipt of compensation.'[86] Nevertheless, Barron notes that over 1,000 compensation cases relating to fatal and non-fatal accidents were heard during 1926, possibly out of the desire to 'avoid costly court cases.'[87]

Subsequent to the dispute, the South Wales Miners' Federation found that many light employment men were not taken on again by the employers and so was forced to attempt to negotiate their re-employment as best it could.[88] The Federation also emphasised its belief that employers continued to have a responsibility to find light work for men injured or impaired in their employment, and utilised test cases and negotiations to successfully secure concessions from the employers. One such concession was that the employers agreed to the payment of half the difference between their pre-accident earnings and unemployment benefit to injured miners who had not secured employment.[89] Here, as in so many other contexts, the miner's trade union acted in the interests of each individual impaired miner and, where they gained any success, made a difference to the living standard and life chances of the miner.

Political strategies and disability

In the 1937 novel *Cwmardy*, by the communist Lewis Jones, one of the characters angrily rejects the idea that government ministers or MPs grasp the realities of life for miners:

> Who is this Home Secretary ... this man who calls us hooligans and savages? Is he a working man? Have he ever worked down a pit? Have his mother been put in a county court because he have been too bad to work for a week or two? Not on your life! ... They claim they own the pits. All right. Let them come and work the coal themselves if they want it. Let them sweat and pant till their bodies twist in knots as ours have. Let them timber holes whose top they can't see and cut ribs in coal like solid steel.[90]

This assertion dramatises the sense of political struggle that is the focus of much of *Cwmardy* and its sequel, *We Live* (1939), by drawing parallels between hard work and disability (panting bodies twisted in knots). It gives voice to a widely held view that there was an enormous gulf between the political class and the people they purported to represent. Historical evidence suggests that this was less marked, and certainly that the interests of disabled miners were indeed represented in Parliament. This was because the miners had long pursued an active and relatively successful political strategy that ensured the return of miners' MPs and the pursuit of miners' goals in Parliament. Moreover, the campaigning and lobbying efforts of the miners' unions, the MFGB and the TUC ensured that miners' concerns were registered in high-level debates and discussions of legislation and official policies, even if those representations were too often marginalised or ignored.

Coalminers were one of the most prominent occupational groups to pursue a parliamentary strategy in any meaningful way during the nineteenth century, and succeeded in returning 'miners' MPs' from the 1870s.[91] Miners realised early that legislative intervention was a particularly effective means of improving working conditions; more importantly, they were enfranchised in large numbers from the 1870s onwards, they were sufficiently concentrated in particular constituencies to wield a considerable influence and they were increasingly organised through their trade unions, so that miners became increasingly aware of their electoral power relative to other types of workers and were able to exert their influence during elections.[92] Thomas Burt and Alexander MacDonald were the first of these miners' MPs – Burt was elected to represent Morpeth, Northumberland in 1874 and served continuously until 1918, while Macdonald represented Stafford from 1874 until his death in 1881.[93] Their number was added to in the years that followed so that, by the second half of the 1880s, there was a small but effective group of miners' MPs that succeeded in making the miners' voice heard on safety legislation, employers' liability and other issues. Prominent among these MPs were Thomas Burt, Ben John Wilson, Ben Pickard, William Crawford and William Abraham, as well as others. This early generation of miners' MPs, before 1900, were members of the Liberal Party and were opposed to the socialism that developed in certain parts of Britain, including some coalfields, from the late 1880s.[94] The Social Democratic Federation, the International Labour Party and the Labour Party came to challenge the Liberal hegemony from the 1890s onwards but had not changed it significantly by the time of the outbreak of the First World War. This was despite the fact that the MFGB had established an electoral fund after 1900 to support miner candidates for parliamentary seats and to assist those individuals elected to the House of Commons in the miners' interests.[95]

This parliamentary strategy was further strengthened with the MFGB's affiliation to the Labour Party in 1908, at which point all the MPs sponsored by the Federation took the Labour Party whip.[96] Gradually, the influence of the miners' interest, in the Commons and within the Labour Party, was extended: there were sixteen MPs supported by the MFGB by 1909, though this had fallen to ten by 1914.[97] By 1924, however, the MFGB sponsored 40 of the 151 Members returned to Parliament under the Labour Party.[98] Within the Labour Party, affiliation in 1908 meant that the MFGB was able to return delegates to the annual party conference and, on the basis of its large membership, was able to send a large bloc that was able to wield a not insignificant influence on party policies.[99] A significant indication of the strength of the miner constituency within the Labour Party was the adoption of nationalisation of the coal industry as an official party policy.

The political strategy of the miners' union movement, through its direct sponsorship of MPs and its influence on Labour Party policy, was further advanced through MFGB's affiliation to the TUC and Scottish unions' relationship with the Scottish Trades Union Congress (STUC). The TUC, especially its Parliamentary Committee, was the political arm of the trade union movement. The Parliamentary Committee was founded in 1872 and was chaired by Alexander MacDonald, the miners' leader.[100] Its specified aim was to take 'any action that may be necessary to secure the repeal of the penal clauses of the Criminal Law Amendment Act, the Truck Act, the getting of a proper Compensation Act, and to watch over the interests of labour generally in the proceedings of Parliament'.[101] In the years that followed, the TUC pursued aims relating to disability according to a particular way of working: the Parliamentary Committee would decide what steps to take, and then a bill or resolution was drafted and passed to a sympathetic MP, or else deputations were sent to government ministers. Only very occasionally were large demonstration meetings held to build public support for any measure or change.[102]

The role of the Parliamentary Committee was transferred to a new General Council in 1921, which then embarked on a more sustained period of negotiation with government and a more moderate approach to industrial matters, especially under Walter Citrine's period as General Secretary from 1926.[103] In addition, the TUC drew on expertise to make its case for improvements to industrial and occupational welfare: Sir Thomas Legge was appointed Medical Officer in 1930 and transformed the TUC's approach to occupational health and welfare issues, including workmen's compensation legislation.[104] At the same time, the economic depression meant that, on the one hand, there was little appetite among resistant employers for statutory interventions and, on the other hand, the labour movement's ability to press for such governmental action was circumscribed.[105]

These various political efforts constituted a technocratic approach to disability, since they largely dealt with the finer points of employers' liability and, more importantly, workmen's compensation, in addition to scientific and medical research into miners' pulmonary disease and nystagmus, with discussions between experts employed or engaged by the TUC and the permanent officials and medical experts of the government.[106] While industrial strategies were waged by the miners' trade unions to support individual miners or particular groups of disabled men, political efforts were, inevitably, undertaken in a different sphere and with different methods. As Bufton and Melling argue, miners' unions devoted more time and effort to fighting the cases of individual miners rather than 'engaging in a generalized public campaign in favour of comprehensive legislation'.[107] Instead, technical expertise was procured by the miners' movement and utilised in the lobbying of and representation to political leaders and government experts.[108]

This is most clear in the numerous activities relating to legislation – resolutions on the system of workmen's compensation might have been passed by miners' meetings, in all coalfields and on a regular basis, but such resolutions fed into MFGB, TUC, STUC and Labour Party efforts in Westminster, whether this be through the introduction of legislation or through efforts to shape legislation as it was being passed by other political parties. Huge amounts of effort and resources went into attempts to influence or amend the Employers' Liability Act of 1880 and the workmen's compensation legislation passed in 1897 and amended in the decades that followed. Apart from the behind-the-scenes lobbying and representation that took place, pressure was also exerted through the rhetoric employed by MPs in the numerous parliamentary debates that took place on these matters, and miners' MPs found themselves in battle with Members who were allied to the coal employers to a greater or lesser degree.[109] In a debate on accidents in mines just after a colliery disaster in Scotland in 1925, for example, Robert Smillie, the Scottish miners' leader and MP for Morpeth, engaged in some typical labourist rhetoric as he lambasted the apathy that tended to follow in the wake of major losses of life in the coal industry:

> we have got so used to slaughter during the War that we are not so easily shocked now. If you take a period of 70 or 90 years in the history of Great Britain prior to the War, you would find that a larger number were killed and injured in the mines than were killed and injured in all our battles during that time. The slaughter has gone on all the time.[110]

Following the passage of the Workmen's Compensation Act in 1897, miners' unions campaigned vigorously for different diseases to be included in the list of conditions covered by the statutory system. This is most evident in relation to efforts from the 1920s onwards to have miners' chest complaints scheduled as an industrial disease under the statutory system.[111] The South Wales Miners' Federation, in particular, has been recognised for engaging in what Michael Bloor describes as 'more than 10 years of political lobbying, legal arguments and epidemiological data gathering' before the compensation amendment of 1943, while McIvor and Johnston have similarly emphasised the crucial role played by the MFGB and the miners' trade union movement more generally.[112] These years were the nadir of the pneumoconiosis crisis, with over 22,000 miners out of work from the disease, 85 per cent of whom were in south Wales.[113] During this time, the MFGB campaigned consistently at local, national and parliamentary level to raise awareness of the effect of the disease. No annual conference of the MFGB passed without resolutions on the workmen's compensation system and, from the 1920s onwards, chest disease being passed; the conference of 1927, for example, maintained that 'miners phthisis, rheumatism, or any other disease which can be proved to have been wholly or partially due to the nature of employment, shall be included in the schedule of diseases'.[114]

While the political campaigns of miners focused on Parliament, those of the women of mining communities were directed more to local government. The organisations that campaigned on behalf of women in mining communities undertook a number of campaigns and initiatives in the period before the First World War – the Women's Co-operative Guild and the Women's Labour League were most prominent in that period – but it is the interwar period that witnessed a significant increase in female activism and influence. Labour women were perhaps the most important groups in the coalfields and, while not able to exert much influence on the direction of party policy on a national level, they succeeded, through local Labour parties, in gaining election to Boards of Guardians and local councils where they were far more able to bring their expertise to bear and make a material difference to the provision of welfare.[115] Women's Co-operative Guild members also sought and gained elected positions on Boards of Guardians, district and county councils, and found their way onto education, health and maternity and child welfare committees. Rose Davies, a prominent Labour activist and member of the Women's Co-operative Guild, and elected as a district and later county councillor in Aberdare from 1925, for example, was the major driving force behind her council's maternity centre.[116]

Even where female activists in the coalfields were not able to gain seats on local councils, they still canvassed local councillors and exerted pressure upon them to improve welfare services for working-class women. The area of provision that received most attention was maternity and child welfare. Feminist campaigners were keen to demonstrate the relative risks faced by women and their husbands and often made the point that miners' wives faced even greater risks to their health and well-being than did their husbands in the notoriously dangerous coal industry. Elizabeth Andrews opined that 'The miner's wife in those days ran greater risks at childbirth than her man in the pit.'[117] Eleanor Rathbone, perhaps the most prominent feminist of the 1920s, estimated that 'A miner's wife runs from three to six times as much danger of death when she has a child as her husband does in going down the pit daily for a year.'[118]

Such feminists were given the opportunity to exert some pressure and bring about improvements by the Maternity and Child Welfare Act of 1918, which stipulated that local councils were to ensure that county council Maternity and Child Welfare committees were to have at least two female members. The Act required them to co-opt female representatives from women's organisations if no female councillors were available. Labour women were keen to remind councils of their obligations in this regard.[119] In the Rhondda valley the local members of the Women's Co-operative Guild utilised their presence on the local Mid-Rhondda Trades and Labour Council (TLC), an organisation that brought various organisations within the labour movement together, to compel district councillors associated with the TLC to use their influence on the council to co-opt working-class women who were members of the local labour movement.[120] Maternity and child welfare was also extremely important on Clydeside and in the surrounding coalfield districts, where motherhood was characterised by female activists as 'the most dangerous of trades'.[121]

Campaigns to develop maternity services intended to improve maternal health and prevent the great toll in reproductive impairment that impacted on mining women. Another important campaign that was partly intended to do the same thing was that in support of the extension of pithead baths to greater numbers of collieries. Branches of the Women's Labour League in south Wales took up the matter of pithead baths from 1912 and a coalfield-wide campaign ensued in the years that followed. This campaign received support from the miners' union, and also from middle-class reformers in the region and, indeed, coal companies such as the Ocean Coal Company.[122] Elizabeth Andrews, the Wales Women's Organiser for the Labour Party, placed the matter of pithead baths at the centre of her testimony to the Sankey Commission into the coal industry in 1919 and thereby succeeded in getting it placed on the political agenda for the rest of the interwar period; the MFGB and the Labour Party itself gave the issue a great deal of prominence and helped to move the movement forward.[123] Miners' leaders Robert Smillie and Frank Hodges noted that without the introduction of pithead baths, miners' wives and mothers would remain 'life-long slaves of the pit'.[124]

Crucially, the report of the Sankey Commission led the government to establish the Miners' Welfare Fund, which took the matter up from 1927 onwards and made grants towards the erection of baths in coalfields across Britain: a few baths were opened in the immediate post-war years and 1920s, but the pace of expansion increased considerably in the 1930s and 1940s; 307 had been erected by the outbreak of the Second World War and this had increased to 348 by the end of the war.[125] When the coal industry was nationalised in 1947, the NCB undertook to ensure that every new pit would be equipped with a baths, and looked to provide all pits still without a baths by that time within seven years.[126] With the extension of such facilities to a greater number of pits, women's campaigning in the coalfields helped to make a material difference to the working lives of women in mining communities and helped to lessen the risks of reproductive impairment. In a sense, perhaps, the campaigns to improve women's reproductive health and lessen the impairment that resulted from childbirth were more successful than the efforts of miners' trade unions to shape the statutory compensation legislation for their members. This was because maternalist politics coincided with official concerns about the size and fitness of the British population and the importance attached to industrial productivity and military preparedness in the defence of Britain and its empire against foreign competitors from the late nineteenth century onwards.

Conclusion

Disability is inherently political. The denial of rights, opportunities and experiences to disabled people and the resultant experience of disability makes this inevitable. This was evident in a number of different contexts in relation to the British coal industry, from the level of personal experience to the highest political stage of the land. As far as the latter is concerned, it is possible to discern a process of politicisation, largely brought about by statutory interventions and official policies, that witnessed disability issues become the matter of party manifestos, parliamentary debates and significant enactments of legislation. Indeed, it might be argued that such politicisation reached its apogee in the 1930s and, especially, 1940s as official attention was increasingly drawn to disability in the coalfields, as scientific and medical research, supported by government, was conducted and as measures such as the Disabled Persons (Employment) Act of 1944 and the National Insurance (Industrial Injuries) Act of 1946, for all their flaws, were passed.

More interestingly, disability was political at the personal, individual level, as disabled miners found themselves enmeshed in unequal power relations with individuals and agencies around them. This was most marked in relation to the coal employers but was not wholly absent from their dealings with their own unions, the bodies that proclaimed to fight their cause. Due to the character of the primary source material that has come down to us, this is a very difficult issue to examine, but historians would be well served by asking what kinds of power were communicated in disability issues and, more importantly, how much of that power was negotiated by disabled people themselves. Disabled people have been largely ignored in the historiography of coal, despite unions' continuous campaigning for their rights and compensation, and the perspectives of disabled miners have rarely figured in accounts of the history of the industry.[127] Nevertheless, while disabled miners occasionally found themselves dissatisfied with their unions, very few seemed to be in any doubt that it was their work that had impaired them and their employers who disabled them through the denial of a just compensation settlement. There is little evidence of any disability consciousness having developed in the coalfields and, instead, miners and their families tended to view disability through the lens of class consciousness. Disability and class consciousness intersect most obviously in coalfields literature, particularly in portrayals of solidarity which use the rhetoric and imagery of disability to achieve their impact. This and other characteristics and traditions of coalfields literature are discussed in our final chapter.

Notes

1 Hansard, 3 May 1922.
2 On the politics of disability, see Michael Oliver, *The Politics of Disablement* (Basingstoke: Macmillan, 1990); David Mitchell and Sharon Snyder, *The Biopolitics of Disability: Neoliberalism, Ablenationalism, and Peripheral Embodiment* (Ann Arbor: University of Michigan Press, 2015).
3 For key works in the comparative coalfield societies literature, see Stefan Berger, Andy Croll and Norman LaPorte (eds), *Towards a Comparative History of Coalfield Societies* (Aldershot: Ashgate, 2005); John McIlroy, Alan Campbell and Keith Gildart (eds), *Industrial Politics and the 1926 Mining Lockout: The Struggle for Dignity* (Cardiff: University of Wales Press, 2004); Stefan Berger, 'Working-Class Culture and the Labour Movement in the South Wales and Ruhr Coalfields, 1850–2000: A Comparison', *Llafur*, 8:2 (2001), pp. 5–40; David Gilbert, *Class, Community, and Collective Action: Social change in two British coalfields, 1850–1926* (Oxford: Clarendon Press, 1992); Roger Fagge, *Power, Culture and Conflict in the Coalfields: West Virginia and South Wales, 1900–1922* (Manchester: Manchester University Press, 1996); Leighton S. James, *The Politics of Identity and Civil Society in Britain*

and Germany: Miners in the Ruhr and South Wales 1890–1926 (Manchester: Manchester University Press, 2008).
4   Scottish Labour Party MP 1922–31 (Coatbridge) and 1935–45 (Bothwell).
5   Labour Party MP 1918–22 (Barnard Castle).
6   Labour Party MP 1919–49 (Chester-le-Street).
7   In 1918 Keating unsuccessfully bid for the Labour parliamentary candidacy; in 1923 he was elected a Labour councillor in Mountain Ash.
8   Contested as Labour Party candidate on South Shields Council 1926, sponsored by the Miners' Lodge. He won a seat on the Taunton Town Council for Labour in 1948, and unsuccessfully stood as the Labour Party candidate for North Devon in 1955.
9   Having previously been both a member of the Communist Party and the Labour Party, he stood as the candidate for the Liberal Party in Neath in 1928.
10 Jack Jones was a CP member 1920–23, chosen as Corresponding Secretary for the South Wales Region, founding a branch at Merthyr Tydfil; Lewis Jones was Welsh organiser for the NUWM, and elected as a CP member of the Glamorgan County Council in 1936.
11 Harold Heslop represented Harton colliery on the council of the Durham Miners' Association; John Swan was elected Agent for the Association in 1923, and later became its General Secretary 1935–45.
12 This is discussed in detail in the second half of Chapter 6.
13 Roy Church and Quentin Outram, *Strikes and Solidarity: Coalfield Conflict in Britain* (Cambridge: Cambridge University Press, 2002).
14 Barry Supple, *The History of the British Coal Industry: Volume 4. 1913–1946: The Political Economy of Decline* (Oxford: Clarendon, 1987); Alan Campbell, Nina Fishman, David Howell (eds), *Miners, Unions, and Politics, 1910–47* (Aldershot: Scolar Press, 1996).
15 James Hinton, *Labour and Socialism: A History of the British Labour Movement, 1867–1974* (Brighton: Harvester Press, 1983), p. 24.
16 John Benson, *British Coalminers in the Nineteenth Century: A Social History* (Dublin: Gill and Macmillan, 1980), pp. 198–9.
17 Alan Campbell, *The Scottish Miners, 1874–1939. Volume Two: Trade Unions and Politics* (Aldershot: Ashgate, 2000), p. 117.
18 Campbell, *The Scottish Miners, 1874–1939. Volume Two*, pp. 15–71.
19 V. L. Allen, *The Militancy of British Miners* (Shipley: Moor Press, 1981), p. 22; Hywel Francis and David Smith, *The Fed: A History of the South Wales Miners in the Twentieth Century* (London: Lawrence and Wishart, 1980), pp. 1–2. The 'sliding scale' was the mechanism utilised in some coalfields by which wages paid to workers rose or fell in direct relation to changes in the price of coal.
20 Benson, *British Coalminers in the Nineteenth Century*, p. 199.
21 On the MFGB, see Keith Gildart, 'The Miners' Federation of Great Britain', in Gildart (ed.), *Coal in Victorian Britain, Part II: Coal in Victorian Society, Volume 6, Industrial Relations and Trade Unionism* (London: Pickering & Chatto, 2012),

pp. 183–92; R. Page Arnot, *The Miners: A History of the Miners' Federation of Great Britain* (London: George Allen & Unwin Ltd, 1949), pp. 90–116; Hinton, *Labour and Socialism*, pp. 45–6; H. A. Clegg, Alan Fox and A. F. Thomson, *A History of British Trade Unions since 1889, Volume 1: 1889–1910* (Oxford: Clarendon Press, 1964), pp. 98–111.
22 Campbell, *The Scottish Miners, 1874–1939. Volume Two*, p. 41.
23 Gildart 'The Miners' Federation of Great Britain', pp. 183–4.
24 Arnot, *The Miners*, pp. 90–116; David Howell, '"All or Nowt": The Politics of the MFGB', in Alan Campbell, Nina Fishman and David Howell (eds), *Miners, Unions and Politics, 1910–47* (Aldershot: Scolar Press, 1996), p. 43.
25 Martin Francis, 'Labour and Gender', in Duncan Tanner, Pat Thane and Nick Tiratsoo (eds), *Labour's First Century* (Cambridge: Cambridge University Press, 2000), p. 192.
26 Brian Harrison, 'Phillips, Marion (1881–1932)', *Oxford Dictionary of National Biography* (23 September 2010),www.oxforddnb.com/view/10.1093/ref:odnb/9780198614128.001.0001/odnb-9780198614128-e-37852 (accessed 28 August 2018); Ursula Masson and Lowri Newman, 'Andrews, Elizabeth (1882–1960)', in Keith Gildart and David Howell (eds), *Dictionary of Labour Biography. Volume XII* (Basingstoke: Macmillan, 2004), pp. 1–11.
27 Gillian Scott, *Feminism and the Politics of Working Women: The Women's Co-operative Guild, 1880s to the Second World War* (London: UCL Press, 1998).
28 Evans and Jones, '"To Help Forward the Great Work of Humanity"', pp. 220–2.
29 Helen Thomas, '"Democracy of Working Women": The Women's Co-operative Guild in South Wales, 1891–1939', *Llafur*, 11:1 (2012), p. 153.
30 Thomas, 'Democracy of Working Women', p. 154.
31 Elizabeth Andrews, *A Woman's Work is Never Done* (Ystrad Rhondda: Cymric Democrat Publishing Society, 1956), pp. 28–31.
32 Keith Gildart, 'Introduction', in Gildart (ed.), *Coal in Victorian Britain. Part II, Coal in Victorian Society. Volume 6, Industrial Relations and Trade Unionism* (London: Pickering & Chatto 2012), pp. xiii–xvi.
33 A point also made by John Benson; Benson, *British Coalminers in the Nineteenth Century*, pp. 206–7. There are some small exceptions to this trend; see, for example, Mark E. Bufton and Joseph Melling, '"A Mere Matter of Rock": Organized Labour, Scientific Evidence and British Government Schemes for Compensation of Silicosis and Pneumoconiosis among Coalminers, 1926–1940', *Medical History*, 49:2 (2005), p. 167 and George R. Boyer, 'What Did Unions Do in Nineteenth-Century Britain?', *Journal of Economic History*, 48:2 (1988), pp. 319–32.
34 Jack Lawson, *Under the Wheels* (London: Hodder & Stoughton, 1934), p. 77.
35 B. L. Coombes, *These Poor Hands: The Autobiography of a Miner working in South Wales, with an Introduction by Bill Jones and Chris Williams* (Cardiff: University of Wales Press, 2002 [1939]), p. 160.
36 South Wales Miners' Federation, *Annual Report of Executive Council, 1936–1937*, p. 44.

37 Gwyn Jones, *Times Like These* (London: Victor Gollancz, 1979), p. 287.
38 Bartrip also speculates that non-unionised workers were at a disadvantage relative to their unionsed colleagues; P. W. J. Bartrip, *Workmen's Compensation in Twentieth Century Britain* (Aldershot: Avebury, 1987), p. 23.
39 On the moral economy of aged and infirm miners, see Ben Curtis and Steven Thompson, '"This is the Country of Premature Old Men": Ageing and Aged Miners in the South Wales Coalfield, c.1880–1947', *Cultural and Social History*, 12:4 (2015), p. 597; for an example of this moral economy in a Scottish context in the middle decades of the twentieth century, see Scottish Oral History Centre Archive, Coal Mining Oral History Project, John Taylor Murphy interviewed by Ian MacDougall, 16 May 1997, comments on the Fife Coal Company. On employer paternalism in the coal industry, see Roy A. Church, *The History of the British Coal Industry, Volume 3: 1830–1913: Victorian Pre-Eminence* (Oxford: Clarendon Press), pp. 274–99.
40 On the unintended consequences of compensation legislation and its role in the lessening of exymployment changes for impaired workers, see Sarah F. Rose, *No Right to be Idle: The Invention of Disability, 1840s–1930s* (Chapel Hill: University of North Carolina Press, 2017).
41 Glamorgan Archives, Powell Duffryn Collection, DPD/2/5/6/206, Applications for tickets for Porthcawl Rest, May–Sept. 1926.
42 D. C. Davies, compensation secretary at Ffaldau Lodge of the Miners' Federation in south Wales was adamant that the entire compensation system before 1948 was weighted very much in the employers' favour; South Wales Miners' Library, Swansea University (hereafter SWML), AUD/382, D.C. Davies oral history interview, 19 June 1976.
43 Instructive here is Michael Bloor, 'The South Wales Miners Federation, Miners' Lung and the Instrumental Use of Expertise, 1900–1950', *Social Studies of Science*, 30:1 (2000), pp. 125–40.
44 South Wales Coalfield Collection, Swansea University (hereafter SWCC), MNA/NUM/L/33/45, Ferndale and Tylorstown Joint Miners' Lodges, Non-Unionist Campaign (Ferndale, c.1932).
45 Durham County Record Office (hereafter DCRO), D/DMA Acc 1004 D 169, Durham Miners' Association, Review of the Work of the Compensation Department for the year 1925, p. 488.
46 Gwent Archives, D.844.20–72, Ebbw Vale and District Miners' Federation, General notices re. injuries and claims, 1898–1914.
47 Will Paynter, *My Generation* (London: Allen and Unwin, 1972), pp. 110–11.
48 K. Brown, 'The Lodges of the Durham Miners' Association, 1869–1926', *Northern History*, 23 (1987), p. 146. Jack Lawson, *A Man's Life* (London: Hodder & Stoughton, 1944), p. 137. For more on mining autobiography, see Keith Gildart, 'Mining Memories: Reading Coalfield Autobiographies', *Labor History*, 50:2 (2009), pp. 139–61.
49 See, for example, The Fabian Society, *The Workmen's Compensation Act What It Means, and How to Make Use of It* (London: Fabian Society, 1900); Harold J.

Finch, South Wales Miners' Federation, *Guide to Workmen's Compensation Act, 1925–43* (Cardiff: South Wales Miners' Federation, 1944).

50 For examples of miners who became compensation secretaries after gaining experience in their own cases, see SWML, AUD/56, Haydn Mainwaring oral history interview (1980); SWML, AUD/222, Dick Cook interview (1974).

51 Harold Heslop, *Last Cage Down* (London: Lawrence Wishart Books, 1984), p. 139.

52 For a history of Methodism in the Durham coalfields, see Robert Moore, *Pit-men, Preachers and Politics: The Effects of Methodism in a Durham Mining Community* (Cambridge: Cambridge University Press, 1974.).

53 Steven Thompson, 'Varieties of Voluntarism in the South Wales Coalfield, circa 1880–1948', in Colin Rochester, George Campbell Gosling, Alison Penn and Meta Zimmeck (eds), *Understanding the Roots of Voluntary Action: Historical Perspectives on Current Social Policy* (Brighton: Sussex Academic Press, 2011), pp. 82–94.

54 On 'friendly arrangements', see North East England Mining Archive and Research Centre, University of Sunderland, NUMDA/6/1/1/1, Durham Miners' Association, Reports of the Compensation Department, Volume I, Arbitration Committee, Report of Proceedings of Arbitration Committee Meeting held in The Coal Trade Offices, Newcastle-on-Tyne on 3 March 1919; Bartrip notes that the Arbitration Committee in the Durham coalfield was one of the few such bodies established in any industry during the first half of the twentieth century; Bartrip, *Workmen's Compensation in Twentieth Century Britain*, p. 19.

55 On the consensus between employers and unions, see John Benson, 'Coalminers, Coalowners and Collaboration: The Miners' Permanent Relief Fund Movement in England, 1860–1895', *Labour History Review*, 68:2 (2003), pp. 181–94; on the different politics in south Wales, see Thompson, 'Varieties of Voluntarism in the South Wales Coalfield'. On Durham, see Brown, 'The Lodges of the Durham Miners' Association', p. 143.

56 DCRO, D/DMA Acc 1004 D 169, Durham Miners' Association, Review of the Work of the Compensation Department for the year 1922, p. 355.

57 Durham Miners' Association, Review of the Work of the Compensation Department during the year 1924, p. 871.

58 Bartrip, *Workmen's Compensation in Twentieth Century Britain*, pp. 22–7, 59–63, 133–6.

59 In addition, this class of 'partial compensation' men, for whom 'light employment' was necessary, ensured that the tendency for workmen's compensation legislation to discourage employers from appointing impaired miners or retaining them in employment was not total; on this matter in a different context, see Sarah F. Rose, *No Right to be Idle: The Invention of Disability, 1840s–1930s* (Chapel Hill: University of North Carolina Press, 2017).

60 Bartrip, *Workmen's Compensation in Twentieth Century Britain*, pp. 153–7.

61 For examples of union recognition of this situation, see SWML, South Wales Miners' Federation, Annual Report of Executive Council, 1935–1936, p. 31; DCRO,

D/DMA 91, Durham Miners Association, Review of the Work of the Compensation Department for the year 1924, p. 869.
62 For an example of coalowners preferring not to take cases to law, see SWCC, Swansea University, MNA/NUM/3/8/10a, South Wales Miners' Federation Rhondda No. 1 District, Monthly Report, 14 October 1901.
63 DCRO, D/DMA Acc 1004 D 169, Durham Miners' Association, Review of the Work of the Compensation Department for the year 1925, pp. 488–9.
64 DCRO, D/DMA Acc 1004 D 169, Durham Miners' Association, Review of the Work of the Compensation Department for the year 1925, p. 489.
65 *The Colliery Workers' Magazine*, 1:4 (April 1923), p. 94.
66 Rodney Lowe, *The Welfare State in Britain since 1945* (London: Macmillan, 1993).
67 For examples, see SWMF Executive Council Minutes, 22 May 1915, 8 June 1915, 10 August 1915, 4 June 1920, 2 August 1924, 24 September 1924, 27 September 1924; SWMF Annual Report of Executive Council, 1940–1941, Report of Compensation Department, p. 45.
68 SWMF Executive Council Minutes, 12 February 1916.
69 National Library of Scotland (hereafter NLS), Dep 304/3, Fife and Kinross Miners' Association, Board Meeting Minutes 24 February 1910.
70 SWCC, MNA/NUM/L/19/4, Caerau Lodge, Committee Meeting Minutes, 8 February 1917.
71 SWCC, Swansea University, MNA/NUM/L/19/4, Caerau Lodge, Committee Meeting Minutes, 13 March 1924.
72 On doctor–patient relations in one coalfield, see Steven Thompson, 'Paying the Piper and Calling the Tune? Complaints against Doctors in Workers' Medical Schemes in the South Wales Coalfield', in Jonathan Reinarz and Rebecca Wynter (eds), *Complaints, Controversies and Grievances in Medicine: Historical and Social Science Perspectives* (London: Taylor & Francis, 2015), pp. 93–108.
73 A good example can be found in SWCC, South Wales Miners' Federation, Rhondda No. 1 District, Monthly Report, 6 May 1918.
74 NLS, Acc 4312/2, National Union of Mineworkers, Minute Book, 1920–1927, 8 January 1927.
75 For examples, see SWCC, MNA/NUM/L/19/3, Caerau Lodge, Committee Meeting Minutes, 2 November 1912; SWCC, 29 November 1912; SWCC, MNA/NUM/L/19/7, Committee meeting minutes, 6 July 1922; SWCC, 28 February 1924.
76 For example, see SWCC, MNA/NUM/3/8/10a, South Wales Miners' Federation Rhondda No. 1 District, Annual Report for 1913, p. 2.
77 NLS, Dep 304/3, Fife and Kinross Miners' Association, Executive Committee Meeting, 23 January 1912; for examples of this in practice, see NLS, Edinburgh, Acc. 4312/12, Mid and East Lothian Miners Association, Executive Committee Minutes, 22 June 1927; ibid., 22 August 1928.
78 For an indicative example of a union confirming the decisions and actions of its officials after a complaint from a member, see SWCC, MNA/NUM/3/1/1, South

Wales Miners' Federation, Executive Council Minutes, 3 February, 10 February, 8 May 1913.
79 SWCC, MNA/NUM/3/8/10a, South Wales Miners' Federation Rhondda No. 1 District, Monthly Report, 4 January 1904.
80 Lewis Jones, *Cwmardy and We Live* (Cardigan: Parthian, 2006), p. 207; B. L. Coombes, *Miners Day* (Harmondsworth: Penguin Books, 1945), p. 113.
81 Heslop, *Last Cage Down*, p. 96.
82 SWCC, Swansea University, SWCC/MNA/NUM/3/8/7(d), Maesteg District, Benefit Fund Rules, 1934.
83 Rhondda No. 1 District, Monthly report, 4 April 1921: Committee Minutes, 7, 21 March 1921.
84 SWMF Executive Council Minutes, 26 February 1912.
85 SWMF Executive Council Minutes, 3 May 1926.
86 John Swan, cited in Hester Barron, *The 1926 Miners' Lockout: Meanings of Community in the Durham Coalfield* (Oxford: Oxford University Press), p. 122.
87 Barron, *The 1926 Miners' Lockout*, p. 122.
88 South Wales Miners' Federation, Council Meeting, 22 January 1927; Council Meeting, 21 February 1927.
89 South Wales Miners' Federation, Council Meeting, 31 December 1926, 18 January 1927.
90 Jones, *Cwmardy and We Live*, p. 268. See Chapter 6 for an extended discussion.
91 On the parliamentary strategies of miners' unions, see Clegg, Fox and Thomson, *A History of British Trade Unions since 1889*, pp. 239–49, 269–304, 364–422; Keith Gildart, 'Labour Politics', in Gildart, *Coal in Victorian Britain, Part II: Coal in Victorian Society, Volume 6*, pp. 385–94.
92 Clegg, Fox, and Thomson, *A History of British Trade Unions since 1889*, p. 271.
93 Clegg, Fox, and Thomson, *A History of British Trade Unions since 1889*, p. 51.
94 Gildart, 'Labour Politics', p. 385; Clegg, Fox and Thomson, *A History of British Trade Unions since 1889*, p. 273.
95 Gildart, 'Labour Politics', p. 388.
96 Gildart, 'Labour Politics', p. 388.
97 Gildart, 'Labour Politics', p. 390.
98 Howell, '"All or Nowt": The Politics of the MFGB', p. 40.
99 Howell, '"All or Nowt": The Politics of the MFGB', p. 39.
100 The Scottish TUC's Parliamentary Committee was also chaired by a miners' representative, Robert Smillie, for a time; see Angela Tuckett, *The Scottish Trades Union Congress: The First 80 Years* (Edinburgh: Mainstream Publishing, 1986), p. 42.
101 Ross M. Martin, *TUC: The Growth of a Pressure Group 1868–1976* (Oxford: Clarendon Press, 1980), p. 43; see also Clegg, Fox and Thomson, *A History of British Trade Unions since 1889*, p. 250.
102 Clegg, Fox and Thomson, *A History of British Trade Unions since 1889*, pp. 252–3.

103 Vicky Long, *The Rise and Fall of the Healthy Factory: The Politics of Industrial Health in Britain, 1914–60* (Basingstoke: Palgrave Macmillan, 2011), pp. 89–91.
104 Long, *The Rise and Fall of the Healthy Factory*, pp. 91, 96–7.
105 Long, *The Rise and Fall of the Healthy Factory*, p. 122.
106 Long, *The Rise and Fall of the Healthy Factory*, pp. 95–6.
107 Bufton and Melling, '"A Mere Matter of Rock"', p. 167.
108 Long, *The Rise and Fall of the Healthy Factory*, pp. 95–6; Bloor, 'The South Wales Miners Federation, Miners' Lung and the Instrumental Use of Expertise'.
109 On the coal employers and their parliamentary strategies, see Quentin Outram, 'Class Warriors: The Coalowners', in McIlroy, Campbell and Gildart, *Industrial Politics and the 1926 Mining Lockout*; Ronald Johnston, *Clydeside Capital, 1870–1920: A Social History of Employers* (East Linton: Tuckwell, 2000), esp. pp. 125–6.
110 *House of Commons Debates*, 31 March 1925 vol. 182 cc1245–1246.
111 This is one of the most important areas of miners' unions' campaigning on occupational health; see, for example, Paul Weindling, 'Linking Self Help and Medical Science: The History of Occupational Health', in Paul Weindling (ed.), *The Social History of Occupational Health* (London: Croom Helm, 1985), p. 17.
112 Michael Bloor, 'No Longer Dying for a Living: Collective Responses to Injury Risks in South Wales Mining Communities, 1900–47', *Sociology*, 36 (2002), p. 100. For more on the campaigning of miners' unions, see Arthur J. McIvor and Robert Johnston, *Miners' Lung: A History of Dust Disease in British Coal Mining* (Aldershot: Ashgate, 2007), pp. 74, 185–200.
113 Francis and Smith, *The Fed*, p. 439.
114 SWCC, MNANUM/3/1/1, Minutes of the SWMF Annual Conference, 1–2 July 1927.
115 Francis, 'Labour and Gender', pp. 196–7.
116 Lowri Newman, '"Providing an opportunity to exercise their energies": The role of Labour Women's Sections in Shaping Political Identities, South Wales, 1918–1939', in Ester Breitenbach and Pat Thane (eds), *Women and Citizenship in Britain and Ireland in the Twentieth Century: What Difference did the Vote Make?* (London: Continuum, 2010), p. 35.
117 Elizabeth Andrews, *A Woman's Work is Never Done*, edited by Ursula Masson (Dinas Powys: Honno, 2006 [1957]), p. 41. More generally, see Jones, 'Counting the Cost Of Coal'.
118 At the same conference at which Rathbone made this statement, Dr J. H. Jenkins, Medical Officer of Health for the Rhondda valleys in south Wales stated his opinion that childbirth was appromiately four times more dangerous than working underground in the coal industry; *Western Mail*, 13 January 1926, pp. 7, 10.
119 Newman, '"Providing an opportunity to exercise their energies"', p. 35.
120 National Library of Wales, MS18148E, Minute book of Mid-Rhondda Trades and Labour Council, 1 February 1918; 7 February 1918. For further evidence of the

importance of maternity and child welfare in Labour women's campaigns, see National Library of Wales, Labour Party Archives, Minutes of the East Glamorgan Women's (Labour) Advisory Council, 1933–44, passim.

121 Annmarie Hughes, '"The Politics of the Kitchen" and the Dissenting Domestics: The ILP, Labour Women and the Female "Citizens" of Inter-War Clydeside', *Scottish Labour History*, 34 (1999), p. 46.

122 Neil Evans and Dot Jones, '"A Blessing for the Miner's Wife": The Campaign for Pithead Baths in the South Wales Coalfield, 1908–1950', *Llafur*, 6:3 (1994), pp. 14–15.

123 Neil Evans and Dot Jones, '"To Help Forward the Great Work of Humanity": Women in the Labour Party in Wales', in Duncan Tanner, Chris Williams and Deian Hopkin (eds), *The Labour Party in Wales 1900–2000* (Cardiff: University of Wales Press, 2000), p. 220.

124 Robert Smillie and Frank Hodges, 'Introduction', in Edgar L. Chappell and J. A. Lovat-Fraser, *Pithead and Factory Baths* (Cardiff: Welsh Housing and Development Association, 1920), p. vii. For a similar perspective, see 'The Miner's Lot', *The Lancet*, 13 August 1938, p. 408.

125 Evans and Jones, '"A Blessing for the Miner's Wife"', p. 19.

126 Evans and Jones, '"A Blessing for the Miner's Wife"', pp. 20–1.

127 For an honourable exception, see McIvor and Johnston, *Miners' Lung*, pp. 237–307.

6

SITES OF STRUGGLE: DISABILITY IN WORKING-CLASS COALFIELDS LITERATURE

In Lewis Jones's dramatic retelling of the Tonypandy 'Riots' of 1910–11 in *Cwmardy* (1937), a young communist challenges the authorities to 'come and work the coal themselves if they want it. Let them sweat and pant till their bodies twist in knots as ours have.' He knows, however, that '[t]hey will do none of these things', and tells the striking men to take heart, for:

> While it is true our bodies belong to the pit, so also is it true that this makes us masters of the pit. It can't live without us. When we are not there to feed it with our flesh, to work life into it with our sweat and blood, it lies quiet like a paralysed thing that can do nothing but moan.[1]

The tributes of flesh and blood demanded by the monstrous mine allude to the routine injuries and accidents which maim, kill or at the very least promise disability as a none-too-distant part of the life course. But the central image of the mine as a 'paralysed thing' turns the normal relationship between mining and disability on its head by projecting a condition so often associated with industrial accidents onto the pit itself. Disability in the form of paralysis and 'moan[ing]' is imagined, rather conventionally, in terms of loss of agency and pain. Yet in this metaphor power lies with an organised collective of embodied workers, including – or especially – those whose bodies are 'twist[ed]' and impaired: by withholding labour they have agency and can 'paralyse' the monstrous machinery of capitalism. In this short, illustrative excerpt from Lewis Jones's novel, we see how the imagery of disability is embedded in metaphors of power, work and resistance; furthermore, by portraying the miner's body as 'twist[ed] in knots', the emblematic worker is a disabled worker.

As we have seen throughout this book, the fiction, poetry, ballads, autobiography and drama written in and about the coalfields offer valuable insights into the way disability was regarded and experienced in these communities.

The preceding chapters have turned to this literature as a historical source to help expand our understanding of disability in work, leisure, politics, welfare and the various medical encounters that went with impairment. Imaginative literature is, however, more than the sum of the scenes and episodes contained within it. To assess the cultural and political meaning(s) of disability in literature (and, by extension, to understand something about the communities from which this writing originates) we need to be aware that literature has its own traditions, formal constraints and innovations. Representations of disability within working-class coalfields writing not only interact with prevailing community understandings of disability, they must also negotiate literary form and convention, imagery and language. As literary theorist Ato Quayson points out, 'not only do the characters [in any given text] organize their perceptions of one another on the basis of given symbolic assumptions, but as fictional characters they are themselves also woven out of a network of symbols and interact through a symbolic relay of signs'.[2] To study the 'network of symbols' and 'relay of signs' in literature is to recognise that understanding the meaning of disability in a text requires looking beyond what happens or what is said (events, dialogue or even plot are of only partial significance). Rather, we must work at the more intricate and sophisticated level of language (signs) and systems of representation (the network of symbols, metaphors, images, textual conventions and cultural assumptions) which carry both pre-existing and new meanings in any literary text. This final chapter, then, delves more deeply into the formal structures and recurring tropes – the images, set pieces and metaphors – in coalfields literature. In a deliberate departure from preceding chapters, it foregrounds the tools and methods of the literary and cultural critic, especially those literary theories developed by disability scholars. We show that while it has been overlooked in literary studies of working-class industrial literature, disability is in fact central to some of the most iconic works of this period.

Working-class writing 1900–48: a brief literary history

This book as a whole covers the period from 1880 to 1948. Late Victorian coalfields literature is fascinating in its own right and we explore some of the representations of disability found in nineteenth-century writing in preceding chapters. In this final chapter, however, we concentrate on the working-class voices which emerged in the twentieth century. In his seminal lecture on 'The Welsh Industrial Novel', Raymond Williams describes the development of industrial writing from early outsider perspectives that portrayed the industrial landscape as a 'panorama of Hell' and towards an insider narrative. That is, the 'movement towards describing what it is like to live in hell, and slowly, as the disorder becomes an habitual order, what it is like to get used to it, to grow up in it, to see it as home'.³ While Williams's account overlooks important examples of industrial literature, particularly by women, it is undoubtedly the case that a new proletarian literature, much of it from the south Wales coalfield and almost all of it written by men, came to dominate and define industrial literature in the first half of the twentieth century.⁴ Fiction, drama and verse poured from the pens of men who had worked as miners or who had been raised in mining communities: writers such as Joe Corrie, James C. Welsh, Tom Hanlin, Harold Heslop, Jack Lawson, John Swan, Sid Chaplin, Lewis Jones, Rhys Davies, Idris Davies, Jack Jones, Glyn Jones, Gwyn Jones, Gwyn Thomas and Bert Coombes.⁵ Coalfields drama by playwrights such as J. O. Francis, Ruth Dodds,⁶ Jack Jones, Emlyn Williams and Joe Corrie also emerged as a major form in the twentieth century, particularly in Wales and Scotland, where it was often performed by amateur as well as professional groups.⁷ In the work produced by these writers disability is generally shown to be the product of capitalist systems, poor industrial conditions and limited welfare provision. Unlike much of the Victorian literature, which attaches moral or religious overtones to impairment, disability is portrayed as both indiscriminate and ubiquitous.

The rise of working-class socialist writers during the 1920s and 1930s was supported by the development of politically left-leaning publishers,⁸ though a buoyant market for industrial writing in the 1930s⁹ that meant authors were also picked up by mainstream publishers.¹⁰ Coalfields writing from Britain in this period thus had a large, often international, audience. Being published in the mainstream could have a politically moderating effect on the final version. The Hunwick-born miner-writer Harold Heslop reported that his novel, *The Gate of a Strange Field* (1929), was cut by about a quarter and the majority of the 'anti-capitalist references [were] deleted'.¹¹ Even left-wing publishers found some texts too unpalatable, and Gollancz rejected Gwyn Thomas's *Sorrow for Thy Sons*, which had been submitted in response to a competition in 1937: 'Gollancz said he liked the fervour of the book, but its facts were so raw, its wrath so pitiless, its commercial prospects were nil unless he could issue a free pair of asbestos underdrawers to very reader. So he had to say no to publication.'¹² Not all interwar writing was by working-class writers. A. J. Cronin's best-selling *The Citadel* (1937) was published by Gollancz, adapted into an Oscar-winning film in 1938 and credited by some as having a significant impact on promoting public support for the establishment of the NHS.¹³ The novel – about a doctor's dissatisfactions with both colliery owners and the compensation system – abounds with images of illness and disability, including a striking portrayal of the industrial landscape of south Wales itself as a 'strange, disfigured country'.¹⁴ One of the most commercially successful novels¹⁵ was Richard Llewellyn's *How Green Was My Valley* (1939), pithily described by Raymond Williams as 'the export version of the Welsh industrial experience'.¹⁶ It contains a textbook version of 'overcoming' disability through willpower and Christian faith, as discussed below. It has never been out of print and was widely translated and distributed, no doubt helped by the 1941 John Ford film, which won five Oscars. Despite the dominance of these stories of individual medical heroism (Cronin) and dubious nostalgia (Llewellyn),[17] several of the more realist and proletarian novels by working-class writers were very successful. For instance, Harold Heslop's debut novel, *Goaf*[18] (in which nystagmus is represented as the 'price' the miner is 'compelled to pay'[19]), first appeared in the Soviet Union as *Pod vlastu uglya* [Under the Sway of Coal] in 1926,[20] selling half a million copies in the cheap edition,[21] before its publication in Britain in 1934 to widespread acclaim in the press.[22]

Of course, publishers issue contracts with a particular audience in mind, and this audience was not necessarily located primarily in the coalfields. An awareness of, perhaps even a goal of reaching, an audience beyond the communities from which they came is evident in the form and narrative focus of the novels of this period. Heavily invested in realism for political reasons (though not necessarily documentary or social realism), working-class writers aimed to portray miners' lives with as much veracity as possible. Personal experience of the subject matter was considered an important marker of authenticity. Bert Coombes famously argued that 'the dust should still be in his throat as he was writing – it seemed to me – then it would be authentic'.[23] Autobiographical writing flourished, with miner-writers such as James Lawson, Harold Heslop and Jack Jones drawing heavily on their own lives in their fiction. Yet it was not all a matter of life underpinning fiction. Coombes's own memoir, *These Poor Hands: The Autobiography of a Miner Working in South Wales* (1939), which remains a major reference point to this day (including in this volume), itself began life as a novel and bears traces of this genesis.[24] As we shall see, realism and autobiography were not the only modes by which writers sought to capture coalfields experiences of injury, incapacitation and disability. Experiments with modernist and surrealist forms became increasingly important, often containing within them a seam of dark humour. We look at these later in the chapter, but first we must turn to the dominant, if diverse, conventions of realism in coalfields writing.

Disability and realism

Realism means many things in literary criticism, but, according to Raymond Williams, in the industrial novel realism rests on the 'assumption' that:

> the lives of individuals, however intensely or personally realized, are not just influenced but in certain crucial ways formed by social relations. Thus industrial

work, and its characteristic places and communities, are not just a new background: a new 'setting' for a story. In the true industrial novel they are seen as formative ... The working society – actual work, actual relations, an actual and visibly altered place – is in the industrial novel central ... because in these working communities it is a trivial fantasy to suppose that these general and pressing conditions are for long or even at all separable from the immediate and the personal.[25]

Social and industrial relations in the 'true industrial novel' (by which Williams means a realist text that reveals 'hidden or underlying forces or movements'[26]) are shown to shape the lives of fictional characters. In turn, these characters' lives and the events in which they are involved in various ways represent the forces of work, capital and history which affect them. Indeed, some writers, including the communist activist Lewis Jones, saw fiction, in his case a form of socialist realism, as the best way to reveal the complexity of coalfield life as influenced by historical movements and social relations. In his foreword to *Cwmardy*, Jones explains:

> the full meaning of life in the Welsh mining areas could be expressed for the general reader more truthfully and vividly, if treated imaginatively, than by any amount of statistical and historical research. What I have set out to do, therefore, is to 'novelise' (if I may use the term) a phase of working-class history.[27]

Similar claims have been made for the importance of realist writing in representing a social model of disability, as theorists David T. Mitchell and Sharon L. Snyder point out: 'Realism promoted a more direct depiction of the political reality of disabled characters, from architecture to attitudes. Realistic depictions, argued social realism, will offer familiarity with an experience that has been understood as thoroughly alien.'[28] It is, of course, an oversimplification to portray literary realism as offering an unmediated and 'authentic' window on the world. Literary realism is carefully and selectively constructed, while, as Tobin Siebers argues, there is a 'temptation to view disability and pain as more real than their opposites. The perception already exists that broken bodies and things are more real than anything else.'[29] That is, the damaged or painful body seems more insistently corporeal: the disabled body is a visible body, while the non-disabled body, according to Maren Tova Linett, appropriates 'the neutral condition of invisibility'.[30] Coalfields realism tends to foreground broken bodies, sometimes in contrast to sculpted, strong or hypermasculine bodies.

The presence of disability in literature is, of course, much more than a 'realistic' (or otherwise) portrayal of impairment and its social consequences. Indeed, disability critics have pointed out that, while disability is a ubiquitous presence in literature, it tends most often to function as a symbol of something else – a versatile metaphor or plot device rather than an exploration of disability itself. Mitchell and Snyder argue that disability is a 'crutch' upon which texts rely for their 'representative power, disruptive potentiality, and analytical insight'.[31] Working-class literature of the coalfields depicts impairment as a product of industry and therefore a ubiquitous and 'realistic' lived experience, while simultaneously using disability as a versatile symbol by which to expose and contest the workings of industrial and capitalist society.

One function of disability and disabled characters in coalfield literature is to act as a nexus via which a range of different forces – economic, social, political, medical – are brought into contact or revealed to underpin the wider social and economic 'disqualification' of the industrial working class.[32] Writing about nineteenth-century 'critical realism',[33] Georg Lukács identifies the importance of a 'typical' character, a 'type' that interacts with different forces within the text:

> The 'centre' figure need not represent an 'average man' but is rather the product of a particular social and personal environment. The problem is to find a central figure in whose life all the important extremes in the world of the novel converge and around whom a complete world with all its vital contradictions can be organized.[34]

This typical figure, as Moyra Haslett explains, is often 'portrayed as passive rather than active, played on by events rather than mastering them', but they bring other characters and factions into contact.[35] Lukács's 'typical' figure is not merely a stereotype, as Fredric Jameson points out; rather, 'the "typical" was what ultimately registered the subterranean movements of History itself'.[36] While coalfields novels are in fundamental ways very different to the nineteenth-century models of which Lukács is thinking, in coalfields literature the impaired worker is often, by several measures, a 'typical' working-class figure around whom economic, medical, political, historical and social narratives converge. Indeed, congenital, work- or age-related disability itself is a locus of meaning through which different social and political forces are made apparent. In this chapter, then, we propose that the person with disabilities in coalfields literature can be seen as the paradigmatic citizen of the colliery districts.

An example of the disabled character as a 'typical' character can be found in the miner known as Big Jim in Lewis Jones's *Cwmardy*. Big Jim's experiences reveal the wider socio-historic and economic contexts in which the characters move. Originally from Welsh-speaking, agrarian Wales, this archetypal big hewer has proudly served as a soldier in the Boer War and, later, the Great War; thus industrial capitalism is shown to operate hand in hand with both imperialism and mechanised total war. Most significantly, from the perspective of our contention that disability is a condition emblematic of the industrial worker, Big Jim's life course over *Cwmardy* and its sequel, *We Live* (1939), exemplifies the *inevitability* of disability as a consequence of mining, due to overwork, lack of economic security and dangerous conditions. Facing premature physical decline and in financially precarious circumstances due to repeated strikes and lockouts, Big Jim struggles to breathe as a result of dust inhalation and is stooped and unsteady from joint-related injuries and strain. The working life of this foot-soldier of capitalist imperialism leads ultimately to physical impairment; disability is presented as the result of his loyal service.[37]

It is not surprising that Lewis Jones and other politically aware writers responded to the commonplace impairments of the coalfields by creating emblematic disabled characters. The figure of the impaired, maimed or 'stunted'[38] wage-labourer within capitalism was a material and symbolic presence from Marx onwards. Marx not only lists disabled people among the 'ragged' paupers who, after orphaned children and the aged, make up the lowest tier of surplus labour, those 'victims of industry, whose number increases with the growth of dangerous machinery, of mines, chemical works, etc.';[39] crucially, he uses disability as a metaphor for *all* industrial workers. The specialisation brought about by division of labour, which capitalism then exploits, 'converts the worker into a crippled monstrosity' where 'the individual himself is divided up' by repetitive and 'automatic motor' tasks.[40] Despite this interest in the fragmented and disabled body in Marx, B. J. Gleeson claims that 'the issue of disablement has been largely neglected in the socialist tradition.'[41] While this may be true in academic studies, it is certainly not true of socialist or communist coalfield writers.

Realist coalfields literature overwhelmingly represents impairment and disability as the product of the material conditions of industrial life, while using disability symbolically to represent the struggles of a working class facing catastrophic levels of unemployment and consequent material deprivation during the interwar period.[42] Disability is thus both an authentic and central element of coalfields experience and a metaphor through which the working classes are presented as 'disqualified'. But working-class coalfields literature, and socialist realism in particular, indicates that the experience of disability may be transformed by socialist organisation(s). To put it slightly differently, the condition of disability in realist coalfields literature operates along vectors of economic disqualification and physical (and mental) impairment; it is alleviated by social solutions, including mutualism and solidarity.

Normalcy, disability and the life course

If disability was an expected, near-universal part of a worker's life course (be they male or female[43]) and if, as we argued earlier, the paradigmatic worker is an impaired worker, coalfields literature implicitly invites us to reconsider what we consider to be 'normal'. The concept of 'normalcy' and its relationship to disability has been a rich ground for disability theory, showing as it does how the apparently invisible 'able' body is reliant on constructing the 'disabled' body as aberrant 'other'. Lennard Davis introduces the idea of normalcy thus:

> Disability is not an object – a woman with a cane – but a social process that intimately involves everyone who has a body and lives in the world of the senses. Just as the conceptualisation of race, class, and gender shapes the lives of those who are not black, poor or female, so the concept of disability regulates the bodies of those who are 'normal'. In fact the very concept of normalcy by which most people (by definition) shape their existence is in fact tied inexorably to the concept of disability, or rather, the concept of disability is a function of normalcy. Normalcy and disability are part of the same system.[44]

The concept of normalcy is taken more explicitly into the realm of ideology in Rosemarie Garland Thomson's formulation of the 'normate', a term which names 'the veiled subject position of cultural self, the figure outlined by the array of deviant others whose marked bodies shore up the normate's boundaries. The term *normate* usefully designates the social figure through which people can represent themselves as definitive human beings.'[45] The normate, broadly constructed, is white, male, able-bodied, educated, middle class and in employment. While the shadow of the normate is discernible in coalfields literature (sometimes in the text as doctor or minister, or as imagined reader), the norm in the context of the coalfields is, arguably, impairment and – in the depression years – widespread 'disqualification' through unemployment, poverty and disability.

Although still bearing ideologically on ideas of valuable masculinity, the characteristics to which 'normalcy' generally refer are challenged by the specific conditions of coalfields life. Realist novels address this by foregrounding the accelerated ageing which is an expected part of the life course of men and women, and thus showing disability to be a near-universal expectation. This typical life course is established by stock scenes and characters portrayed at pivotal moments: the boy's first day down the pit; the young woman contemplating marriage; the ground-down wife and mother struggling to feed a family on inadequate funds; the weak or worn-out miner; the man killed or maimed in the prime of life. As Edward Slavishak has said of nineteenth-century Pennsylvanian colliers, men operated in a 'culture of risk in which every minute might be their last and in which every worker's able-bodied prime preceded a future life of disability.'[46] The decline of Big Jim, over the course of *Cwmardy* and *We Live*, from gigantic hewer in the prime of life to an increasingly disabled – yet still working – miner exemplifies the normal life course, from vigorous breadwinner to a bowed and breathless worker.

The process of decline and premature ageing[47] begins directly on entry to the pit in childhood: 'round here they are only children till they are twelve. Then they are sent away over the hills to the mine, and in one week they are old men,' remarks one character in Emlyn Williams's play *The Corn is Green* (1938).[48] In James C. Welsh's novel *The Underworld* (1920), Robert is warned by his mother: 'look how quick a miner turns auld, Rob. He's done at forty years auld ... but meenisters an' schoolmaisters, an' folk o' that kin', leeve a gey lang while.'[49] In the same novel, the ageing effects of the industry are conveyed via the assembled bodies of miners at a union meeting: 'eyes glad with expectancy, and eyes dulled with long years of privations and brutal labour; limbs young and supple and full of energy, and limbs stiff and sore, crooked and maimed.'[50] The structure of the sentence, with its list of juxtapositions, holds up a distorted mirror to the men: youth will rapidly become age; health and strength will be dulled, maimed and broken. In another James C. Welsh novel, *The Morlocks* (1924), the description of a man as 'old' is qualified in terms of diminished life expectancy under pit conditions:

> An old man, named Wattie Wotherspoon, acted as bottomer on the shift, as such jobs, supposed to be easy and having light duties, were generally held by old men.
>
> Not that Wotherspoon was so very old in years; for as he himself said, he 'wasna a deidly auld man'; but owing to the effects of black damp, coal dust, and insufficient air, in the days before legislation was seriously, and in a way more humanely, applied to coal-mining, he had suffered, and paid the price of coal in giving years of his life.[51]

Women – working in houses that serviced the mines – were also subject to early physical decline. Indeed, as Ben Curtis and Steven Thompson point out, 'physical impairment among women servicing the coal industry as wives and mothers was ... unusually high.'[52] Coalfields writers were alert to this, and a prematurely aged woman's body is a recurring image in interwar coalfields writing.[53] These 'breaking' bodies are often introduced at the start of the fiction in order to set the wider social scene, drawing on well-established conventions of using female figures as allegories; here they symbolise the privations of coalfield communities as a whole.

The first glimpse of Siân in the first chapter of *Cwmardy* is typical: 'she removed the shawl that hid her haggard face and big-boned body, with its slightly stooping shoulders. Care-dulled eyes made her look older than she really was.'[54] Premature age and the disabilities that go with it are the result of women's service of industry – reproduction, and also the cooking, cleaning, washing and care of the men who work the pit, not to mention the stress and hunger of managing a home in impoverished conditions during strikes or lockouts. In the first chapter of another Welsh novel, *Times Like These* (1936) by Gwyn Jones, Polly Biesty, though

> not quite so old as her husband, [was] in the sad years called 'breaking.' It is the aptest word for the state – when her body, like a hard-worked machine, was at every point giving way to strain. Her hair was white, beautiful, a good setting for her pleasant, care-marked face. She moved heavily, almost lurchingly, when things were at their worst with her.[55]

Lennard Davis argues that 'the imperatives of industrialism and capitalism redefined the body ... the human body came to be seen as an extension of the factory machinery.'[56] Polly's domestic labour is explicitly portrayed as industrial work via the imagery of mechanisation; her lurching body is the rather more human consequence of servicing the industrial machine.

The overlap between industrial and domestic labour which results in inevitable disability, and often an early death, is perhaps most forcefully portrayed in 'Nightgown' (1942), a short story by Rhys Davies. The plot concerns a woman who becomes progressively impaired in the service of her husband and five 'big' sons with ravenous appetites. Feeding the men while starving herself in order to buy a satin nightgown that is far beyond her means, she is slowly, metaphorically, devoured by her service to them (and, by extension, the colliery). Dressed in men's cast-offs, her body starts to mimic that of a worn-out collier. She goes about her work 'in a slower fashion, her face closed and her body shorter, because her legs had gone bowed'.[57] As we have seen, bowed legs are a deformation of the body particularly associated with mining (see Chapter 2). The accompanying aches which she feels in her failing body are similarly portrayed in the language of a mining accident: 'She felt as if the wheels of several coal waggons had gone over her body, though there was no feeling in her legs.' Eventually, while cooking a meal for the men on the range, she collapses and her 'black-faced' body is discovered by the men on their return.[58] The blackness is from the soot on the frying pan, but recalls the distinctive face of the collier covered in coal dust.

Broken and disabled female bodies portrayed in coalfields writing literally and figuratively represent the relentless toil and poverty of all industrial workers. In their representations of prematurely aged women and men, coalfields writers both 'normalise' the incidence of disability in middle age (that is, they show that it is the usual and expected life course in these communities) and provide a 'diagnosis' – that disability is caused by poverty and overwork – which is, it is implied, common to all working-class people in the coalfields. Rather than being the aberration, a debilitated and impaired body is the paradigmatic body of coalfields literature. This doesn't necessarily undermine the theory that disability and normalcy produce each other, because disability is pictured here both as 'normal' (in that sense of ubiquitous) *and* as a symptom of social injustice. It is a sign of the unjust capitalist system which needs to be challenged. Yet, in the universe of the fiction the relationship between disability and normalcy is not wholly oppositional; rather, there is an implicit acknowledgement that we are all only *temporarily* able-bodied. By making disability a normal part of the life course, coalfields literature reveals that the borders between 'able-bodied' and disabled are both blurred and easily crossed.

Disability humour

Representations of disability are, as we glimpsed at the start of this chapter, closely bound up with power struggles. In coalfields literature the comedy of disability – or disability humour – is used to expose and disrupt power relations. Of our time, Dan Goodley and Geert van Hove claim: 'Disability is the last taboo for comedy, parody and pastiche.'[59] This was not the case in the early twentieth century, and much coalfields writing includes comic scenes which revolve around disability where the person with the disability is frequently the wit rather than the butt of the joke. An impairment is deployed to confound or outwit the able-bodied or 'normate', and in its later form a dry, often bitter, humour uses the 'incongruity' of disability to drive home the deprivations of coalfields society.

Novels of the north-east of England in particular draw on the trope of the 'canny collier', a clever, abrasive trickster character who outwits authority.[60] A colliery worker with a wooden leg, who knows he cannot join up, tricks a recruiting officer out of the King's shilling in Ramsay Guthrie's *Kitty Fagan: A Romance of Pit Life* (1900). In the same novel an 'infirm' and deaf miner who is being evicted for being a union member uses his inability to hear to delay the bailiffs who are legally required to read an eviction notice. Towards the end of the first lengthy reading, Neddy interrupts to ask a friend 'what's he jabberin' aboot.'[61] On the second reading he asks '[a]re ye speakin', mister … [b]ecause if ye are, an' it's onythin particular-like, ye'll have to speak up a wee bittie.'[62] On the third reading he pretends to be delighted and thanks the bailiff for offering him a job at the pit. Thus the canny Durham miner inverts the ableist humour which laughs at miscommunication arising from a hearing impairment, to turn the tables on the bailiff.

Current understanding of disability humour often turns on questions of who is making the joke, on whether this is an 'insider' joke made by people with impairments to others in the know, or perhaps intended to puncture ableist assumptions. Often such jokes waver on a knife edge even when the person telling the joke is themselves disabled. Robert 'Bob' McLeod (1876–1958), from Musselburgh in Scotland, was a poet and song-writer with impairments resulting from a mining accident. He used humour in his writing and performances in ways which both challenge and sometimes repeat prevailing prejudices about disability, convalescence and ideas of 'malingering'. When Bob McLeod's leg and hip were crushed and his foot partially amputated he took up writing poems and songs during the year he spent in hospital. One humorous poem, set in hospital at Christmas time, called 'Takkin' a Rest', turns disability into a 'rest':

> I'm expectin' tae get oot then,
> But my feet they will be tender;
> So ye'll hae tae gae up tae the smith,
> And order a little fender.[63]

> The doctor says I'll need it much,
> For my leg is a little shorter;
> I tellt him it was short before,
> He said Mac, you're a corker.

> So freends, aa dear ye'll think I'm queer,
> But I hae done my best;
> I've just noo got my paarich,[64]
> So I'm gaun tae hae a rest.[65]

As well as a reference to his enforced idleness, the title of this poem, 'Takkin' a Rest', is both a satirical reference to the lack of rest afforded to overworked miners and an allusion to the suspicion of malingering which could attend compensation payouts (see Chapter 3). In performances of his work, much of it written in the same distinctive voice of a male collier,[66] McLeod often appeared in drag, a decision which his daughter claimed was in part an attempt to hide a 'crippled leg'.[67] This complex interplay of disability, comedy and cross-dressing suggests the flexibility and intersectionality of disability humour, which would repay a longer study than is attempted here.

In the politically charged interwar period, when the dangers of the mines were equalled by a debilitating economic depression, a bitter, sardonic humour reached its peak in the satirical wit of Gwyn Thomas. Humour dependent on dark irony became 'one of the characteristic notes of working-class writing in the 1930s', according to Simon Dentith, who identifies 'a particular tone of voice, which can be described provisionally as one of sardonic worldly wisdom, characterized often by ironic understatement or by the choice of telling anecdote'.[68] This idiom was, according to Dentith, 'a characteristic resource of the speech communities from which the novelists emerged.'⁶⁹ It is a claim corroborated by some of its major writers. Sid Chaplin described the Durham coalfields as 'an oral society'⁷⁰ and Gwyn Thomas identified a similar working-class south Wales oral tradition to which he attributed his humour: 'I think my humour shows the way in which the intellect of the working-class [sic] might have developed their world.'⁷¹ Thomas's humour repeatedly riffs upon vectors of class, disability and poverty,⁷² and he sees it as arising from the conditions in which he grew up: 'there was enough incongruity between the way my people lived in the Rhondda of my early manhood, and the way in which they would have wanted to live, to have nourished at least 10,000 humourists of the first rank.'⁷³ Thomas claimed that the vast majority of Welsh writers 'are the survivors of great historic mutilations, and like most survivors our spirit and pens are erratic'.⁷⁴ This embodied metaphor of 'mutilations' (first industrialisation, followed by the crushing economic depression of the interwar years) is suggestive of the way Thomas sees disability as part of the condition of the depressed industrial areas. In his devastating one-liners the physical impairments of colliery work are aligned with the economic deprivations of low pay: 'His father's toil had been so excessive as to make him stoop like a victim of curvature. That had been just as well, because his father's wages were so low it would have been impossible to count them standing up straight.'⁷⁵ Notice that it is poor pay that undermines this man's dignity, not his stooped body, though the disabled body stands for the status of the exploited working man. Thomas's humour is not one of resignation, however, but of resistance: his humour gave him an idiom in which to address the experience – embodied, economic, political – of interwar south Wales. Dai Smith argues that Thomas's 'key discovery was that it was through humour that he could transcend the limitation of that realism which, by its bogus claim that to name things is to describe them, had entombed so much proletarian reality within its gloomy documentation'. As Smith points out, 'the laughter was always a prelude to thought, never a release from responsibility'.⁷⁶

Modernism from the coalfields

Thomas's humour, which edges into the grotesque, the gothic and the surreal, has much in common with other modernist strains of coalfield writing.⁷⁷ Indeed, to represent realism as the only or most apposite literary form of working-class coalfields communities is to tell only part of the story. In the late 1930s and 1940s writers experimented with modernism, including oral or folk forms. Modernism's interest in fragmentation of the self and its challenge to totalising or linear narratives has been seen as pertinent to disability, while representation of disability demanded a reconsideration of form, voice and authenticity. Moreover, modernist representations of disability take nothing for granted. Ato Quayson, in his typology of disability in literature, has described 'disability as enigma or hermeneutical impasse',[78] and this is foregrounded in modernist writing. In *Bodies of Modernism*, Marven Tova Linett characterises 'modernism's understanding of disability not as a given, but as a question'.[79] In modernist coalfields literature disability is linked to images of fragmentation and surreal, often comic, dislocation and absurdity; in its more sombre moments, the questions raised are often connected to religion or metaphysics.

'Hangman's Assistant' (1946) by David Alexander[80] is a fine example of coalfields modernism which fuses the comic and the surreal. The characters in this short story influenced by Franz Kafka are assailed by apparently intractable and inexplicable forces; disability, by turns uncanny and absurd, is an important element in all this. Arriving at work, the protagonist, Twm Pant, is told by the under-manager that he is to assist with a hanging. Once he realises that this is not 'a leg pull' he demurs, citing his conditions of employment: 'Light pick and shovel work, that's what my certificate says. I've got silicosis and hanging a man is outside my grade. I'll take it to the lodge committee.'[81] Conceding defeat, the under-manager sends another man, Dai, instead while Twm is made to empty a barrel of something unpleasant and dubious (what, we do not learn). The hangman – a sinister and shapeshifting figure – arrives, limping as he makes his way towards Twm down the railway track. He terrifies Twm by briefly turning into a 'huge yellow tiger'[82] before heading off to the stables to hang Ianto Lewis for an unspecified crime: 'I don't know – something he did about twenty years ago. They just found out about it.'[83] Dai, Ianto and the hangman disappear into the building and, one soft thud later, Twm assumes the deed is done. But soon Ianto emerges from the stables 'as if nothing had happened'[84] and walks away (an ironic nod to the trope of the resurrected miner, perhaps, of which more below). The hangman emerges, spots Dai this time, and shouts 'There he is – there he is!'[85] whereupon Dai runs for his life with the hangman and his noose in pursuit. The story ends as 'they bec[o]me merged into the grey-black mass of the slagheap beyond the trees.'[86]

Banal bureaucracy, unexplained persecution and a sense of guilt and entrapment pervade the story, suggesting the unseen hand of an inexorable force. This, coupled with Alexander's absurd and sinister use of comedy, recalls Milan Kundera's assessment of Kafka that 'A joke is only a joke if you're outside the bowl; by contrast, the Kafkan takes us inside, into the *guts* of a joke, into the horror of the comic.'[87] The comedy and the horror in 'Hangman's Assistant' derive in large part from the presence of disability in the story. The initial exchange between Twm, the labourer, and the 'under-manager' who is assigning tasks is mediated by their respective disabilities. Twm, as we have seen, has a 'certificate' which specifies the type of work he can do, given his siliocosis (light surface work was often assigned to miners with impairments); thus he is able to use the threat of the lodge (the miners' union) to demand his rights. The under-manager is a figure of fun, 'furious' at Twm's response, he is also 'full of silicosis', his frustration causing him to choke: 'His face became purple, then blue, and finally settled back to its normal grey.'[88] From comedy, disability turns to horror with the arrival of the hangman: "Then coming down the track from the powder magazine he saw a man with a limp.' On closer inspection Twm realises that this asymmetrical gait is due to the man's walking one foot on the rail sleeper and the other in the gap. But the suggestion of disability is reinforced in the ensuing description: 'He walked as if he had one short leg, swaying from side to side like a rocking ship.'[89] In some Christian iconography and folk tale the devil is portrayed with a limp, while in Greek and Christian mythology lameness is connected both with punishment and with negative moral qualities.[90] The sinister purpose of the limping hangman certainly evokes a sense of foreboding and dread in Twm. The lopsided gait and the shapeshifting qualities of the hangman are also reproduced in the style of the writing. The swaying of the hangman in particular mimics the 'lack of symmetry and formal balance'[91] which Tyrus Miller ascribes to late modernist texts and which Linett sees reflected in the 'lack of symmetry and balance ... in the bodies of characters'[92] in modernist writing's concern with deformity (of body and art). A comic play on the officiousness of petty management and organised labour, the story is also a modernist retelling of the superstitious sense of the inescapable and inscrutable 'fate' which hangs over the individual miner and the community as a whole in coalfields culture.[93]

Not all coalfields modernism was as surreal or absurd as Alexander's European-influenced comedy. Writers searching for a way of getting closer to the language as well as the experiences of their communities experimented with finding a form suited to the oral traditions of coalfields culture. Modernist writers had long been fascinated by oral storytellers, including Irish, Welsh and Scottish authors James Joyce, Caradoc Evans and Lewis Grassic Gibbon, who incorporated the idiom and qualities of speech and folk tale into their distinctive narrative voices. An industrial branch of oral-modernist writing was pursued by the versatile Durham short story writer and poet Sid Chaplin.[94] His interest in orality was to find an 'authentic' (yet not necessarily realist) mode of writing to create a working-class narrative that did justice to the collective voice of a people and their way of life. Recalling his immersion in an oral mining culture, Chaplin wrote:

> Later I discovered the reality behind it all; the dust and darkness, the laming and maiming, the bitter waters and blood and sweat that mingles with comradeship on the coalface. And a pitman with his lamp face down in the dust so that his face was in the shade said, 'Ah mind, Ah mind once ...' All this becomes part of the pattern of my living, and the pattern of my stories.

I am the spokesman, the story-teller. The stories themselves bear my signature, but by the nature of that pattern they belong to many people.[95]

Here, disability – 'the laming and maiming' – is closely tied up with the 'pattern' of Chaplin's stories of the pit. The miner's lamp lying 'face down' in the dust is suggestive of the embodied miner himself, while the tableau foregrounds the senses so often invoked in descriptions of the mine. The darkness in which the representative voice holds additional power mimics blindness – a recurring image to describe conditions underground – while the attention given to the miner's voice suggests not only the importance of a collective memory but also the primacy and sensitivity of hearing in the mines that was a crucial early warning system for roof falls. Chaplin's stories draw on a particularly male form of folk story imbued 'with the essential inner core in the talk of men going to and from the coal',[96] although he also uses the fragmented perspective of children and acknowledges women storytellers, such as the source for his story about a rebellious miner's daughter 'What Katie Did' (1946).[97] Far from being the preserve of a metropolitan elite, then, coalfields modernism is attuned to a collective working-class narrative tradition. Modernist writers also drew heavily on that other oral tradition of the coalfields: Christian religion.

Resurrections: Christianity and disability

The miner resurrected is a recurring image in a range of coalfields literature, including some of Chaplin's short stories.[98] Resurrection, and the miner as a Christ-like martyr, use suffering and sacrifice to dignify and magnify the injuries and disabilities sustained by colliers. One such story, 'The Kiss' (1936) by Glyn Jones, in which a collier comes back from the dead to make contact with his maimed brother, offers a complex example of the miner-as-Christ. The protagonist seems to have been buried in a roof fall and emerges from this tomb after a few days bearing wounds akin to stigmata: the 'centres of his palms worn into holes'.[99] The resurrected collier goes home to a brother whose hand has been crushed and swollen out of all recognition. The man unwinds the mass of bandages 'with great care and tenderness',[100] slowly uncovering a hand that is 'a shapeless black mass of stinking flesh,'[101] to the horror of their anguished mother, who cannot bear to witness the injury uncovered. His 'love-acts' are described as a 'Eucharistic task'[102] and the story concludes with the resurrected collier '[kissing] the putrid flesh of his brother's hand'.[103] It is an act of love and union and a bearing of witness which transcends the revulsion and horror inspired in the men's mother (and the reader) by the crushed hand.[104] He refuses his brother's abjection in a symbolic act of inclusion and acceptance.

Christianity, as outlined by Nancy Eiesland in *The Disabled God*, has not always been an inclusive creed. Taking as a paradigmatic example her own exclusion from Eucharist by ministers who, though well-meaning, did not accommodate the physically disabled within the ritual of the sacrament, Eiesland outlines the stigmatisation and disempowering narratives of traditional Christian theology. Yet, in medieval Christianity the disabled or impaired body could be seen as 'an *alter Christus* (another Christ) – that is, an individual who truly embodied the suffering of Christ'.[105] Eiesland explores a symbolism in which Christ's incarnate corporeality and crucifixion are seen as proof of God's love and acceptance of *all* bodies, including the disabled body: 'The disabled God is not only the One from heaven but the revelation of true personhood, underscoring the reality that full personhood is fully compatible with the experience of disability'.[106] In the nonconformist traditions of the north-east England and south Wales coalfields in particular, Christianity was an important if waning force in the early twentieth century (as discussed in Chapter 4). The suffering and disabled miner as Christ is a recurring image in coalfields literature and art, and not limited to modernist forms. Miners' hands bear stigmata-like injuries, as we saw in 'The Kiss', sometimes directly connected to working conditions, as in the wounds received through use of a bad shovel in Chaplin's *The Thin Seam* (1950). Christ himself is reimagined as a collier in some texts: the poet Idris Davies pictures 'Jesus crawling in the local mine'[107] and imagines how 'embarrassed' the ministers of 'Bethel' would be 'if Christ / Came with pick and shovel to the colliery yard / Seeking a stent ....'[108] Here, the 'true' Christ is aligned with the workers against an organised religion perceived to have betrayed the workers, a position not uncommon in the work of socialist writers.[109]

Disability was important in this rivalry between Christianity and socialism or communism that was played out in modernist, realist and romantic coalfields writing in the 1930s and 1940s. Gwyn Thomas saw nonconformity as a conservative rather than radical force, framing the chapel as a bystander to protest marches in *Sorrow for Thy Sons* or in league with the coalowners in his modernist-grotesque novella *The Dark Philosophers*. In both, the chapel is responsible for exacerbating poverty which in turn results in disability, illness or death, as discussed in Chapter 4. In stark and revealing contrast, the chapel enjoys a prominent place in the south Wales colliery district portrayed in the wildly popular 'historical' novel *How Green Was My Valley*. A brilliantly nostalgic and highly problematic epic set in an imagined south Wales mining valley where nonconformity is the glue that holds society together, its treatment of disability is tied to the clichéd trope of 'overcoming'. The young hero, Huw, is confined to bed for five years following an accident in a river. Over months and painful years, he learns to walk again, healed by the nonconformist minister who sets a regime of increasingly challenging walks on one of the iconic hillsides so important to Welsh industrial novels.[110] In the Hollywood version directed by John Ford, the lengthy recovery is condensed into one short scene on a mountain strewn with daffodils (one of Wales's national emblems), which symbolically links the nation with the restoration of an able(ist) body. In the novel, the minister tells Huw 'never mind what all the doctors have got to say ... Nature ... is the handmaiden of the Lord' – what Huw truly needs, in his view, is 'faith'.[111] Huw duly regains his mobility, overcoming his disability through a mixture of faith and determination.

Rejecting such narratives of individual tragedy and the miraculous 'resolution' of disability, left-wing writers such as Lewis Jones and Gwyn Thomas saw solidarity and organised labour as the means by which disability could be 'overcome', or at least the limitations of impairment ameliorated. In the politicised world of working-class fiction, Christian faith was eschewed in favour of a model of interdependency and inclusivity based on mutualism and worker solidarity.

Solidarity and interdependency: marching and the socialist rhetoric of disability

Community solidarity and mutualism pivot on images of disability in a number of major coalfields texts, driving the plot and providing a rich imagery by which writers can convey a substantial sense of what solidarity means in the coalfields communities. Representations of organised marches, processions and mass protests provide a good example of this. These are recurring features of the literature of the 1930s and were an iconic part of the workers' movements of the period. Before turning to literary representations, it is worth noting the historical genesis of the interwar organised protest march in which disability groups were central.

The first coordinated march – that is, one in which participants from multiple starting points converged on London – was led by the National League of the Blind of Great Britain and Ireland (NLB) in 1920.[112] The marchers were blind male workers who were staking a claim to rights within a wider labour movement. They carried a banner declaring 'Fellow workers, we want the right hand of comradeship', and reported to the press that they sought the same respect and treatment accorded the railwaymen or the miners.[113] One of the speakers and leader of the north-eastern contingent, D. B. Lawley, was introduced in terms of his credentials as a former miner before blindness had forced him to give up this work. In this way, the NLB march of 1920 aligned itself with the aims and rhetoric of other workers' movements, with a similar emphasis on the importance of rights to state support, rather than private charity. These alliances were at times strained; the NLB organised a second march in 1936 where they refused the National Unemployed Workers' Movement's (NUWM) offer of cooperation. Matthias Reiss has argued that:

> this form of political expression outside of Parliament had been discredited by the NUWM's extensive use of it. The NUWM's numerous marches had featured mass demonstrations, clashes with the police and workhouse authorities, as well as raids on government buildings and Parliament. This, together with the NUWM's reputation as a Communist front organisation, had tainted the Hunger Marches as a means of political protest.[114]

The 1936 march was less successful in regard to publicity and public support than that of 1921, which the NLB pamphlet *Golden Jubilee* attributed to the loss of their novelty value in the public imagination.[115]

It would be inaccurate, however, to imply that the NUWM's organised hunger marches and other forms of industrial protest in this period involved only the straightforwardly 'able-bodied'. Disability was evoked as a motivating factor in some marches, and could be a consequence of participation, yet organised care on some marches could apparently, if less frequently, result in improved health. Participants in such marches in the 1930s were sometimes selected for their likely ability to endure considerable physical demands, as Ellen Wilkinson recalled in the case of the 1936 Jarrow March, where 200 of the strongest, yet still malnourished, men were chosen.[116] The recognition that malnourishment combined with the demands of the march could lead to temporary or permanent disablement led the March Committee to arrange for medical attendance, which, according to Wilkinson, actually led to improved health for many of the men. Less organised groups did not fare so well, and a long march could exacerbate underlying illness or weakness.[117] The possibility that a protest march could lead to illness or disablement was supported in some of the fiction where marchers are portrayed departing the coalfields. A concern for the welfare of the protesters is reflected in a comic scene in Rhys Davies's novel *Jubilee Blues* (1938), in which a wife rushes out to demand that her husband wears his patched 'under-pants':

> 'Wait!' she reproached shrilly, 'you'll get your pleurisy back. Come in by here to the Jubilee lobby now and put 'em on.' Of welfare-centre origin, the pants were now patched like a crazy pavement. The other men were grinning, but the women were sympathetic to their sister, muttering and nodding their heads to each other. Who had to nurse and slave for men when they were ill?[118]

Conversely, physical disability could appear as the *only* reason a person might be prevented from joining his comrades, as we see in a remark in *Cwmardy* (mentioned in Chapter 5) which makes disability the barometer of total community involvement. A mass meeting is called 'at which all the adults in the valley, with the exception of the bedridden, attended'.[119] Lewis is indicating that no one who is able to move stays away, while simultaneously acknowledging the existence of the many people who were sick or disabled in the town.

As we have indicated in earlier chapters, disability was itself a major concern of the labour movement, and worker disability was foregrounded on some protest marches. In a 1952 NUM march, a banner of the Gwendraeth Great Mountain Lodge laments the 'Hundreds of Miners from one village disabled' by 'Pneumoconiosis / The Deadly Dust' (Figure 6). It includes the following verse:

> They toiled to dig the Nations' [sic] Coal
> And breathed the deadly dust,
> Betrayed once more, denied the 'dole'
> By those who held their trust
> They are not here amidst the throng
> Their health is too impaired,
> We march for them to right the wrong
> So that they may be spared.[120]

The statement of solidarity and activism on behalf of miners 'too impaired' to march themselves draws on the rhetoric of pity (the banner is headed 'Mountain

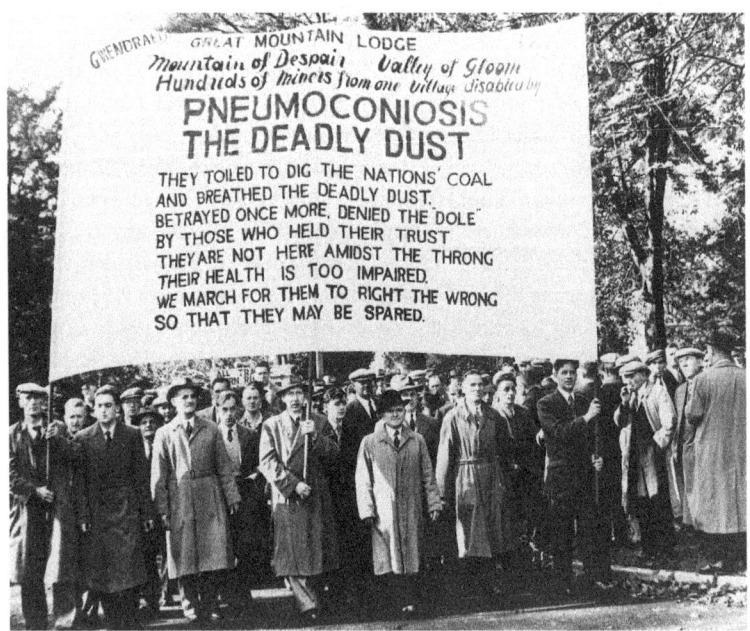

6 Pneumoconiosis banner in NUM march, 1952

of Despair' and 'Valley of Gloom') and isolation ('they are not here amidst the throng'). Yet the protest is also a clear gesture of mutualism and an effort to convince the state of its duty towards men who 'dig the nations' [sic] coal'.

Mass gatherings of protest, not to mention community celebration and commemoration, have long and diverse histories which predate the organised London marches of the interwar period. In the literature and iconography of the coalfields, community solidarity and protest are evoked via a range of mass gatherings, from military procession to riot, funeral marches to carnival, and disability is an important element in all these.[121] In a 1911 plate in the *Labour Leader*, entitled 'The Toll of Industry' (Figure 7) a drawing shows massed ranks

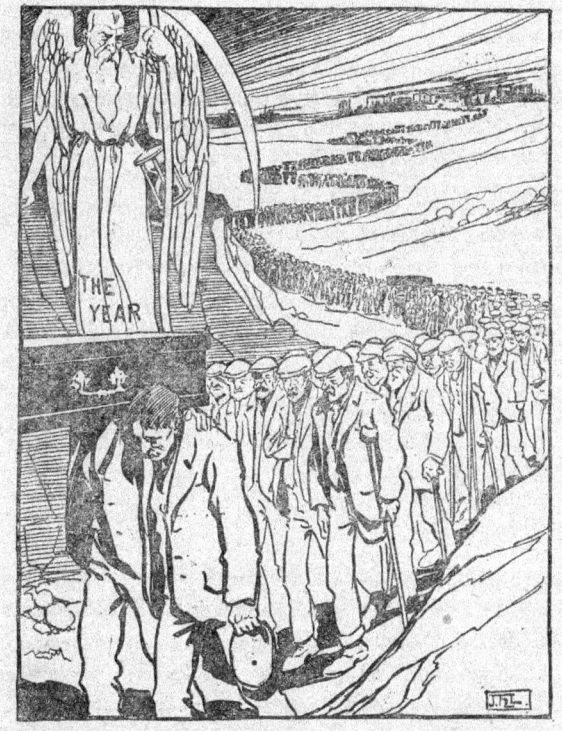

7 'The Toll of Industry': a plate from *The Labour Leader*, 1911

of men, many with crutches, following coffins which are carried at intervals on the shoulders of fellow workers.[122] The columns of men stretch in a winding ribbon back into the distance, apparently issuing without end from a distant and almost indiscernible industrial township. The scene is somewhere between a funeral procession and a protest march, over which the angel of death solemnly looks. The accompanying caption states that the image is 'an accurate portrayal of the annual toll of industry' where for every death, 100 people are disabled. The full caption reads:

> During the year 1910, 3,474 persons were killed and 379,902 were disabled whilst at work. This means that if a procession were formed of the victims of industry, it would stretch 43½ miles with a corpse every twenty yards. Between each corpse 100 disabled workpeople would be marshalled, marching five abreast, and if the widows and orphans followed in the procession it would then be 45½ miles long. In each hundred disabled workpeople there would be approximately 45 miners, 41 factory workers, and 14 persons from the following occupations – railwaymen, seamen, dockers, quarrymen and those employed on works of construction.[123]

In this symbolic procession, the disabled marchers represent the wider community of workers and their families.

This function of workers with disabilities as *general representatives* of colliers and their families recurs in literary works, where those maimed by poor safety in the mines are joined by ranks of those literally and figuratively disabled by the poverty of unemployment. A verse by Idris Davies in *Gwalia Deserta* (1938) imagines a march arriving in London:

> And we come to the gates of Londinium,
> Begging with broken hands,
> Boys bach, boys bach all together,
> Out of the derelict lands.[124]

In this poem, London is imagined as a fortified, gated city to which the miners with 'broken hands' come begging 'all together', and these three conditions – disablement, poverty and solidarity – are repeatedly used to characterise marchers in coalfields literature and iconography.

In fiction and poetry, bodily metaphors and the actual or symbolic presence of people with disabilities on marches were not only used to represent collective injury and travail, they epitomised community and worker solidarity. Yet portrayals of disability could also be used to complicate and challenge the propagandist rhetoric of working-class might. Take the following passage from Gwyn Thomas's *Sorrow for Thy Sons*. It comes near the end of the novel and describes a great protest march in Rhondda against the backdrop of mass unemployment and the Means Test. It is written in Thomas's characteristically terse comic style and is worth quoting at length:

> The people in front of Hugh and Alf began to move. The brothers fell into step. That was not an easy job. Three of the four men in the rank in front of them walked with a limp. It was hard to say which leg they were going to put forward next. Hugh stopped for a moment and looked back. Their own contingent was six or seven thousand strong. It stretched too far back around too many corners to be seen as a whole ...
>
> A young boy, the son of one of the limping men, walked by Alf's side playing a harmonica as broad as his face. The boy had a loose, undisciplined mouth and dribbled a good deal, but the music he produced was sprightly. He worked on three tunes: a Welsh folk song reset to a rhythm basis, a tune of the American Civil War and an anthem of the international class war. At interval's [sic], the boy's father turned round with a handkerchief in his hand and wiped the boy's mouth.
>
> Hugh looked once more at the vast body of demonstrators who were advancing down the mountain road half a mile away ...
>
> 'It's significant,' he said. 'Watching this is like listening to great music, only greater, much greater. Wonderful people! When they can come onto the streets at a few days' notice with ranks as firm and solid as these, there's nothing they can't achieve. I'll never forget this moment. Here is the final answer to all that goddamn poetic loneliness I've fed on like a swine ever since I grew to full height. Fifty thousand of the oppressed banding together against a common injury. Strong faces. Strong bodies marching. Strong voices singing. Strong wills. Strong arms to snatch us out of our dirty, brooding, fornicating little closets and plant us up on high, where the air is clear and worth drinking. From a point like this, life's immediate purposes seem so far away as to look like a straight, simple line without a twist or break in any part of it. I feel ... I feel like an eagle.'
>
> 'Speak quieter. If the police hear you talking like that I'll spend tonight bailing you out.'
>
> Silence, except for the sound of feet and the boy's harmonica. Hugh noticed that a lot of feet made sloppy sounds as they reached the floor, as if the soles were leaving the uppers.[125]

In keeping with the rest of the novel – whose opening pages and subsequent chapters dwell on numerous impaired, disabled or disfigured characters – this passage is reliant on the language of embodiment. There is a stark contrast between the imagery of the crooked, asymmetrical and 'undisciplined' bodies of the people and the 'strong' unbroken ranks of the march in abstract as articulated by Hugh. The ironic clash between the two visions is used to make several different but related arguments about the workers, disability and solidarity.

Despite the fact that the organised march is presented as a potentially meaningful and effective way of protesting against conditions in the Rhondda valleys during the Depression, Hugh's representation of the massed people is treated with suspicion. His soaring rhetoric of 'strong marching bodies' is juxtaposed with the child with an unspecified disability and with the individual workers whose bodies are deformed by work and unemployment, poverty and squalid living conditions. The contrast between wholeness and fragmentation, extreme strength and vulnerable imperfection, set up in this passage recalls the juxtaposition deliberately presented between fascist and modernist art in Germany in 1937, at about the same time the novel was written (c.1936). In *Disability Aesthetics* Tobin Siebers analyses the Nazi aesthetics of the 'Great German Art' exhibition (*Grosse Deutsche Kunstausstellung*) of 1937, as juxtaposed to so-called 'Degenerate Art' (*Entartete Kunst*), which was shown in a popular exhibition in Germany in the same year. The 'Great German Art' produced almost uniform figures of physical 'perfection', as against the abstract and 'deformed' figures of modernist art which Hitler and his Ministry for Culture interpreted in terms of disability and illness. Siebers explains that:

> The Great German Art works to achieve qualification for the German people by designing a specific though imaginary human type based on the healthy and able body. This type was proposed as the norm, and deviation from it tended to justify disqualification and oppression.[126]

Hugh's eagle-perspective sees the people become a single 'vast body', made of 'firm' and 'solid' ranks. It is a 'body' constructed via military imagery of power, discipline and uniformity. Hugh's speech relies on repetition of the word 'strong', repeated so often that it becomes absurd: 'Strong faces. Strong bodies marching. Strong voices singing. Strong wills. Strong arms …'. The imagery of muscular strength supporting determination ('strong wills') recalls fascist rhetoric, from the 'single will' which would direct German culture via the 'National Chamber of Culture' established in 1933,[127] through to iconic Nazi propaganda such as *Triumph of the Will* (1934). The Great German Art sees strength in discipline of mind and body: it 'refuses variation by embracing an idea of human form characterized by exaggerated perfection and striking regularity.'[128] The trajectory of Hugh's rhetoric is similarly towards the perfect, pure and regular, away from the 'dirty, brooding, fornicating' life in the 'little closets' of the town, and up to the 'high' 'clear' 'air'. From this perspective (which exaggerates the familiar spatial tropes of the Welsh industrial novel – a space of epiphanies and meditations – which we have already encountered as a healing space in the discussion of *How Green Was My Valley* above), Hugh sees 'life's immediate purposes' as a '*straight*, simple line *without a twist or break* in any part of it' (emphasis added).

Hugh is attempting to represent a political or ideological purpose in terms of an abstraction, but the purity of an unbroken and untwisted line again draws our attention to the contrast between exaggerated bodily perfection and the imperfect and impaired bodies of the miners.

In fact, the marching ranks are of course made up of limping men who are perpetually out of step. As individuals, the people are dribbling, hobbling or so poorly shod as to make them walk with difficulty: their feet make 'sloppy sounds' on the floor 'as if their soles were leaving the uppers' (the nearly departed soles invoke the homonym 'souls', suggesting the men are being pushed to the brink of mortality). Individual impairment in this novel rarely demands the explicit explanation or narrative that Mitchell and Snyder argue is usually required of disability (though part of the plot is driven by the slow decline of Alf's girlfriend due to tuberculosis). Rather, disability here is collective: most of the figures we see are impaired in some way, and the causes – industry and poverty – are everywhere evident. Here, as elsewhere in Thomas's acerbic oeuvre, poverty and disability are mutually reinforcing. In this sense, Thomas 'pictures disability as the measure of the evils'[129] of poverty and unemployment as well as the poor safety record of mining. In so doing he arguably 'stigmatizes' disability as an allegorical symbol of the problems against which the men are marching.[130] Yet there is much more to this scene than the stigmatisation of disability purely as 'lack' that needs supplement,[131] or ill-health that needs a medical solution.

If we look at the young boy, we see a figure who is impaired but not apparently disabled. His participation in the march invites us to consider the idea of interdependence, as linked to community solidarity. Once more, the contrasts set up by Gwyn Thomas in this passage offer a way in. The quasi-military discipline of the 'vast body' of men is implicitly aligned with individual corporeal discipline, but this is undone by the 'loose, *undisciplined* mouth' of the boy who 'dribbles'. Disability is often constructed as a 'failure to control the body',[132] by which measure the uncontrolled, undisciplined mouth is a disability (though, as Susan Wendell argues, the disabled body actually exposes the 'myth[ical]' nature of control over the body). In Thomas's fiction the boy is not abject or 'other' due to his impairment, he is not even apparently 'disabled' by his 'undisciplined' mouth. Rather, he is routinely cared for by another marcher (his father), while at the same time he performs culturally and politically significant tunes which unify the marchers. The tunes themselves – Welsh, American and international socialist – tell us something about the wider allegiances of the community, thus this 'body' of men with the boy at the centre represent the cultural as well as political identities of the group. His repurposed Welsh folk song is a nod to the residual ethnic and linguistic roots of the area reworked for the modern industrial era; the tune from the American civil war signals a republican radicalism (and perhaps an implicit alignment of the cause of the colliers with anti-slavery); the 'international socialist anthem' firmly locates the marchers in a transnational class war.

This passage, then, enacts a kind of disability aesthetics of its own, drawing into question the high-flown imagery of bodily perfection espoused by Hugh in his propagandist version of the power of unity and organised political action. If there is some stigmatisation of disability (it is the undesirable consequence of poverty and exploitation), disability is simultaneously a productively 'complicating feature' (Mitchell and Snyder's term) of this passage. In contrast to Hugh's 'strong bodies', Thomas's humorous picture of out-of-step marchers and the musician, a dribbling boy cared for by his limping father, is an unsentimental but much warmer and more attractive portrayal of cohesive community solidarity than the uniform ranks of Hugh's quasi-fascistic vision, one in which people with impairments are figuratively and practically a part. Crucially, it is also one that challenges or blurs the lines between conventional binaries of disabled/able-bodied (or 'normal'), carer and recipient of care, thus evoking the idea of *interdependence* – a contemporary disability studies term, but one anticipated by Thomas's vision of community solidarity.

Interdependency and collective strength

The question of dependency is an important one in understanding disability as a socially constructed concept, as Michael Davidson explains:

> For many able bodied persons, disability *is synonymous* with dependency, the former framed as a condition of tragic limit and loss requiring regimes of care and rehabilitation. For disability activists who have fought long and hard to achieve a degree of autonomy dependency conjures up the specter of paternalism that has historically marked living with a physical or cognitive impairment.[133]

Against the received image of a disabled individual isolated and rendered miserable by their lack of independence, disability theory has come to stress the *dependency* or *interdependency* of us all – impaired or not. Lennard Davis argues that 'if we redefine our notions of independence to include the vast networks of assistance and provision that make modern life possible – no one can live without being dependent on these – then the seeming state of exception of disability turns out to be the unexceptional state of existence.'[134] Thus, once we return disability to its social context (and stop treating it as an individual aberration or medical problem), as the social model of disability proposes, we recognise that much disablement is social in its origin. And once we focus on social interactions which are disabling or enabling, we also see that *all* people are enabled or disabled by a complex network of social and material relations.

Coalfields literature foregrounds themes of (inter)dependency, emphasising the role and value of mutual support which challenges 'independence as the unspoken, untheorized norm'.[135] Community solidarity is a form of interdependence and is a source of pride: 'you will never see a miner refuse help to another who is sick or injured, for it may be his own turn next', claims Bert Coombes in *These Poor Hands*.[136] Mutualism, the support of sick and disabled workers through the contributions of all, is seen as an important achievement of the industrial communities in coalfields writing, even as the strains of caring or being cared for (with attendant financial, emotional, physical and psychological stresses on both sides) are acknowledged in realist fiction and biography. While personal care is generally, though not exclusively, the domain of women, interdependency is traced beyond the domestic sphere, emphasising that individualism is an illusion. Thus 'the notion of dependency leaves the relatively narrow domain of caring labour that is associated with the fulfilment of basic needs and enters a wider social domain in which our social dependencies become important in the constitution of our identities'.[137] One of the ways that families and the wider community provide support is in raising donations for the injured miner and his family, known as a 'lift'. This could be quite a substantial amount of money, and is the source of dramatic tension in many coalfields stories.

In Joe Corrie's *Black Earth* the paralysed miner, Jack, squanders all the family's 'lift' money on gambling, much to the distress of his wife.[138] In Rhys Davies's short story 'The Benefit Concert' (1946),[139] money is raised for a good-quality prosthetic leg for an ex-miner, but the local chapel hypocritically keep the vast majority of the money, using £1 on the leg and keeping £100 to redecorate their place of worship. In James C. Welsh's *The Underworld*, the desire to provide mutual support is ideologically pitted against the manager's suspicion of disabled people as malingerers: 'I ha'e been considerin' for a while ... about puttin' a stop to this collectin' business at the office on pay Saturdays, for it just encourages some men to lie off work when there's no' very muckle wrong wi' them; after they get the collection they soon start work again.'[140] In the end, a miner raises the lift despite a ban, with donations collected along political lines – there is a gulf between those whose 'will to give was often greater than the means'[141] and class traitors who put themselves first, 'the "belly-crawlers" ... who "kept in" with the management by carrying tales, and generally acting as traitors to the other men'.[142]

Thus, the idea of the strong 'body' of the collective is not after all in conflict with images of the impaired bodies which make up the procession in *Sorrow for Thy Sons* and other texts. Rather, it is the marching people's daily acts of mutual care and a recognition of interdependence which *comprise* that solidarity. Thomas's marchers find power in communal action: 'banding together against a common injury'. This phrase evokes ubiquitous bodily suffering as well as the more figurative injury of unemployment, but also suggests power – and possibly healing – through an inclusive unity. Lewis Jones uses similar imagery, ultimately stretching the bounds of realism for symbolic ends in *We Live*. As Mary fights for 'Unity in Action' her health briefly improves and the bowed body of her father-in-law, Big Jim, who has also joined the struggle, momentarily becomes upright.

Mary is a leading figure in the local communist party. Despite her poor health – she has tuberculosis (TB) – she has been organising the women of each street to march in unison: 'as a contingent with its own banner, and not in the usual straggling individual manner'.[143] On seeing the women, children and unemployed men of Sunnybank 'lined up with a red banner at their head', Mary temporarily forgets her 'chest'[144]. At the same time her bright eyes, a symptom associated with TB, become a symbol of hope and are mirrored by the whole crowd.[145]

> Mary forgot her chest … as she looked behind her at the ranks of men and women who were ready to march. Each pair of eyes gleamed as brightly as her own and every mouth wore a smile, even the little babies', clutched tightly to their mothers' bodies in heavy woollen shawls.[146]

The same march sees Big Jim and Siân, his wife, take their places at the head of the procession, despite being somewhat frail and unable to keep in step. Proud of his reputation for quasi-mythical masculine strength (and his military past as a soldier), Big Jim tries to cover up signs of his impairments:

> Big Jim, failing to walk erect, pretended he was doing so by stretching his head unnaturally far back and twirling his moustache arrogantly. But, not noticing where he was going, he stumbled against a stone in the roadway and would have fallen had not Siân gripped him tightly.[147]

The comic unreliability of the ageing body undercuts Big Jim's characteristic arrogance and bluster, but there is also an emphasis on mutual care and support which we saw among Gwyn Thomas's marchers. As Big Jim's life testifies, colliers are able to gain meaningful power only through collective action: 'power did not depend alone on bulk'.[148]

Yet the power of the collective as it is represented in this novel rests on more than the fruits of organisation and mutual care: an element of physical transformation occurs repeatedly in Jones's writing, a restorative or healing effect of collective action. Only a page after Jim's stumble as he tries to compensate for his stoop, 'Siân and Big Jim … *walked silent and erect*, like soldiers'[149] (emphasis added). They are pictured 'right at the head of the demonstration, with the blood-red banner streaming directly behind them';[150] perhaps the tableau now demands an upright couple. Elsewhere, however, physical strength is directly drawn from the power of the mass, as in this scene where Len – Mary's husband and Big Jim's son – joins a demonstration:

> Len momentarily felt himself like a weak straw drifting in and out with the surge of bodies. Then something powerful swept through his being as the mass soaked its strength into him, and he realised that the strength of them all was the measure of his own, that his existence and power as an individual was buried in that of the mass now pregnant with motion behind him. The momentous thought made him inhale deeply and his chest expanded, throwing his head erect and his shoulders square to the breeze that blew the banners into red rippling slogans of defiance and action.[151]

Blurring the lines between metaphor and actuality, Len – who has lung disease – finds his chest expanding and his shoulders 'squared', gaining health and an embodied masculinity via the solidarity of the mass (though it is typical of the complex gendering in the novel that this more masculine stance is afforded by the 'pregnant' motion of the crowd).

The reciprocal relationship between personal health and collective politics is explicitly articulated by Lewis in a scene in which the sick or disabled individual is shown to stand a better chance within the community than without. Mary and her activist husband, Len, reject medical advice that she should go to a sanatorium:

> 'If you were penned up in a home, away from the workers, out of the struggle, you would die as quickly and surely as though you were poisoned. Your life does not exist only in your body, but in what your body and brains do for the struggle in which your father reared you.' He broke down for some minutes and buried his wet face on her shoulder, eventually raising it to continue, without looking at her. 'If I thought there was the least hope you would be cured or even get a little better by going to the sanatorium, I would gladly tell you to go. You believe that, don't you, comrade?' he asked pleadingly.
> She answered with a nod, knowing he was putting her own ideas into words without being aware of it himself.[152]

Mary's physical existence is bound up with her political activism, in which her impairment is subsumed, and thus her disability is in some degree mitigated by the collective strength of the 'body' of the Party.

Conclusion

Disability in coalfields literature, as elsewhere, is a site of struggle. The phrase, borrowed from Mitchell and Snyder, refers to multiple struggles; the fight for disability rights on the one hand,[153] but also cultural and literary battles over representation and meaning. Though it has been neglected in the study of coalfields literature, coalfields writers, following Marx, used disability as an urgent metaphor through which the working class as a whole are presented as 'disqualified' and via which socialist solutions of solidarity and interdependency were presented. In the writing discussed here, disability is presented as a direct consequence of male and female bodies worn out in the service of the industrial machine, compounded by economic disadvantage. The disabled body as created by capitalism, and the body which most workers would sooner or later inherit, could, however, be shielded and included in the community by an ethical mutualism to be achieved by political solidarity, or so the rhetoric went. In its aesthetic and ethical engagement with disability, coalfields writing draws on humour, religion, political theory and the daily experience of gendered work. It adopted and adapted different literary forms, in particular realism in which representative workers' lives rendered the economic, political, social forces of industrial life apparent. Disability, and the representative disabled worker, is at the centre of coalfields writing in part because of the way in which work, medicine, welfare and politics – those daily concerns of coalfields life – were brought into sharp relief by the experience, while the imagery of disability was a powerful tool in the rhetoric of working-class struggle. In the hands of modernist writers it was possible to show how the marked, maimed or impaired body was not only a daily feature of coalfields life but also spoke to an aesthetic which, with its emphasis on fragmentation, framed 'disability' as fundamental to the human condition. Indeed, when we look *at* rather than *through* disability in coalfields literature it becomes plain that, rather than being a marginal experience or occasional rhetorical device, it is the fulcrum on which much of this writing pivots.[154]

Notes

1 Lewis Jones, *Cwmardy and We Live* (Cardigan: Parthian, 2006) pp. 268–9.
2 Ato Quayson, *Aesthetic Nervousness: Disability and the Crisis of Representation* (New York: Columbia University Press, 2007), p. 18.
3 Raymond Williams, 'The Welsh Industrial Novel', in *Who Speaks for Wales? Nation, Culture, Identity*, edited by Daniel Williams (Cardiff: University of Wales Press, 2003), p. 96.
4 Between 1920 and 1950 we have found examples of at least 26 coalfields novels published set in south Wales, as compared to 10 set in north-east England and 7 set in Scotland. There were also at least 19 active writers (novelists, short-story writers, poets or dramatists) who wrote about the south Wales coalfields, compared to 8 for north-east England and 6 for Scotland.

5 Rhys Davies, Glyn Jones and Gwyn Jones were raised in mining communities but did not work as miners themselves. Gwyn Jones's father was a miner, Rhys Davies and Glyn Jones both had mothers who were trained as teachers, while their fathers were a shopkeeper and postal worker, respectively.

6 Women writing on heavy industry were rare at this time, although middle-class female novelists had played an important part in nineteenth-century coalfields literature. Ruth Dodds (1890–1976) was a Gateshead playwright who joined the Gateshead ILP Players at its foundation in 1919 (they were the Progressive Players from 1924). She wrote *The Pitman's Pay* (1920), winning first prize in the Sheffield Playgoers Society, although they would not perform the play because of its political content in favour of trade unions. Dodds was Secretary of the Gateshead branch of the National Union of Women's Suffrage Societies (from 1914), a Labour Councillor (elected 1929) and editor of the *Gateshead Labour News*, writing under the byline 'Redcap'. See Ros Merkin, 'No Space of Our Own? Margaret Macnamara, Alma Brosnan, Ruth Dodds and the ILP Arts Guild', in Maggie Gale and Viv Gardner (eds), *Women, Theatre and Performance* (Manchester: Manchester University Press, 2000), pp. 180–97.

7 Dave Russell finds 'little evidence of a strong local or regional dialect drama [in north-east England] before the twentieth century, although it certainly existed and systematic research is once again absent here'. *Looking North: Northern England and the National Imagination* (Manchester: Manchester University Press, 2004), p. 150.

8 For example, The Labour Publishing Co., The Forward Press, Independent Labour Party Publications, Lawrence and Wishart (initially associated with the Communist Party), Victor Gollancz and Michael Joseph Ltd.

9 See Michael J. Dixon, 'The Epic Rhondda: Romanticism and Realism in the Rhondda Trilogy', in Meic Stephens (ed.), *Rhys Davies: Decoding the Hare* (Cardiff: University of Wales Press, 2001); Huw Osborne, *Rhys Davies* (Cardiff: University of Wales Press, 2009).

10 Including Routledge, William Heinemann, Putnam & Holden, Hamish Hamilton and Hodder & Stoughton.

11 Harold Heslop, '13-XI-1930 Morning Session: Heslop', *Literature of the World Revolution: Second International Conference of Revolutionary Writers* (Moscow: International Union of Revolutionary Writers, 1931), p. 226.

12 Gwyn Thomas, *A Few Selected Exits* (1968), quoted in Dai Smith, 'Introduction' to Gwyn Thomas, *Sorrow for Thy Sons* (London: Lawrence and Wishart, 1986), p. 7.

13 S. O'Mahony, 'A. J. Cronin and The Citadel: Did a Work of Fiction contribute to the Foundation of the NHS?', *The Journal of the Royal College of Physicians of Edinburgh*, 42 (2012), pp. 172–8. Christopher Meredith questions this claim, pointing out idealisation of the individual hero in the novel and its pessimism about collective structures put in place by mining communities. Christopher Meredith, 'Cronin and the Chronotope: Place, Time and Pessimistic

Individualism in The Citadel', *North American Journal of Welsh Studies*, 8 (2013), pp. 50–65.
14 A. J. Cronin. *The Citadel* (London: Vista, 1996), p. 7.
15 John Harris, '"A Hallelujah of a Book": How Green Was My Valley as Bestseller', in Tony Brown (ed.), *Welsh Writing in English: A Yearbook of Critical Essays*, 3 (1997) pp. 42–62.
16 Williams, 'The Welsh Industrial Novel', p. 108.
17 Richard Llewellyn's links with the mining communities he mythologised were very distant. A. J. Cronin was a doctor, originally from Scotland, who was appointed Medical Inspector of Mines surveying medical regulations in collieries, as well as writing reports on the correlation between dust inhalation and lung disease. He worked in the Tredegar coalfields, the same mining district from which Aneurin Bevan drew inspiration when proposing plans for the NHS. Nicklaus Thomas-Symonds, *Nye: The Political Life of Aneurin Bevan* (London: I. B. Tauris & Co., 2015), p. 39.
18 Goaf is a pitmatic word for the mined-out spaces in a pit, also called the waste.
19 Harold Heslop, *Goaf* (London: The Fortune Press, 1934), p. 129.
20 Also referred to as 'The Price of Coal' and 'The Wilderness of Toil'. In 1930, Harold Heslop was invited to be the British representative at the Karkov Conference of Revolutionary and Proletarian Writers, and spoke about emergent proletarian/working-class writing in Britain.
21 Translated into Russian by Zinaida Vengerova-Minskaia. Gustav H. Klaus. *The Literature of Labour: Two Hundred Years of Working-Class Writing* (Brighton: The Harvester Press, 1985), p. 95.
22 It was praised by the *Sunday Sun* and *Manchester Guardian*; the *Daily Herald* claimed that 'it should be illegal for miner-owners *not* to read *Goaf*. See Heslop, *Out of the Old Earth* (Newcastle-upon-Tyne: Bloodaxe Books, 1994), p. 23.
23 Bill Jones and Chris Williams, *B. L. Coombes* (Cardiff: University of Wales Press, 1999), p. 60.
24 Barbara Prys-Williams, *Twentieth-Century Autobiography* (Cardiff: University of Wales Press, 2004).
25 Williams, 'The Welsh Industrial Novel', p. 103.
26 Raymond Williams, *Keywords*, 2nd edn (London: Fontana Press, 1988), p. 261.
27 Lewis Jones, *Cwmardy* (London: Lawrence & Wishart, 1937), n.p.
28 David Mitchell and Sharon Snyder, 'The Uneasy Home of Disability in Literature and Film', in Gary Albrecht, Katherine D. Seelman and Michael Bury (eds), *Handbook of Disability Studies* (London: Sage Publications, 2001), p. 199.
29 Tobin Siebers, 'Disability in Theory: From Social Constructionism to the New Realism of the Body', in Lennard J. Davis (ed.), *The Disability Studies Reader*, 2nd edition (New York and London: Routledge, 2006), p. 180.
30 Marven Tova Linett, *Bodies of Modernism: Physical Disability in Transatlantic Modernist Literature* (Ann Arbor: University of Michigan Press, 2017), p. 11.
31 David T. Mitchell and Sharon L. Snyder, *Narrative Prosthesis: Disability and the Dependencies of Discourse* (Ann Arbor: University of Michigan Press, 2000), p. 49

32 Mitchell and Snyder, *Narrative Prosthesis*, p. 49.
33 That is, realist texts critical of bourgeois society.
34 Georg Lukács, 'Narrate or Describe', in *Writer and Critic and Other Essays*, edited and translated by Arthur Kahn (London: Merlin Press, 1970), p. 142.
35 Moyra Haslett, *Marxist Literary and Cultural Theories* (Basingstoke: Macmillan), p. 91.
36 Fredric Jameson, *The Antinomies of Realism* (London and New York: Verso Books, 2015 [2013]), p. 144, fn.11.
37 Though not directly related to physical impairment, Big Jim is also a representative of Welsh-speaking Wales whose poor grasp of English is disabling when he finds himself in court as a witness to a fatal accident in the mine. Despite the workers' efforts, a fellow collier is blamed for what is really corporate negligence.
38 Karl Marx, *Capital: The Process of Capitalist Production*, translated from the third German edition by S. Moore and B. Aveling (New York: International Publishers, 1967), p. 257.
39 Karl Marx, *Capital: A Critique of Political Economy*, Volume I, trans. Ben Fowkes (New York: Penguin, 1976), p. 797.
40 Marx, *Capital: A Critique of Political Economy*, Volume I, p. 481.
41 B. J. Gleeson, 'Disability Studies: A Historical Materialist View', *Disability & Society*, 12:2 (1997), p. 194.
42 In 1936, 56.9 per cent of all miners were unemployed, and miners with disabilities were more likely to be unemployed; see Chapter 1.
43 Throughout this book we have included women's work in the home as part of a wider definition of industrial labour. This approach is supported by the use in coalfields fiction of industrial imagery to portray 'women's work' in colliery homes.
44 Lennard Davis, *Enforcing Normalcy: Disabiltiy, Deafness and the Body* (London and New York: Verso, 1995), p. 2. Tobin Siebers, among other critics, points out that disability is the 'trope by which assumed inferiority of these other minority identities achieved expression', *Disability Aesthetics*, p. 24.
45 Rosemarie Garland Thomson, *Extraordinary Bodies: Figuring Physical Disability in American Culture and Literature* (New York: Columbia University Press, 2017 [1997]), p. 8.
46 Edward Slavishak, *Bodies of Work: Civic Display and Labor in Industrial Pittsburgh* (Durham, NC and London: Duke University Press, 2008), p. 161.
47 See Ben Curtis and Steven Thompson, '"This Is the Country of Premature Old Men": Ageing and Aged Miners in the South Wales Coalfield, c.1880–1947', *Cultural and Social History*, 12:4 (2015), pp. 71–88.
48 Emlyn Williams, *The Corn is Green: A Comedy in Three Acts* (London: Heinemann, 1956), p. 15.
49 James C. Welsh. *The Underworld: The Story of Robert Sinclair, Miner* (London: H. Jenkins, 1920), p. 69.
50 Welsh, *The Underworld*, p. 56.
51 A 'bottomer' is someone who operates winding gear at the bottom of the shaft. James C. Welsh, *The Morlocks* (London: Herbert Jenkins Ltd, 1924), p. 120.

52 Curtis and Thompson, '"This Is the Country of Premature Old Men"', p. 27.
53 See Alexandra Jones, '"Her Body [was] Like a Hard-Worked Machine": Women's Work and Disability in Coalfields Literature, 1880–1950', *Disability Studies Quarterly*, 37:4 (2017).
54 Jones, *Cwmardy and We Live*, p. 14.
55 Gwyn Jones, *Times Like These* (London: Victor Gollancz, 1979), pp. 21–2.
56 Lennard Davies, *Enforcing Normalcy*, pp. 86–7.
57 Rhys Davies 'Nightgown', in Rhys Davies, *Collected Stories: Volume I*, edited by (Llandysul: Gomer Press, 1996), p. 243.
58 Davies 'Nightgown', p. 243.
59 Dan Goodley and Geert Van Hove, 'Disability Studies, People with Learning Disabilities and Inclusion', in Dan Goodley and Geert Van Hove (eds), *Another Disability Studies Reader? People with Learning Difficulties and a Disabling World* (Antwerp: Garant, 2005), p. 22.
60 This type of humour appears to be linked to the ballad tradition of telling amusing escapades of coalfields people, such as Tommy Armstrong's 'Wor Nannies a Maisor'. As Welsh author Ernest Rhys comments in the preface to his stories set in the Durham coalfield: 'one must turn to the Border Ballads, to Johnnie Armstrong or Dick of the Cow, to recover any traces of a humour like theirs'; Ernest Rhys, *Black Horse Pit* (London: Robert Holden & Co. Ltd, 1925) p. 6.
61 Ramsay Guthrie, *Kitty Fagan: A Romance of Pit Life* (London: Christian Commonwealth Publishing, 1900), p. 66.
62 Guthrie, *Kitty Fagan*, p. 66.
63 McLeod is referring to the prosthetic boot or leg irons he needed following his injury that would have been made by the local blacksmith.
64 Parish relief, a form of financial aid.
65 Robert McLeod, *Robert McLeod: Cowdenbeath Miner Poet, An Anthology by Arthur Nevay*, edited by Margaret Bennett (Fife: Grace Not Publications, 2015), p. 62.
66 There were exceptions such as 'My Man's on the Buroo', a poem in the voice of a miner's wife.
67 McLeod, *Robert McLeod*, p. 14.
68 Simon Dentith, 'Tone of Voice in Industrial Writing in the 1930s', in Gustav Klaus and Stephen Knight (eds), *British Industrial Fictions* (Cardiff: University of Wales Press, 2000), p. 100.
69 Dentith, 'Tone of Voice', p. 99.
70 Sid Chaplin, *The Leaping Lad and Other Stories*, edited by Geoffrey Halson (Harlow: Longman Group Ltd, 1970 [1946]), p. 2.
71 Quoted in Dai Smith, *Aneurin Bevan and the World of South Wales* (Cardiff: University of Wales Press, 1993), p. 140.
72 Raymond Williams sees this Welsh wit as a protective mechanism in 'Welsh Culture', *Who Speaks for Wales? Nation, Culture, Identity*, edited by Daniel Williams (Cardiff: University of Wales Press, 2003), p. 9.
73 Quoted in Smith, *Aneurin Bevan and the World of South Wales*, p. 140.

74 Quoted in Smith, *Aneurin Bevan and the World of South Wales*, p. 140.
75 Gwyn Thomas, *Sorrow for Thy Sons* (London: Lawrence and Wishart, 1986), p. 67.
76 Smith, *Aneurin Bevan and the World of South Wales*, p. 145.
77 See Laura Wainwright, '"Hellish Funny": The Grotesque Modernism of Gwyn Thomas and Rhys Davies', in *New Territories in Modernism: Anglophone Welsh Writing 1930–1949* (Cardiff: University of Wales Press, 2018).
78 Ato Quayson, *Aesthetic Nervousness: Disability and the Crisis of Representation* (New York: Columbia University Press, 2007), p. 217, fn.13. Quayson gives Franz Kafka's *Metamorphosis* as an example of this form.
79 Linett, *Bodies of Modernism*, p. 3.
80 David Alexander Williams, or 'Dai Alex' as he was known, was a colliery carpenter and a communist whose writing often focuses on occupational illness and disability.
81 Dai Alexander, 'Hangman's Assistant', in Gwyn Jones and Islwyn Ffowc Elis (eds), *Classic Welsh Short Stories* (Oxford: Oxford University Press, 1992), p. 76.
82 Alexander, 'Hangman's Assistant', p. 77.
83 Alexander, 'Hangman's Assistant', p. 74.
84 Alexander, 'Hangman's Assistant', p. 78.
85 Alexander, 'Hangman's Assistant', p. 78.
86 Alexander, 'Hangman's Assistant', p. 78.
87 Milan Kundera, *The Art of the Novel* (New York: Harper & Row, 1993 [1968]), p. 104. Original italics.
88 Alexander, 'Hangman's Assistant', pp. 75–6.
89 Alexander, 'Hangman's Assistant', p. 77.
90 Livio Pestilli, *Picturing the Lame in Italian Art from Antiquity to the Modern Era* (London: Routledge, 2016).
91 Tyrus Miller, *Late Modernism: Politics, Fiction and the Arts Between the World Wars* (1999), quoted in Linett, *Bodies of Modernism*, p. 145.
92 Linett, *Bodies of Modernism*, p. 145.
93 Jane Aaron has commented that 'the lack of opportunity to find employment as anything other than a coalminer (or his wife) created a sense of a doomed or haunted community, sacrificed to the needs of Westminster and the British Empire'; Jane Aaron, *Welsh Gothic* (Cardiff: University of Wales Press, 2013), pp. 6–7.
94 Ernest Rhys's interlinked short stories, *Black Horse Pit*, are similarly influenced by the oral culture of the Durham coalfields, but though published in 1925 they have more in common with George Moore's proto-modernist *The Untilled Field* (1905) than the more overtly modernist techniques being developed by Chaplin in the 1940s.
95 Sid Chaplin and Geoffrey Halson (eds), *The Leaping Lad and Other Stories* (Harlow: Longman Group Ltd, 1970 [1946]), p. 8.
96 Chaplin, *The Leaping Lad*, p. 4.
97 Sid Chaplin, 'What Katie Did', in Chaplin, *The Leaping Lad*, pp. 126–35.

98 See, for instance, 'Easter 1927' in *The Leaping Lad*.
99 Glyn Jones, 'The Kiss', in *The Collected Stories of Glyn Jones*, edited by Tony Brown (Cardiff: University of Wales Press, 1999), pp. 41–8.
100 Jones, 'The Kiss', p. 47.
101 Jones, 'The Kiss', p. 48.
102 Jones, 'The Kiss', p. 47.
103 Jones, 'The Kiss', p. 48.
104 The homoerotic dimensions of this story, which pays such detailed attention to the unwinding of the bandages and the unrecognisable flesh, are discussed in Tony Brown, 'Glyn Jones and the Uncanny', *Almanac: A Yearbook of Welsh Writing in English: Critical Essays*, 12 (2007/08), pp. 89–114. Disability, religion and homoeroticism are not uncommon bedfellows in portrayals of working-class bodies in coalfields literature, as in this image of a body being sacrificed to and sanctified by toil in Harold Heslop's *The Earth Beneath* (1946): 'It seemed nothing could prevent those muscles from being shaped into a vision that would have blessed Michael Angelo; nothing could prevent those muscles being made like iron in this unholy cathedral of pitiless toil. And as this toil ate those muscles of the flesh it made them lovely.' Harold Heslop, *The Earth Beneath* (London: T. V. Boardman and Company, 1946), p. 71.
105 Pestilli, *Picturing the Lame*, p. 3.
106 Nancy Eiesland, *The Disabled God: Toward a Liberatory Theology of Disability* (Nashville, TN: Abingdon Press, 1994), p. 100.
107 Idris Davies, *Gwalia Deserta* (London: J. M. Dent & Sons Ltd., 1938), p. 13.
108 Idris Davies, 'Cwrdd Mawr', in *The Complete Poems*, edited by Dafydd Johnston (Cardiff: University of Wales Press, 1994), p. 217. The title means, literally, 'Big Meeting' and refers to a large event in the chapel.
109 On Davies and his relationship with Christianity, see M. Wynn Thomas, *In the Shadow of the Pulpit: Literature and Nonconformist Wales* (Cardiff: University of Wales Press, 2011), pp. 172–9 and Daniel G. Williams, *Black Skin, Blue Books: African Americans and Wales, 1845–1945* (Cardiff: University of Wales Press, 2012), esp. pp. 114–17. Peter Lord discusses Christ and Christian iconography in industrial art from Wales in *The Visual Culture of Wales: Industrial Society* (Cardiff: University of Wales Press, 1998), particularly that of Archie Griffiths (see pp. 189–99).
110 Williams, 'The Welsh Industrial Novel', p. 104.
111 Richard Llewellyn, *How Green Was My Valley* (London: Penguin Books, 1991), p. 80.
112 The NLB was founded in 1893 as a Trade Union focused on rights for blind workers.
113 Mathias Reiss, 'Forgotten Pioneers of the National Protest March: The National League of the Blind's Marches to London, 1920 and 1936', *Labour History Review*, 70:2 (2005), pp. 133–65.
114 Reiss, 'Forgotten Pioneers', p. 154.
115 Reiss, 'Forgotten Pioneers', p. 154.

116 Ellen Wilkinson, *The Town that Was Murdered* (London: Victor Gollancz Ltd, 1939), p. 200.
117 Wilkinson, *The Town that Was Murdered*, p. 203.
118 Rhys Davies, *Jubilee Blues* (London: Heinemann, 1938), p. 274. The scene is perhaps based on one Davies witnessed and described in his non-fiction account of men assembling to march to London in *My Wales* (London: Jarrolds, 1937). Davies writes: 'a woman … bawled to her son: " -and 'bove all, keep the flannel on your chest; don't you come back to me with another London cough"' (p. 137). We are grateful to John Boaler for identifying both Davies quotations.
119 Jones, *Cwmardy and We Live*, p. 207.
120 'Pneumoconiosis banner in NUM March, 1952', https://museum.wales/picture-library/item/977/Pneumoconiosis-banner-in-NUM-March-1952-bw-photo/, accessed 23 September 2018.
121 In one early novel, a riot that takes place in response to a disabled and despised manager's mishandling of the workers is transformed into a near atrocity as soldiers prepare to fire on the unarmed rioters. It then becomes a protest march fuelled by Christian hymns, all in the space of a couple of chapters. See Irene Saunderson, *A Welsh Heroine* (London: Lynwood & Co., 1910).
122 *The Labour Leader* was a socialist newspaper that originated from a relaunch of *The Miner* in 1888, a monthly paper founded by Keir Hardie. It was purchased by the ILP in 1904 and was renamed a number of times in its near-hundred-years' publication history; it was the *New Leader* from 1922, the *Socialist Leader* from 1946, and *Labour Leader* again from 1975. It ceased publishing in 1986. Safety in the heavy industries was a hot topic in contemporary politics; this plate is from the same year as the passing of the Coal Mines Act 1911, which improved safety regulations in mining.
123 *Labour Leader*, 8 December 1911.
124 Idris Davies, 'Gwalia Deserta', XXVII, in Dafydd Johnston (ed.), *The Complete Poems of Idris Davies* (Cardiff: University of Wales Press, 1994), p. 15. We are grateful to John Boaler, a research student at Swansea University, for drawing this stanza to our attention.
125 Thomas, *Sorrow for Thy Sons*, pp. 250–1.
126 Siebers, *Disability Aesthetics*, p. 31.
127 Toby Clark, *Art and Propaganda in the Twentieth Century* (London: George Widenfeld and Nicholson Ltd), p. 61.
128 Siebers, *Disability Aesthetics*, p. 32.
129 Siebers, *Disability Aesthetics*, p. 37.
130 Siebers makes a parallel case in respect of using disability to represent the evils of warfare in *Disability Aesthetics*, p. 37.
131 Disability has been defined as 'lack' by Mitchell and Snyder: 'the deficient body, by virtue of its insufficiency, serves as a baseline for the articulation of the normal body. Disability as lack is to be corrected by prosthesis – a supplement which normalises and completes', *Narrative Prosthesis*, p. 7. In industrial fiction, disability

is also linked to excess: excess of work in particular, though in the end this results in lack of health and strength.
132 Susan Wendell, *The Rejected Body* (New York and London: Routledge, 1996), p. 60.
133 Michael Davidson, 'Introduction', *Journal of Literary and Cultural Disability Studies*, 1:2 (2007), p. i. Emphasis in the original.
134 Lennard J. Davis, 'Dependency and Justice', *Journal of Literary and Cultural Disability Studies*, 1:2 (2007), p. 4.
135 Davidson, 'Introduction', p. iii.
136 Coombes, *These Poor Hands*, p. 165.
137 Eva Feder Kittay and Ellen K. Feder cited in Alice Hall, *Literature and Disability* (London: Routledge, 2016), p. 69.
138 'Lift' was a term for the donations of money raised for an injured miner by collecting from fellow miners. The physical connotations of the word – to lift a fellow worker over a hurdle – suggest embodied aid.
139 Rhys Davies, 'The Benefit Concert', in Rhys Davies and Meic Stephens (ed. and intro.), *Collected Stories: Volume II* (Llandysul: Gomer Press, 1996), pp. 17–25.
140 Welsh, *The Underworld*, p. 17.
141 Welsh, *The Underworld*, p. 20.
142 Welsh, *The Underworld*, p. 20.
143 Jones, *Cwmardy and We Live*, p. 743.
144 Jones, *Cwmardy and We Live*, p. 744.
145 On TB and its cultural associations, see Susan Sontag, *Illness as Metaphor* (New York: Farrar, Strauss and Giroux, 1978).
146 Jones, *Cwmardy and We Live*, p. 744.
147 Jones, *Cwmardy and We Live*, p. 744.
148 Jones, *Cwmardy and We Live*, p. 549.
149 Jones, *Cwmardy and We Live*, p. 745.
150 Jones, *Cwmardy and We Live*, p. 745.
151 Jones, *Cwmardy and We Live*, p. 751.
152 Jones, *Cwmardy and We Live*, p. 739.
153 Disability studies invites us to consider disability as a 'site of struggle' where disability is 'the result of the interaction between impairment and physical and attitudinal environments'; Mitchell and Snyder, *Narrative Prosthesis*, p. 24.
154 The words are paraphrased from Ato Quayson's discussion in *Aesthetic Nervousness*, pp. 34, 208.

Conclusion

The coal industry has a central place in the economic, political and industrial relations history of modern Britain. No industry compares with its fundamental role in providing so much employment, generating as much economic activity and giving rise to trade unions and a powerful Labour Party that were to play such significant roles in British politics and the evolution of the British state. Another important characteristic of the coal industry now needs to be recognised: it is clearly crucial to the modern history of disability in Britain. No other industry posed the same variety or severity of risks to its workers or generated as large a number of disabled individuals on a daily basis. No other industry was required to organise itself to quite the same degree to respond to the lives and fates of people impaired in its ordinary functions. No other industry left such a legacy of ill-health, impairment and chronic sickness during the twentieth century. Former coalfield communities across Britain continue to suffer the legacy of nineteenth- and twentieth-century coal capitalism and continue to face high levels of impairment and disability in their post-industrial situation.[1]

That the coal industry impaired such large numbers of people was evident to miners, doctors, journalists, writers, social surveyors, government inspectors and commissioners, even employers at times. The large-scale disasters that took hundreds of lives at a time received most of the attention and pricked the conscience of the broader public, but it was also evident to anyone who looked that impairment and disability were common features of mining communities. For even the most casual observer of any coalmining community, the results of industrial impairment were immediately obvious. Whether it was to the *Morning Chronicle* correspondent in the 1850s, to the socialist missionaries in the 1890s or to a Polish sociologist in the 1940s, the ubiquity of disability in mining communities was immediately obvious, and an evident shock to such individuals who visited mining communities for the first time.[2] The inhabitants of mining communities, of course, considered it a normal aspect of everyday life and, apart from writers who looked to portray or communicate something of the reality of life in such places for an outside audience, were much less likely to comment upon it in quite the same ways.

This did not mean that disability as a result of industrial accident or chronic disease was simply passively accepted by coalfields workers. For the people of mining communities, the toll of impairment, disease and disability gave rise to new forms of organisation and to a particular political activism, both of which placed disability at their core and attempted to assist the victims of coal exploitation. Friendly societies, workers' medical schemes, disablement funds, provident societies, artificial limb funds, blind charities, permanent provident funds, convalescent institutions, truss schemes and other such organisations were numerous in mining communities and touched the lives of a significant proportion of the population. Alongside such schemes, miners' trade unions placed impairment at the heart of their industrial relations activities and, unlike sleeping car porter brotherhoods in America, never wavered from their belief that impairment was caused by dangerous working conditions and uncaring employers, rather than by worker carelessness.[3] If, as one historian has claimed, the South Wales Miners' Federation devoted as much of its time and resources to compensation matters as it did to wages and working conditions, then it is clear that disability was one of the core concerns of miners' unions.[4] In fact, injury and occupational disease were central components of a critique of coal capitalism that lay at the heart of trade union organisation from the mid-Victorian period through to the mid-twentieth century. They also stood right at the heart of the campaign to end private ownership in the industry and to replace it with nationalisation during the three or four decades prior to 1947.[5] In each case, some of the political rhetoric drew upon tropes of pity as well as fraternity and justice, and had negative consequences for the perceptions of disabled people and understandings of disability. More generally, the labour movement in British coalfields attempted to undermine the idea of disability as a matter of individual morality and reframe it as a matter of political economy.[6]

This politicisation of disability is one of the distinctive features of coalfields literature in the same period. At the level of structure as well as content, this politico-ethical trope is central to the emergence of both a new industrial realism and coalfields modernism. While disability, following well-established literary and cultural conventions, could be used as a synechdoche for immorality or a plot device to deliver religious redemption, in the hands of miner-writers disability was a powerful metaphor for the marginalised working class and a litmus test for the solidarity and mutualism espoused by socialist principles. Rather than being primarily a marker of the abnormal against which 'normalcy' could be defined, disability is the presented as both symptom of the deprivations and demands of industry *and* a feature of the daily lived experiences of a mutually supportive community.

Apart from the centrality of disability to daily life and the politics of coalmining communities, it is also evident that the coal industry was crucial in the employment of disabled people. This fact goes right to the heart of one of the major shibboleths of disability studies. According to certain seminal works in disability studies in the 1970s and 1980s, the commodification of labour brought about by industrialisation served to disable and oppress people with bodily impairments through the denial of productive work in the economy and their isolation in the home or in institutions.[7] The situation in the coal industry, however, was far more complex than any such sociological model would recognise. This was partly a product of the nature of the coal industry, since it offered a range of different jobs and tasks to be completed by workers, some of which were suitable for workers with quite severe impairments, such as work in the lamp-room at the pithead. The coal industry thus employed a type of disabled worker quite different from those being trained for low-paid manual labour at workhouses and segregated special education institutions: one that remained integrated in coalfield communities.[8] Periods of labour shortage, such as during the two world wars, also worked to increase the possibilities for employment as impaired former miners were reabsorbed into the workforce.

The employment of impaired miners was also a product of a moral economy within the industry in which employers, to a greater or lesser degree, recognised that they had a responsibility to old and infirm miners who had lost their strength and health in their employ. Certainly, this moral economy came under pressure from the workings of the compensation system that discouraged the employment of impaired workers, who now came to be seen as a 'bad risk', but it did survive throughout these decades and into the period of nationalisation under the NCB. Most importantly of all, the employment of disabled workers was enshrined in the compensation system enacted in 1897, since the category of 'partially disabled', requiring 'partial compensation', placed an expectation for disabled miners to be provided with 'light employment' if the employer wished to avoid the cost of 'full compensation'. This was not an absolute right, of course, and employers used various tactics or loopholes in the legislation to avoid this requirement, or else varied in their estimations of the costs of different responses to 'partially disabled' miners. Nevertheless, the statutory compensation system did help to ensure that large numbers of impaired miners continued to be employed in the industry right through the first half of the twentieth century.

The extent to which the coal industry was disabling, therefore, is extremely complex. Each impaired miner found himself in a unique position as far as his bodily capacity, the attitude of his employer and the possibility of moving to other jobs in the pit were concerned. Given the existence of piece rates at the coalface or different grades of pay for various groups of underground and surface workers, and the varied levels of status attached to these, all impaired miners were disabled to a greater or lesser degree, as impairment affected their ability to work and to earn a livelihood. Nevertheless, it would be wrong to conclude that all men impaired by their work in the coal industry suffered social isolation or economic marginalisation, even if this was the experience of a significant proportion of them. This is especially the case for the types of chronic and progressive conditions associated with old age and infirmity, on the one hand, and occupational disease such as pneumoconiosis, on the other. In such instances, the extent of impairment could intensify gradually over a period of time and bring about small changes in an individual's capacity to carry out his work. Thus the history of the coal industry, with experiences such as these in mind, offers an interesting insight for disability studies scholars interested in isolation, marginalisation and oppression. It presents a challenge to blanket narratives of exclusion, but also places a responsibility on historians of other industries, perhaps, to see if the coal industry was alone in its employment of disabled people in industrial Britain.

While the compensation system ensured some sort of place for impaired men in the industry, it also performed a far more significant role than that in coalfield society, and, indeed, in British society more generally, from 1897 onwards. In fact, it might be argued that the compensation legislation passed in 1897, and amended on a number of occasions up to 1946, was fundamental to the creation of disability in British society. Establishing eligibility for compensation payments through medical diagnosis and, possibly, legal judgement created a category of disabled workmen that possessed certain rights in law. Deborah Stone's work posits disability as 'a juridical and administrative construct of state policy'.[9] As Gleeson insists, this is just a construct and it tells us nothing about the lived reality of the disabled person's experiences of disability. Nevertheless, this designation of disability was extremely powerful, since, while it did not prevent poverty and was certainly not a permanent designation, it helped to determine access to compensation payments that were of real importance to the impaired miner and his family and could prevent reliance on the hated Poor Law.

Equally important, the compensation system, and especially its adversarial character, ensured that a vast bureaucratic and legal machinery developed to administer the scheme, and that trade unions and employers' organisations devoted a significant amount of their time and resources to the administration of disability. Coal companies and employer organisations spent huge sums of money on mutual indemnity policies to spread the risk of their compensation liabilities, while miners' trade unions devoted significant amounts of their finite resources to securing compensation payments for disabled members. Both sides purchased medical and scientific expertise to assist them in their battles over individual legal cases and utilised a number of different political and industrial strategies in attempts to influence the passage of legislation. In all these ways, therefore, disability was one of the fundamentally important organising principles of coalfield society and conditioned the industrial and political strategies of unions and employers. The fact that many of those fights continue even after the closure in December 2015 of Kellingley, the last deep coal mine in Britain, speaks to the ultimate failure of both the state and employers to create a consistent model of adequate, liveable compensation for disabled members of the industry. Few things, possibly not even wages or working conditions, matched disability in importance in coalfield society.

One of the corollaries of this centrality of disability in coalfield society was that, relative to other groups of disabled people, in other times or places, disabled people in mining communities – at least, those affected by impairments resulting from paid work (mainly men) – were empowered by the considerable power exerted on their behalf by miners' trade unions. This power was not absolute, of course, and trade unions invariably came up against the greater power held by employers in the industry. In addition, trade unions could decide, as a result of a paucity of resources or a calculation as to the likely success of a particular case, not to put its full weight behind an individual's cause. Nevertheless, that unions campaigned for better working conditions to lessen the incidence of impairment, that they negotiated alternative jobs at the colliery, that they fought compensation cases through the courts and that they aided members to access welfare, medical and rehabilitation services, meant that disabled people in mining communities gained a powerful advocate that was able to make at least some improvements in people's lives.

The women of mining communities had fewer resources on which to draw in their battles for representation and improvement, but certain circumstances meant that the smaller scale of their campaigns was not necessarily a hindrance to their hopes of making progress. In particular, the maternalist politics pursued through the women's sections of the Labour Party, and conducted in the sphere of local government, coincided with national concerns over maternity and reproductive health. The growing 'toll of motherhood' in the 1930s, in particular, led to significant efforts to improve maternity services and lessen maternal mortality and morbidity, but it was arguably the development of sulphonamide drugs from the mid- to late 1930s that made the biggest impact here.

That such advocacy, for disabled men and disabled women, was based upon a medical model of disability is undeniable. Unions, similar to other organisations within the labour movement, looked to gain access to more and better medical and rehabilitation services, while women's organisations sought solutions to the problems of women's reproductive impairment through maternity services that were highly medicalised. Neither of these two broad political efforts gave much attention to the social factors that disabled impaired miners and women in the community. What efforts there were to ameliorate the social exclusion and isolation experienced by disabled people in mining communities tended to come in informal ways, through the small-scale, everyday support and assistance given by friends, neighbours and local organisations. Such practical forms of support, whether visits to the homes of impaired miners, assistance to attend a local rugby game or help to old miners to complete their work underground, do not necessarily register in the historical record to any great degree, but they were practical manifestations of a communal spirit that looked to lessen hardship and improve life, even if only to small degrees. More study is required of unions as organisations of disability advocacy and with the potential to push for access to work and workers' rights for disabled people, much as recent research has explored disability-led organisations of the era such as the radical National League of the Blind.[10]

Nevertheless, despite such efforts, social isolation and marginalisation were still the experience of the majority of disabled people in mining communities. For the paraplegic miners confined to their beds, no number of visits from friends and former work colleagues could transform the desperate isolation of their daily lives, while even those miners with only early-stage chest diseases found their working capacity compromised, their earning ability lessened and their status impacted. More fundamentally, any degree of impairment that required a man to finish work, whether through injury or chest disease, removed that man from the sphere of work and cut him off from the source of a great deal of his identity, his social relations with friends and work colleagues and his status as a respectable working man who provided for his family. Other means were available to him to retain his authority as the head of the household and to retain social contact with others in the community, but it was clear that his life was changed significantly by his impairment. The ubiquity of disability meant that coalfield communities were arguably less disabling than other types of communities across Britain, but impairment was nevertheless a life-changing event with far-reaching, disabling consequences for everyday life.

Notes

1 Mike Foden, Steve Fothergill and Tony Gore, *The State of the Coalfields: Economic and Social Conditions in the Former Mining Communities of England, Scotland and Wales* (Sheffield: Centre for Regional Economic and Social Research, Sheffield Hallam University, 2014).
2 Jules Ginswick (ed.), *Labour and the Poor in England and Wales 1849–1851: The Letters to The Morning Chronicle. Vol. III The Mining and Manufacturing Districts of South Wales and North Wales* (London: F. Cass, 1983), p. 49; 'Socialist Campaign in South Wales', *Commonweal*, 27 August 1887, quoted in Ken John, 'Sam Mainwaring and the Autonomist Tradition', *Llafur*, 4:3 (1986), p. 65; Ferdynand Zweig, *Men in the Pits* (London: Society of Friends, 1948), p. 5.

3 John Williams-Searle, 'Cold Charity: Manhood, Brotherhood, and the Transformation of Disability, 1870–1900', in P. Longmore and L. Umansky (eds), *The New Disability History: American Perspectives* (New York: New York University Press, 2001), pp. 157–86.
4 Dot Jones, 'Workmen's Compensation and the South Wales Miner, 1898–1914', *Bulletin of the Board of Celtic Studies*, 29:1 (1980), pp. 133–155.
5 For examples, see *The Eight Hours Movement (Coal Mines): Proceedings at a Joint Conference of representative coal owners and the Miners' Federation of Great Britain held at the Westminster Palace Hotel, London, S.W., on the 21st January, and the 11th February, 1891* (1891), pp. 10–11, 42–3; Coal Industry Commission, *Vol. I: Reports and Minutes of Evidence on the First Stage of the Inquiry*, Cmd. 359, (London: HMSO, 1919), xi, Evidence of William Straker and Vernon Hartshorn, pp. 322, 362–3.
6 Sarah F. Rose, *No Right to be Idle: The Invention of Disability, 1840s–1930s* (Chapel Hill: University of North Carolina Press, 2017).
7 B. J. Gleeson, 'Disability Studies: A Historical Materialist View', *Disability & Society*, 12:2 (1997), pp. 179–202.
8 Anne Borsay, *Disability and Social Policy in Britain since 1750: A History of Exclusion* (Basingstoke: Palgrave Macmillan, 2005), p. 96.
9 Gleeson, 'Disability Studies: A Historical Materialist View', p. 189.
10 Mathias Reiss, *Blind Workers against Charity: The National League of the Blind of Great Britain and Ireland, 1893–1970* (London: Palgrave Macmillan, 2015).

Select bibliography

Primary sources

Manuscripts

Durham County Record Office
D/DCNA – Durham County Nursing Association, records, 1918–81
D/DCOA – Durham Coal Owners' Association Records, 1872–1947
D/DCOMPA – Durham Coal Owners' Mutual Protection Association Records, 1897–1957
D/DMA – National Union of Mineworkers, Durham Area Records, 1847–1948

Glamorgan Archives
DBLI RH – Rhondda Institution for the Blind, 1920–87
DPD – Powell Duffryn Ltd, Steam Coal Company Corporate, Financial and Production Records, 1802–1959
DXEL – The Rest Convalescence Home, Porthcawl Records, 1862–2003

Gwent Archives
CSW.BG.B – Bedwellty Board of Guardians Records, 1849–1930
CSW.BG.P – Pontypool Board of Guardians Records, 1836–1930
D.2472 – Ebbw Vale Workmen's Medical Society Records, 1896–1971
D.914 – Ebbw Vale Workmen's Medical Society Records, 1905–46
D.3246 – Tredegar Workmen's Medical Aid Society Records, 1873–1995

The National Archives, Kew, London
BT 189 – Board of Trade: Coal Controllers Advisory Board Minutes, 1917–20
BX 3 – Coal Industry Social Welfare Organisation: Miscellania, 1921–58
COAL 43 – National Coal Board: Medical Department: Papers, 1947–87
FS 15, 28 – Registry of Friendly Societies, 1787–1965
PIN 12 – Home Office and Ministry of National Insurance and its Successors, Workmen's Compensation, Correspondence and Papers 1900–79
POWE 1 – Miners' Welfare Committee and Commission 1921–52
POWE 10 – Ministry of Power and predecessors and successors: Establishments Division: Correspondence and Papers, 1887–1973

National Archives of Scotland, Edinburgh
CB 19 – Scottish Workers' Compensation Scheme, Directors' Minute Books, 1912–14
FS 4 – Friendly Societies, 3rd Series
SC 21 – Dunfermline Sheriff Court, 1811–1984
SC 67 – Stirling Sheriff Court, 1605–1989

National Library of Scotland
ACC 4312 – Minute Books of the National Union of Mineworkers, Lothians Area, 1894–1946
DEP 304 – Fife and Kinross Miners Association Minutes, 1901–13

NHS Greater Glasgow and Clyde Archives
HB 47 – Glasgow Ophthalmic Institution, minutes, registers, reports, 1870–1967

North East Mining Archive and Research Centre
NUMDA – Durham Miners' Association and National Union of Mineworkers, Durham Area

Northumberland Archives
NRO 263 – Northumberland and Durham Coal Owners Association Records

Richard Burton Archives, Swansea University
SWCC – South Wales Coalfield Collection

Scottish Oral History Centre, Strathclyde University
SOH 6 – Coal Mining Oral History Project, 1999

South Wales Miners Library, Swansea University
AUD – Oral History collection, 1910–80

Tyne and Wear Archives Service
CH/MPR – Northumberland and Durham Miners Permanent Relief Fund Friendly Society Records, 1862–1995
HO/SRI – Sunderland Royal Infirmary Records, 1800–1973

West Glamorgan Archives Service
D/D SHF – Ladies Samaritan Fund, Singleton Hospital, Swansea, Minutes, Accounts, Reports and Correspondence, 1909–86

Newspapers and periodicals

Aberdare Times
Amman Valley Chronicle
British Medical Journal
The Cambrian
Cardiff Times
Colliery Guardian
Colliery Workers' Magazine
Y Darian
Evening Express

Evening Telegraph
Glasgow Herald
Y Goleuad
Y Gwladgarwr
Labour Woman
The Miner
Monmouth Guardian
Morpeth Herald
The Newcastle Courant
Northern Echo
Picture Post
Scottish Medical Journal
South Wales Daily Post
The Times

UK statutes

Employers' Liability Act, 1880
Workmen's Compensation Act, 1897
Blind Persons Act, 1920
Disabled Persons (Employment) Act, 1944

Other published sources

Aaron, Jane and Ursula Masson (eds), *The Very Salt of Life: Welsh Women's Political Writings from Chartism to Suffrage* (Dinas Powys: Honno, 2007).

Andrews, Elizabeth, *A Woman's Work Is Never Done: Being the Recollections of a Childhood and Upbringing amongst the South Wales Miners and a Lifetime of Service to the Labour Movement in Wales* (Rhondda: Cymric Democrat Publishing Society, 1957).

Barnett, Henry Norman, *Accidental Injuries to Workmen, with Reference to Workmen's Compensation Act, 1906. With Article on Injuries to the Organs of Special Sense* (London: Rebman, 1909).

Campbell, George L., *Miners' Insurance Funds: Their Origin and Extent* (London, 1880).

Campbell, George L., *Miners' Thrift and Employers' Liability* (Wigan: Strowger and Son, 1891).

Campbell, Janet M., *Maternal Mortality* (London: HMSO, 1924).

Chaplin, Sid, *The Leaping Lad and Other Stories*, edited by Geoffrey Halson (Harlow: Longman Group Ltd, 1970 [1946]).

Chaplin, Sid, *The Thin Seam* (London: Phoenix House, 1950).

Chelmsford, Viscount, *The Miners' Welfare Fund* (London: HMSO, 1927).

Coombes, B. L., *These Poor Hands: The Autobiography of a Miner working in South Wales*, with an Introduction by Bill Jones and Chris Williams (Cardiff: University of Wales Press, 2002 [1939]).

Coombes, B. L., *I Am A Miner* (London: Fact, 1939).
Coombes, B. L., *Those Clouded Hills* (London: Cobbett Publishing Co., 1944).
Coombes, B. L., *Miners Day* (Harmondsworth: Penguin Books, 1945).
Corrie, Joe, *Black Earth* (London: Routledge, 1939).
Corrie, Joe, *Plays Poems and Theatre Writings*, edited by Linda MacKenney (Edinburgh: 7:84 Publications, 1985).
Cronin, A. J., *The Stars Look Down* (London: New English Library, 1978 [1935]).
Cronin, A. J., *The Citadel* (London: Vista, 1996 [1937]).
Cronin, A. J., *Adventures in Two Worlds* (London: Victor Gollancz, 1952).
Davies, Idris, *Gwalia Deserta* (London: J. M. Dent & Sons Ltd., 1938).
Davies, Idris, *The Complete Poems of Idris Davies*, edited by Dafydd Johnston (Cardiff: University of Wales Press, 1994).
Davies, Rhys, *A Time to Laugh* (Cardigan: Parthian, 2014 [1937]).
Davies, Rhys, *Jubilee Blues* (London: Heinemann, 1938).
Davies, Rhys, *Collected Stories: Volume I*, edited by Meic Stephens (Llandysul: Gomer Press, 1996).
Davies, Rhys, *Collected Stories: Volume II*, edited by Meic Stephens (Llandysul: Gomer Press, 1996).
Dodds, Ruth, *The Pitman's Pay: A Historical Play in Four Acts* (London: The Labour Publishing Company, 1923).
Francis, J. O., *Change: A Glamorgan Play in Four Acts* (4th edn) (London and Cardiff: Samuel French, 1920 [1913]).
Gilmore, Hugh, *The Black Diamond* (London: Thomas Mitchell Primitive Methodist Publishing House, 1880).
Grant, J. C., *The Back-to-Backs* (London: Chatto and Windus, 1930).
Guthrie, Ramsay, *Kitty Fagan: A Romance of Pit Life* (London: Christian Commonwealth Publishing, 1900).
Guthrie, Ramsay, *Black Dyke* (London: Charles H. Kelly, 1904).
Hanlin, Tom, *Once in Every Lifetime* (New York: The Viking Press, 1945).
Hanlin, Tom, *Yesterday Will Return* (New York: The Viking Press, 1946).
Hanlin, Tom, *Miracle at Cardenrigg* (New York: Random House, 1949).
Heslop, Harold, *The Gate of a Strange Field* (London: Brentano, 1929).
Heslop, Harold, *Goaf* (London: The Fortune Press, 1934).
Heslop, Harold, *Last Cage Down* (London: Lawrence Wishart Books, 1984 [1935]).
Heslop, Harold, *The Earth Beneath* (London: T. V. Boardman, 1946).
Horner, Arthur, *Incorrigible Rebel* (London: McGibbon & Kee, 1960).
Hugh-Jones, Philip and C. M. Fletcher, *The Social Consequences of Pneumoconiosis among Coalminers in South Wales* (London: HMSO, 1951).
Hughes, T. Rowland, *William Jones* (Llandysul: Gwasg Gomer, 1991 [1944]).
Hughes, T. Rowland, trans. Richard Ruck, *William Jones* (Aberystwyth: Gwasg Aberystwyth, 1953).
Jones, Glyn, *The Collected Poems of Glyn Jones*, edited by Meic Stephens (Cardiff: University of Wales Press, 1996).

Jones, Glyn, *The Collected Stories of Glyn Jones*, edited by Tony Brown (Cardiff: University of Wales Press, 1999).
Jones, Gwyn, *Times Like These* (London: Victor Gollancz, 1979 [1936]).
Jones, Jack, *Rhondda Roundabout* (London: Hamish Hamilton, 1949 [1934]).
Jones, Jack, *Black Parade* (Cardigan: Parthian, 2009 [1935]).
Jones, Jack, *Unfinished Journey* (London: Hamish Hamilton, 1937).
Jones, Jack, *Bidden to the Feast* (London: Corgi Books, 1968 [1938]).
Jones, Lewis, *Cwmardy and We Live* (Cardigan: Parthian, 2006 [1937 and 1939]).
Keating, Joseph, *Son of Judith* (London: George Allen, 1900).
Keating, Joseph, *My Struggle for Life: With an Introduction by Paul O'Leary* (Dublin: University College Dublin Press, 2005 [1916]).
Lawson, Jack, *Under the Wheels* (London: Hodder & Stoughton, 1934).
Lawson, Jack, *A Man's Life*, Black Jacket edn (London: Hodder & Stoughton, 1944).
Lindsay, Harry, *Rhoda Roberts: A Welsh Mining Story* (London: Chatto and Windus, 1895).
Llewellyn, Richard, *How Green Was My Valley* (London: Penguin Books, 1991 [1939]).
Lloyd, Ellis, *Scarlet Nest* (London: Hodder and Stoughton, 1919).
McLeod, Robert, *Robert McLeod: Cowdenbeath Miner Poet, An Anthology by Arthur Nevay*, edited by Margaret Bennett (Fife: Grace Not Publications, 2015).
Medical Research Council, 'Chronic Pulmonary Disease in South Wales Coalminers', *Medical Studies*, 1942.
Miners' Welfare Commission, *Mining People* (London: HMSO, 1945).
Miners' Welfare Commission, *Miners' Welfare in War-Time: Report of the Miners' Welfare Commission for 6 ½ years to June 30th 1946* (London: HMSO, 1946).
Orwell, George, *The Road to Wigan Pier*, New Ed (London: Penguin Classics, 2001 [1937]).
Raine, Allen, *A Welsh Witch: A Romance of Rough Places* (London: Hutchinson & Co., 1902).
Rice, Margery Spring, *Working-Class Wives: Their Health and Conditions* (London: Virago, 1989 [1939]).
Rhys, Ernest, *Black Horse Pit* (London: Robert Holden, 1925).
Rosen, George, *The History of Miners' Diseases : A Medical and Social Interpretation* (New York: Schuman's, 1943).
Swan, John, *The Mad Miner* (London: Houghton, 1933).
Thomas, Gwyn, *The Dark Philosophers* (Cardigan: Parthian, 2006 [1946]).
Thomas, Gwyn, *Where Did I Put My Pity?* (London: Progress, 1946).
Thomas, Gwyn, *Sorrow for Thy Sons* (London: Lawrence and Wishart, 1986).
Thomson, Robert Tickell, *The Workmen's Compensation Act, 1897. A Plea for Revision* (London: Effingham Wilson, 1901).
Welsh, James C., *The Underworld: The Story of Robert Sinclair, Miner* (London: Herbert Jenkins, 1920).
Welsh, James C., *The King and the Miner: A Contrast* (London: ILP Publication Department, 1923).
Welsh, James C., *The Morlocks* (London: Herbert Jenkins, 1924).
Wilkinson, Ellen, *The Town that Was Murdered* (London: Victor Gollancz Ltd, 1939).

Williams, Emlyn, *The Corn is Green: A Comedy in Three Acts* (London: Heinemann, 1956 [1938]).
Williams, Enid M., *The Health of Old and Retired Miners in South Wales* (Cardiff: University of Wales Press Board, 1933).
Wilson, Arnold Talbot and Hermann Levy, *Workmen's Compensation* (London: Oxford University Press, 1939).

Online collections

The British Newspaper Archive, http://www.britishnewspaperarchive.co.uk/.
Hansard, 1803–2005, http://hansard.millbanksystems.com/.
The Statistical Accounts of Scotland, 1791–1845, http://edina.ac.uk//stat-acc-scot.
Turner, David, Steven Thompson, Kirsti Bohata, Vicky Long, Arthur McIvor, Mike Mantin, Daniel Blackie, Ben Curtis, Angela Turner, Victoria Brown, Alexandra Jones, Anne Borsay, Disability and Industrial Society, 1780–1948: A Comparative Cultural History of British Coalfields: Statistical Compendium, http://doi.org/10.5281/zenodo.183686.
UK Parliamentary Papers (Proquest), http://parlipapers.proquest.com/.
Welsh Newspapers Online, http://newspapers.library.wales/.

Secondary sources

Allen, V. L., *The Militancy of British Miners* (Shipley: Moor Press, 1981).
Bartrip, P. W. J., *Workmen's Compensation in Twentieth Century Britain* (Aldershot: Avebury, 1987).
Baynton, Douglas C., 'Disability and the Justification of Inequality in American History', in Paul K. Longmore and Lauri Umansky (eds), *The New Disability History: American Perspectives* (New York: New York University Press, 2001), pp. 33–57.
Benson, John, *British Coalminers in the Nineteenth Century: A Social History* (Dublin: Gill and Macmillan, 1980).
Benson, John, 'Coalminers, Coalowners and Collaboration: The Miners' Permanent Relief Fund Movement in England, 1860–1895', *Labour History Review*, 68:2 (2003), pp. 181–94.
Benson, John (ed.), *Coal in Victorian Britain* (London: Pickering & Chatto, 2012).
Berger, Stefan, 'Working-Class Culture and the Labour Movement in the South Wales and Ruhr Coalfields, 1850–2000: A Comparison', *Llafur*, 8:2 (2001), pp. 5–40.
Berger, Stefan, Andy Croll and Norman LaPorte (eds), *Towards a Comparative History of Coalfield Societies* (Aldershot: Ashgate, 2005).
Bloor, Michael, 'The South Wales Miners Federation, Miners' Lung and the Instrumental Use of Expertise, 1900–1950', *Social Studies of Science*, 30:1 (2000), pp. 125–40.
Bohata, Kirsti and Alexandra Jones, 'Welsh Women's Industrial Fiction 1880–1910', *Women's Writing* 24:4 (2014), pp. 499–516.

Borsay, Anne, 'Returning Patients to the Community: Disability, Medicine and Economic Rationality before the Industrial Revolution', *Disability and Society*, 13 (1998), pp. 645–63.

Borsay, Anne, *Disability and Social Policy in Britain since 1750: A History of Exclusion* (Basingstoke: Palgrave Macmillan, 2005).

Bourke, Joanna, *Working Class Cultures in Britain, 1890–1960: Gender, Class, and Ethnicity* (London: Routledge, 1994).

Bruley, Sue, *The Women and Men of 1926: A Gender and Social History of the General Strike and Miners' Lockout in South Wales* (Cardiff: University of Wales Press, 2010).

Bruley, Sue, 'The General Strike and Miners' Lockout of 1926 in South Wales: Oral Testimony and Public Representations', *Welsh History Review*, 26 (2012), pp. 271–96.

Bufton, Mark W. and Joseph Melling, '"A Mere Matter of Rock": Organized Labour, Scientific Evidence and British Government Schemes for Compensation of Silicosis and Pneumoconiosis among Coalminers, 1926–1940', *Medical History*, 49:2 (2005), pp. 155–78.

Bufton, Mark W. and Joseph Melling, 'Coming up for Air: Experts, Employers, and Workers in Campaigns to Compensate Silicosis Sufferers in Britain, 1918–1939', *Social History of Medicine*, 18:1 (2005), pp. 63–86.

Buxton, N. K., *The Economic Development of the British Coal Industry from Industrial Revolution to the Present Day* (London: Batsford Academic, 1978).

Campbell, Alan, *The Scottish Miners, 1874–1939* (Aldershot: Ashgate Publishing Limited, 2000).

Campbell, Alan, Nina Fishman and David Howell (eds), *Miners, Unions and Politics, 1910–47* (Aldershot: Scolar Press, 1996).

Carr, Griselda, *Pit Women: Coal Communities in Northern England in the Early Twentieth Century* (London: Merlin Press, 2001).

Church, Roy A., *The History of the British Coal Industry Volume 3: 1830–1913: Victorian Pre-Eminence* (Oxford: Clarendon Press, 1986).

Colls, Robert, *The Collier's Rant: Song and Culture in the Industrial Village* (London: Croom Helm, 1977).

Cooter, Roger, *Surgery and Society in Peace and War: Orthopaedics and the Organization of Modern Medicine, 1880–1948* (Basingstoke: Macmillan, 1993).

Cronin, Jenny, 'The Origins and Development of Scottish Convalescent Homes, 1860–1939' (unpublished doctoral thesis, Glasgow University, 2003).

Curtis, Ben, *The South Wales Miners: 1964–1985* (Cardiff: University of Wales Press, 2013).

Curtis, Ben and Steven Thompson, '"A Plentiful Crop of Cripples Made by All this Progress": Disability, Artificial Limbs and Working-Class Mutualism in the South Wales Coalfield, 1890–1948', *Social History of Medicine*, 27:4 (2014), pp. 708–27.

Curtis, Ben and Steven Thompson, '"This Is the Country of Premature Old Men": Ageing and Aged Miners in the South Wales Coalfield, c.1880–1947', *Cultural and Social History*, 12:4 (2015), pp. 587–606.

Daunton, M. J., 'Miners' Houses: South Wales and the Great Northern Coalfield, 1880–1914', *International Review of Social History*, 25:2 (1980), pp. 143–75.

Daunton, Martin, 'Down the Pit: Work in the Great Northern and South Wales Coalfields, 1870–1914', *Economic History Review*, 34:4 (1981), pp. 578–97.

Davies, Alan, A. J. Cronin: *The Man Who Created Dr Finlay* (London: Alma Books, 2011).

Dentith, Simon, 'Tone of Voice in Industrial Writing in the 1930s', in Gustav Klaus and Stephen Knight (eds), *British Industrial Fictions* (Cardiff: University of Wales Press, 2000), pp. 99–111.

Digby, Anne, *The Evolution of British General Practice, 1850–1948* (Oxford: Oxford University Press, 1999).

Dixon, Michael J., 'The Epic Rhondda: Romanticism and Realism in the Rhondda Trilogy', in Meic Stephens (ed.), *Rhys Davies: Decoding the Hare* (Cardiff: University of Wales Press, 2001), pp. 40–53.

Eiesland, Nancy, *The Disabled God: Toward a Liberatory Theology of Disability* (Nashville, TN: Abingdon Press, 1994).

Fagge, Roger, *Power, Culture and Conflict in the Coalfields: West Virginia and South Wales, 1900–1922* (Manchester: Manchester University Press, 1996).

Finkelstein, Victor, *Attitudes and Disabled People: Issues for Discussion* (New York: International Exchange of Information in Rehabilitation, 1980).

Fox, Pamela, *Class fictions: Shame and Resistance in the British Working-Class Novel, 1890–1945* (Durham, NC and London: Duke University Press, 1994).

Francis, Hywel and David Smith, *The Fed: A History of the South Wales Miners in the Twentieth Century* (London: Lawrence and Wishart, 1980).

Garland Thomson, Rosemarie, *Extraordinary Bodies: Figuring Physical Disability in American Culture and Literature* (New York: Columbia University Press, 1997).

Garside, W. R., *The Durham Miners, 1919–1960* (London: Allen & Unwin, 1971).

Gier-Viskovatoff, Jaclyn J. and Abigail Porter, 'Women of the British Coalfields on Strike in 1926 and 1984: Documenting Lives Using Oral History and Photography', *Frontiers: A Journal of Women Studies*, 19 (1998), pp. 199–230.

Gilbert, David, *Class, Community, and Collective Action: Social Change in Two British Coalfields, 1850–1926* (Oxford: Clarendon Press, 1992).

Gildart, Keith, 'Mining Memories: Reading Coalfield Autobiographies', *Labor History*, 50 (2009), pp. 139–61.

Gildart, Keith (ed.), *Coal in Victorian Britain, Part II: Coal in Victorian Society, Volume 6, Industrial Relations and Trade Unionism* (London: Pickering & Chatto, 2012).

Gleeson, B. J., 'Disability Studies: A Historical Materialist View', *Disability & Society*, 12:2 (1997), pp. 179–202.

Gleeson, Brendan, *Geographies of Disability* (London: Routledge, 2002).

Gooday, Graeme and Karen Sayer, *Managing the Experience of Hearing Loss in Britain, 1830–1930* (London: Palgrave Pivot, 2015).

Goodley, Dan and Geert Van Hove, 'Disability Studies, People with Learning Disabilities and Inclusion', in Goodley and Van Hove (eds) *Another Disability Studies Reader? People with Learning Difficulties and a Disabling World* (Antwerp: Garant, 2005), pp. 13–26.

Gramich, Katie, 'The Masquerade of Gender in the Stories of Rhys Davies', in Meic Stevens (ed.) *Rhys Davies: Decoding the Hare* (Cardiff: University of Wales Press, 2001), pp. 205–15.

Greasley, David, 'Fifty Years of Coal-Mining Productivity: The Record of the British Coal Industry before 1939', *Journal of Economic History*, 50:4, pp. 877–902.

Griffin, Emma, *A People's History of the Industrial Revolution* (New Haven & London: Yale University Press, 2013).

Hackett, Nan, *British Working-Class Autobiographies: An Annotated Bibliography* (New York: AMS Press, 1985).

Hall, Alice, *Literature and Disability* (London: Routledge, 2016).

Hall, Kim Q. (ed.), *Feminist Disability Studies* (Bloomington: Indiana University Press, 2011).

Hall, Valerie G., *Women at Work, 1860–1939: How Different Industries Shaped Women's Experiences* (Woodbridge: Boydell Press, 2013).

Harrison, Barbara, *Not Only the Dangerous Trades: Women's Work and Health in Britain 1880–1914* (London: Taylor & Francis, 2005).

Hayes, Jeanne and Elizbaeth "Lisa" M. Hannold, 'The Road to Empowerment: A Historical Perspective on the Medicalization of Disability', *Journal of Health and Human Services Administration*, 30:3 (2007), pp. 352–77.

Hinton, James, *Labour and Socialism: A History of the British Labour Movement, 1867–1974* (Brighton: Harvester Press, 1983).

Hopkins, Chris, *English Fiction in the 1930s* (London: Continuum, 2006).

Howard, William S., 'Miners' Autobiographies, 1790–1945: A Study of Life Accounts by English Miners and their Families' (unpublished doctoral thesis, Sunderland Polytechnic, 1991).

James, Leighton S., *The Politics of Identity and Civil Society in Britain and Germany: Miners in the Ruhr and South Wales 1890–1926* (Manchester: Manchester University Press, 2008).

Jameson, Fredric, *The Antinomies of Realism* (London and New York: Verso Books, 2015 [2013]).

John, Angela V., *By the Sweat of Their Brow: Women Workers at Victorian Coal Mines* (London: Croom Helm, 1980).

John, Angela V., 'Scratching the Surface. Women, Work and Coalmining History in England and Wales', *Oral History*, 10 (1982), pp. 13–26.

Jones, Alexandra, '"Her Body [was] Like a Hard-Worked Machine": Women's Work and Disability in Coalfields Literature, 1880–1950', *Disability Studies Quarterly*, 37:4 (2017), DOI: http://dx.doi.org/10.18061/dsq.v37i4.6103, n.p.

Jones, Bill and Chris Williams, *B. L. Coombes* (Cardiff: University of Wales Press, 1999).

Jones, Dot, 'Counting the Cost of Coal: Women's Lives in the Rhondda, 1881–1911', in Angela V. John (ed.), *Our Mothers' Land: Chapters in Welsh Women's History 1830–1939* (Cardiff: University of Wales Press, 1991), pp. 110–33.

Jones, Dot, 'Workmen's Compensation and the South Wales Miner, 1898–1914', *Bulletin of the Board of Celtic Studies*, 29:1 (1980), pp. 133–155.

Kirby, M. W., *The British Coalmining Industry, 1870–1946: A Political and Economic History* (London: Macmillan, 1977).
Klaus, H. Gustav (ed.), *The Socialist Novel in Britain: Towards the Recovery of a Tradition* (Brighton: The Harvester Press, 1982).
Klaus, H. Gustav, *The Literature of Labour: Two Hundred Years of Working-Class Writing* (Brighton: The Harvester Press, 1985).
Klaus, H. Gustav and Stephen Knight (eds), *British Industrial Fictions* (Cardiff, University of Wales Press, 2000).
Knight, Stephen, *A Hundred Years of Fiction: Writing Wales in English* (Cardiff: University of Wales Press, 2004).
Kudlick, Catherine J., 'Disability History: Why We Need Another "Other"', *The American Historical Review*, 108:3 (2003), pp. 763–93.
Kudlick, Catherine, 'Comment: On the Borderland of Medical and Disability History', *Bulletin of the History of Medicine*, 87:4 (2013), p. 540–99.
Lewis, Jane, 'Family Provision of Health and Welfare in the Mixed Economy of Care in the late Nineteenth and Twentieth Centuries', *Social History of Medicine*, 8:1 (1995), pp. 1–16.
Linett, Marven Tova, *Bodies of Modernism: Physical Disability in Transatlantic Modernist Literature* (Ann Arbor: University of Michigan Press, 2017).
Linker, Beth, 'On the Borderland of Medical and Disability History: A Survey of the Fields', *Bulletin of the History of Medicine*, 87:4 (2013), pp. 499–535.
Long, Vicky, *The Rise and Fall of the Healthy Factory: The Politics of Industrial Health in Britain, 1914–60* (Basingstoke: Palgrave Macmillan, 2011).
Longmore, Paul K. and Laurie Umansky (eds), *The New Disability History: American Perspectives* (New York: New York University Press), pp. 1–32.
Lord, Peter, *The Visual Culture of Wales: Industrial Society* (Cardiff: University of Wales, 1998).
Mantin, Mike, 'Coalmining and the National Scheme for Disabled Ex-Servicemen after the First World War', *Social History*, 41:2 (2016), pp. 155–70.
Marx, Karl, *Capital: The Process of Capitalist Production*, translated from the third German edition by S. Moore and B. Aveling (New York: International Publishers, 1967).
Marx, Karl, *Capital: A Critique of Political Economy*, Volume I, trans. Ben Fowkes (New York: Penguin, 1976).
McClintock, Anne, *Imperial Leather: Race, Gender, and Sexuality in Colonial Contest* (London: Routledge, 1995).
McIlroy, John, Alan Campbell and Keith Gildart (eds), *Industrial Politics and the 1926 Mining Lockout: The Struggle for Dignity* (Cardiff: University of Wales Press, 2004).
McIvor, Arthur, *A History of Work in Britain, 1880–1950* (Basingstoke: Palgrave, 2001).
McIvor, Arthur, 'Miners, Silica and Disability: The Bi-National Interplay between South Africa and the United Kingdom, c1900–1930s', *American Journal of Industrial Medicine*, 58 (2015), pp. 23–30.
McIvor, Arthur and Ronald Johnston, *Miners' Lung: A History of Dust Disease in British Coal Mining* (Aldershot: Ashgate, 2007).

Mercier, Laurie and Jaclyn Gier, 'Reconsidering Women and Gender in Mining', *History Compass*, 5 (2007), pp. 995–1001.

Meredith, Christopher, 'Cronin and the Chronotope: Place, Time and Pessimistic Individualism in *The Citadel*', *North American Journal of Welsh Studies*, 8 (2013), pp. 50–65.

Mitchell, David and Sharon Snyder, *Narrative Prosthesis: Disability and the Dependencies of Discourse* (Ann Arbor: University of Michigan Press, 2000).

Mitchell, David and Sharon Snyder, 'The Uneasy Home of Disability in Literature and Film', in Gary Albrecht, Katherine D. Seelman and Michael Bury (eds), *Handbook of Disability Studies* (London: Sage Publications, 2001), pp. 195–218.

Moore, Robert, *Pit-Men, Preachers and Politics: The Effects of Methodism in a Durham Mining Community* (Cambridge: Cambridge University Press, 1974).

Morgan, W. John, 'The Miners' Welfare Fund in Britain 1920–1952', *Social Policy & Administration*, 24:3 (1990), pp. 199–211.

O'Leary, Paul, *Immigration and Integration: The Irish in Wales, 1798–1922* (Cardiff: University of Wales Press, 2002).

O'Mahony, S., 'A. J. Cronin and *The Citadel*: Did a Work of Fiction Contribute to the Foundation of the NHS?', *Journal of the Royal College of Physicians of Edinburgh*, 42 (2012), pp. 172–8.

Oliver, Michael, *The Politics of Disablement: A Sociological Approach* (Basingstoke: Palgrave Macmillan, 1990).

Osborne, Huw, *Rhys Davies* (Cardiff: University of Wales Press, 2009).

Powell, Martin A., 'How Adequate was Hospital Provision before the NHS? An Examination of the 1945 South Wales Hospital Survey', *Local Population Studies*, 48 (1992), pp. 22–32.

Powell, Martin A., 'Coasts and Coalfields: The Geographical Distribution of Doctors in England and Wales in the 1930s', *Social History of Medicine*, 18:2 (2005), pp. 245–63.

Prys-Williams, Barbara, *Twentieth-Century Autobiography* (Cardiff: University of Wales Press, 2004).

Quayson, Ato, *Aesthetic Nervousness: Disability and the Crisis of Representation* (New York: Columbia University Press, 2007).

Reiss, Mathias, 'Forgotten Pioneers of the National Protest March: The National League of the Blind's Marches to London, 1920 and 1936', *Labour History Review*, 70:2 (2005), pp. 133–65.

Rose, Sarah F., *No Right to be Idle: The Invention of Disability, 1840s–1930s* (Chapel Hill: University of North Carolina Press, 2017).

Scott, Gillian, *Feminism and the Politics of Working Women: The Women's Co-operative Guild, 1880s to the Second World War* (London: UCL Press, 1998).

Shakespeare, Tom, 'The Sexual Politics of Disabled Masculinity', *Sexuality and Disability*, 17:1 (1999), pp. 53–64.

Shakespeare, Tom, 'The Social Model of Disability', in Lennard J. Davis (ed.), *The Disability Studies Reader*, 5th edn (New York and London: Routledge, 2017), pp. 195–203.

Sheppard, Lisa and Aidan Byrne, 'A Critical Minefield: The Haunting of the Welsh Working Class Novel', in John Goodridge and Bridget Keenan (eds), *A History of British Working Class Literature* (Cambridge: Cambridge University Press, 2017), pp. 367–84.

Siebers, Tobin, 'Disability in Theory: From Social Constructionism to the New Realism of the Body', in Lennard J. Davis (ed.), *The Disability Studies Reader*, 2nd edn (New York and London: Routledge, 2006), pp. 173–83.

Siebers, Tobin, *Disability Aesthetics: The Aesthetics of Human Disqualification* (Ann Arbor: University of Michigan Press, 2010).

Slavishak, Edward, *Bodies of Work: Civic Display and Labor in Industrial Pittsburgh* (Durham, NC: Duke University Press, 2008).

Smith, Dai, 'A Novel History', in Tony Curtis (ed.), *Wales: The Imagined Nation, Essays in Cultural and National Identity* (Bridgend: Poetry Wales Press, 1986), pp. 129–58.

Smith, Dai, *Aneurin Bevan and the World of South Wales* (Cardiff: University of Wales Press, 1993).

Stone, Deborah, *The Disabled State* (Basingstoke: Macmillan, 1985).

Sturdy, Steve, 'The Industrial Body', in John V. Pickstone and Roger Cooter (eds), *Companion to Medicine in the Twentieth Century* (London: Routledge, 2003), pp. 217–34.

Supple, Barry, *The History of the British Coal Industry Volume 4: 1913–1946: The Political Economy of Decline* (Oxford: Clarendon, 1987).

Thomas, Helen, '"Democracy of Working Women": The Women's Co-operative Guild in South Wales, 1891–1939', *Llafur*, 11:1 (2012), pp. 149–169.

Thomas, M. Wynn, *Transatlantic Connections: Whitman U.S., Whitman U.K.* (Iowa City: Iowa University Press, 2005).

Thomas, M. Wynn, *In the Shadow of the Pulpit: Literature and Nonconformist Wales* (Cardiff: University of Wales Press, 2011).

Thompson, Steven, 'Varieties of Voluntarism in the South Wales Coalfield, circa 1880–1948', in Colin Rochester, George Campbell Gosling, Alison Penn and Meta Zimmeck (eds), *Understanding the Roots of Voluntary Action: Historical Perspectives on Current Social Policy* (Brighton: Sussex Academic Press, 2011), pp. 82–94.

Thompson, Steven, 'The Friendly and Welfare Provision of British Trade Unions: A Case Study of the South Wales Miners' Federation', *Labour History Review*, 77 (2012), pp. 189–210.

Thompson, Steven, 'The Mixed Economy of Care in the South Wales Coalfield, c.1850–1950', in Donnacha Seán Lucey and Virginia Crossman (eds), *Healthcare in Ireland and Britain from 1850: Voluntary, Regional and Comparative Perspectives* (London: Institute of Historical Research, 2015), pp. 141–60.

Turner, Angela and Arthur McIvor, '"Bottom Dog Men" : Disability, Social Welfare and Advocacy in the Scottish Coalfields in the Interwar Years, 1918–1939', *Scottish Historical Review*, 96:2 (2017), pp. 187–213.

Turner, David M., '"Fraudulent" Disability in Historical Perspective', *History and Policy* (2012), http://www.historyandpolicy.org/papers/policy-paper-130.html, accessed 5 January 2013.

Turner, David M. and Daniel Blackie, *Disability in the Industrial Revolution: Physical Impairment in British Coalmining, 1780–1880* (Manchester: Manchester University Press, 2018).

Vicinus, Martha, *The Industrial Muse: A Study of Nineteenth Century British Working-Class Literature* (London: Croom Helm, 1974).

Wainwright, Laura, *New Territories in Modernism: Anglophone Welsh Writing, 1930–1949* (Cardiff: University of Wales Press, 2018).

Weindling, Paul (ed.), *The Social History of Occupational Health* (London: Croom Helm, 1985).

Wendell, Susan, *The Rejected Body* (New York and London: Routledge, 1996).

White, Carol and Sian Rhiannon Williams (eds), *Struggle or Starve: Women's Lives in the South Wales Valleys between the Two World Wars* (Dinas Powys: Honno, 1998).

Williams, Daniel G., *Black Skin, Blue Books: African Americans and Wales, 1845–1945* (Cardiff: University of Wales Press, 2012).

Williams, Raymond, *Who Speaks for Wales? Nation, Culture, Identity*, edited by Daniel G. Williams (Cardiff: University of Wales Press, 2003).

Wilson, Nicola, *Home in British Woking-Class Fiction* (Farnham: Ashgate, 2015).

Index

accidents
  fatal 34–5
  non-fatal 1–4, 24, 34–5, 41, 80, 100, 167, 220, 249
  time of day 29
  rates of 51, 113–14
  see also compensation
age 45, 50, 52, 53, 68, 88, 116, 117, 148–9, 157, 165, 172, 205, 216–17, 238, 252
  premature aging 27, 38, 162, 217, 218–20
Alexander, David 'Dai' 245
  'Hangman's Assistant' 224–5
amputation 35, 43, 74–5, 77, 80, 118, 129, 159, 165, 222
Andrews, Elizabeth 30, 33, 65, 117, 182, 200
  A Woman's Work is Never Done 117, 200
Armstrong, Thomas 'Tommy' 55, 160
arthritis 4, 116
  see also rheumatism

Barnett, Henry Norman 41, 128
baths
  in the home 32–3
  pithead 32–3, 183, 200–1
Baynton, Douglas C. 3–4
'beat' diseases 4, 26, 35–7, 73, 122, 124
begging 129, 159, 116, 232
Benson, John 27, 113, 115, 120, 170, 181, 204, 206
Blackie, Daniel 5, 7
blindness 41, 44, 81, 109, 119, 133, 159, 160, 164, 165, 226, 228–9, 250, 254
  see also eyes and eyesight
British Deaf-Mute 76
bonesetters 86

Borsay, Anne 6, 116
British Medical Association 70
Bruley, Sue 6
Burt, Thomas 196

Campbell, Alan 161, 180
Campbell, George L. 114
Campbell, Dame Janet M. 38
capitalism 106, 192, 211, 216–17, 220, 240, 249, 250
care and carers 7, 12, 236, 237
  convalescent homes 87–8
  in the home 109, 143–5, 154–8, 171, 220
  male carers 145–6, 171
  on marches 229, 235–6
  professional healthcare 70–5, 78–80, 87, 90, 93
  as solidarity 237–8
  see also interdependence
Carr, Griselda 6, 143, 154, 156
Chaplin, Sid 213, 223, 225–6, 245
  The Leaping Lad and Other Stories 128, 226
  The Thin Seam 25–6, 227
charity 81, 87–8, 105, 108–10, 116–17, 167–8, 229, 250
childbirth 33, 38–40, 94, 209
children 31, 39, 40, 70, 71, 94, 118, 119, 144, 148–50, 151–2
  child welfare 183, 199–200, 210
  disabled 87, 144, 167, 168, 227–8, 233–6
  employment of 19–20, 23–4, 30, 149, 218
Citrine, Walter 197
coal companies
  Ashington Coal Company 61, 79
  Blaenclydach Colliery Company 1

coal companies (cont.)
    Consett Iron Company 45
    Dowlais Iron Company 85
    Duffryn Coal Company 186
    Ebbw Vale Steel, Iron and Coal
        Company 46
    Fife Coal Company 77, 126
    Ocean Coal Company 44, 109, 200
    Tredegar Iron and Coal Company 119
coal industry 189, 249
    growth and decline 19–20, 46
    historiography 5
    nationalisation 12, 18, 53, 63, 69, 92,
        93, 181, 197, 201, 250, 251
    as place of employment for disabled
        people 40–54, 250, 251
coalfields
    Ayrshire 20
    Clackmannan 20
    communities 7, 42, 64, 108, 141, 153,
        182, 219, 223, 228, 249, 251,
        254
    Dunbartonshire 20
    Durham 29, 35, 71, 123, 223
    Fife 20, 29, 31, 163
    geological differences between 22, 35
    Great Northern (north-east England)
        19
    Lanarkshire 20, 24, 49, 79, 86
    Lancashire 8
    Lothians 20
    north-east of England 7–8, 19, 20, 45,
        79, 113, 115, 125, 156, 166, 167,
        180, 187, 188, 227
    north Wales 8
    Northumberland 29, 35, 71, 180
    Renfrewshire 20
    Scotland 20, 79, 188
    Scottish coalfields 7–8, 20, 30–1, 71,
        79, 142, 180
    south Wales 7–8, 19–20, 31, 51, 70,
        82–3, 115, 123, 155, 182, 188,
        213, 227
    Staffordshire 8
    Stirling 20
    variations in employment practices
        between 22, 26, 28–9
    Yorkshire 8, 112
coalminers
    body of 66–9
        bow legs 67, 220
        homoeroticism 246
        strength 22, 67–8, 90, 144, 146–7,
            185, 233–4
        see also disability
    as Christ 226–7, 246
    as a "race" apart 67
    as writers 7, 16, 21–2, 28, 31, 214,
        250
coalmining
    and mechanisation 4, 23, 24–6, 38,
        48, 220
coalmining communities see mining
    communities
coalmining occupations 22–4
    bottomer 22–3, 219, 243
    hewing 22, 23, 27, 37–8, 147, 216,
        218
    hierarchy of occupations 22–4, 87,
        146–7, 251
    'light work' 30, 42–6, 47, 48, 49, 51,
        53, 61, 89, 90, 92, 119, 127, 186,
        188–9, 190, 194–5, 206, 219,
        224–5, 251
    putting 22, 23, 41
    surface work 4, 23, 36, 40, 42, 46–9,
        52, 53, 59, 99, 191, 251
class struggle 2, 5, 181, 235–6, 240
collieries
    Blaenclydach 1
    Caerau 191
    Chopwell 45
    Dechmont 120
    Gelli 53
    Hartley 112
    Harton 203
    Hetton 43
    Houghton 127

Kinneil 150, 153
Markham 119
Colliery Guardian 29, 44, 85, 131
compensation 1–2, 40–1, 50, 53, 108, 121–32, 179, 181, 183–202, 251–3
  and 'light work' 42–54
  and occupational disease 36–7, 82
  and poor relief 119
  and union recruitment 151–2
  see also legislation
convalescence 66, 74, 80, 87–8, 150, 156–7, 186, 250
  Ayrshire District Miners' Convalescent Home, Kirkmichael 88
  North Eastern Counties Friendly Societies Convalescent Home 111
  The Rest Convalescent Home, Porthcawl 87
  Schaw Auxiliary Home, Glasgow 80
  Talygarn Rehabilitation Centre 88, 89
Coombes, B. L. (Bert) 25, 28, 36, 44, 73, 74, 125, 130, 161, 162, 164, 169, 171, 184, 193, 213, 214
  These Poor Hands 25, 138, 214, 237
Corrie, Joe 21, 130, 213, 237
  Black Earth 145, 148, 154
Cronin, A.J. 35, 96, 124, 214, 242
  Adventures in Two Worlds 70
  The Citadel 35, 70–1, 73, 124, 213, 241
  The Stars Look Down 59
cross-dressing 220, 222
crushing 25, 35, 44, 74, 80, 166, 222, 226
Curtis, Ben 219

Davies, Idris 21, 213, 227
  Gwalia Deserta 232
Davies, Rhys 213, 241
  'The Benefit Concert' 75, 167, 237
  Jubilee Blues 128, 165, 229

My Wales 247
'Nightgown' 220
'The Pits are on the Top' 138
A Time to Laugh 70
The Withered Root 99
Davis, Lennard 9, 218, 220, 236–7
Deaf Chronicle 76
deafness and hearing loss 41, 76, 109, 164, 221
  and hearing aids 76
Dentith, Simon 222
disability
  aesthetics 10, 234, 236, 240
  and art 10, 225, 227, 234, 246
  as disqualification 153, 173, 216, 217, 218, 234
  and ethnicity 7, 141
  humour 5, 160–1, 168, 214, 221–3, 224–5, 240, 244
  and life course 211, 216–21
  and marriage 153–5, 173
  medical model of 5, 65–6, 72, 78, 93–4, 253
  and medicalisation 64–94
  and modernism 223–6, 250
  and neglect in labour history 5, 65–6, 217
  and neglect in literary criticism 212, 240
  'overcoming' 1–2, 41, 90, 213, 227–8
  and realism 214–17, 223, 238, 240, 250
  as site of struggle 3, 13, 239–40, 248
  social model of 5, 65–6, 141–2, 215, 236–7
  as tragedy 2, 5, 129, 132, 147, 172, 227–8
disabled people
  and authorship 8, 11, 68, 117, 157–8, 175, 222
  and historical records 3, 8–10, 147–8, 166, 168
disasters, mining 4, 34–5, 59, 66, 112–13, 160, 166, 249

doctors 1, 38, 66, 69–73, 75–6, 77, 78, 94, 97, 124, 126, 130, 156, 184, 228
  company 31, 53, 69, 93, 189, 191
  quack 76
  see also compensation
Dodds, Ruth 213, 241
Dűckershoff, Ernst 159, 163, 167, 169
  How the English Workman Lives 159
Durham 19, 26, 29, 32, 34, 35, 39–40, 43, 45, 50, 59, 71, 75, 79, 84–5, 90, 108, 110, 111, 112, 113, 114, 116, 118, 120, 122, 123, 124, 127–8, 147, 155, 172, 179, 180, 181, 186, 187, 188, 189, 206, 221, 223, 225, 244, 245

Eiesland, Nancy 227
employers 40–1, 45, 48, 49, 82, 88–9, 185–6
  and compensation legislation 121–31, 184, 186, 188–91, 194–5, 251–3
  Mining Association of Great Britain 181
  Northumberland Coal Owners' Mutual Protections Association 125
  and the permanent provident fund movement 112–13
  Scottish Mine Owners' Defence and Mutual Insurance Association 79
Eos Wyn *see* Young, Edward
explosions 4, 24, 35, 43, 59, 113
eyes and eyesight 40, 41, 64, 80–1, 128
  injury to 44, 164
  miners' nystagmus 4, 36, 42, 47, 48–50, 72, 73, 80, 81, 83–5, 86–7, 93, 102, 119, 122, 124, 127–8, 184, 191, 198, 214
  symbolism 112, 219, 238
  see also blindness

family 143–53
  daughters 144, 149–50, 172
  role in social welfare 106, 131–2
  sons 144, 148–50, 172
  fate and fatalism 225
Finkelstein, Victor 6
Fletcher, C. M. 73
Foucault, Michel 104
Francis, J. O. 213
friendly societies 69–70, 71, 74, 75, 87, 89, 105, 110–15, 120, 131, 151–2, 158, 250

Garland Thomson, Rosemarie 9, 160–1, 218
gender 5, 141, 143–6, 147, 149–50, 152–3, 154, 163, 218, 239, 240
  see also masculinity
Gilmore, Hugh 55, 176
  The Black Diamond 116, 166
Gleeson, Brendan 11, 140–1, 155, 158, 162, 170, 217, 252
Goodley, Dan 221
Grant, J. C.
  The Back-to-Backs 161, 171, 173
Guthrie, Ramsay 55
  Black Dyke 99, 145
  Kitty Fagan 99, 221

Hanlin, Tom 117, 176, 213
  Miracle at Cardenrigg 59
  Once in Every Lifetime 117
  Yesterday Will Return 23–4, 68, 173
Hardie, Keir 27, 112, 247
Haslett, Moyra 216
healers, unorthodox 85–6
  see also bonesetters
hernia 4, 80
Heslop, Harold 21, 35, 59, 116, 172, 179, 203, 213, 214, 242
  The Earth Beneath 99, 112, 147, 246
  The Gate of a Strange Field 67–8, 116, 213

INDEX

Goaf 214, 242
Last Cage Down 35, 187–8, 193
Pod vlastu uglya 214
home 174
  as a liminal space 155–8
  and social relations 140, 141, 142–55, 170
  as a woman's workplace 30, 32–3, 243
hospitals 78–81
  accident cases 80
  Ashington Hospital 79
  Bath Mineral Hospital 75
  Blantyre Cottage Hospital 79
  Bristol Eye Hospital 75
  Bristol Royal Infirmary 75
  cottage 75, 78, 79
  and disabled people 66, 78
  Edinburgh Royal Infirmary 75
  Ellison Hall Infirmary 79
  Glasgow Ophthalmic Hospital 81
  Glasgow Royal Infirmary 80
  Horden Cottage Hospital 79
  Manchester Royal Infirmary 89
  miners' 79
  and occupational disease 80
  pattern of provision 78–9
  Randolph Wemyss Memorial Hospital 79
  Royal Infirmary, Glasgow 89
  Royal Victorian Infirmary, Newcastle 80
  Sheffield Royal Infirmary 89
  Sunderland Royal Infirmary 79, 80
  voluntary 75, 78
  Western Infirmary, Glasgow 89
  and workers' influence 80
housing 30–3, 40, 57, 142–3, 161, 183
Hughes, T. Rowland 132–3
  William Jones 107, 124

industrial relations 2, 5, 12–13, 42, 45, 46, 51, 142, 179–95, 215, 249–50
  strikes 194–5
    General Strike 1926 116, 167, 180

    lockout (1921) 194
    lockout (1926) 116, 192, 195
interdependence 142, 155, 228, 235, 236–40
Ireland and Irish 7, 166, 225
  see also religion, Catholicism

Jameson, Fredric 216
John, Angela 6, 46
Jones, Glyn 213, 241, 246
  'The Kiss' 226, 227
Jones, Gwyn 213, 241
  Times Like These 185, 220
Jones, Jack 21, 31, 74, 179, 203, 213, 214
  Bidden to the Feast 99, 145
  Black Parade 59, 74, 99, 165
  Rhondda Roundabout 21
  Unfinished Journey 21, 145
Jones, Lewis 21, 25, 179, 195, 203, 213, 215–17, 228, 238
  Cwmardy 25, 59, 68, 193, 195–6, 211, 215, 216–17, 218, 219
  We Live 68, 196, 217, 218, 238–9

Kafka, Franz 224
Keating, Joseph 176, 179
  Son of Judith 59

The Labour Leader 231, 247
lameness and limping 111, 129, 130, 153, 160, 224–6, 233, 235–6
Lawley, D. B. 228
Lawson, Jack 50, 179, 183, 213
  A Man's Life 187
  Under the Wheels 50, 183
Legge, Sir Thomas 197
legislation
  Blind Persons Act (1920) 109
  Coal Mines Act (1911) 29, 247
  Disabled Persons (Employment) Act (1944) 89, 201
  Employers' Liability Act (1880) 40, 105, 121–31, 198

legislation (cont.)
  Industrial Injuries Act (1946) 69,
    105, 122, 129, 131, 201
  Local Government Act (1929) 117
  Maternity and Child Welfare Act
    (1918) 200
  Mines Regulation Act (1908) 28
  Mining Industry Act (1920) 163–4
  National Insurance (Industrial
    Injuries) Act (1946) 131, 201
  Pneumoconiosis etc (Workmen's
    Compensation) Act (1979)
    101
  Poor Law Amendment Act (1834)
    110, 115–16
  Poor Law Amendment (Scotland)
    Act (1845) 135
  Workmen's Compensation Act
    (1897) 40–2, 45, 48, 105, 115,
    121–31, 189, 199
  Workmen's Compensation Act
    (1906) 84, 128
    Amendment (1923) 188, 189
  Workmen's Compensation (Silicosis)
    Act (1918) 82
leisure 163–9
Levy, Hermann 129
Lindsay, Harry 55, 176
  Rhoda Roberts 59, 112, 166
literature
  and authenticity 214, 215, 217, 223,
    225
  autobiography 4, 7, 6, 9, 16, 21, 70,
    72, 124, 145, 146, 169, 187, 205,
    211, 214
  ballads 3, 9, 21, 29, 159–61, 244
  drama 112, 128, 211, 213, 240, 241
  folk tale 223, 225, 226
  as historical source 9–10, 212
  industrial novel, the 212–15, 234
  and methodology 9–11, 211–12,
    223
  modernism 9, 214, 223–6, 227, 240,
    245
  and oral culture 223, 225–6
  poetry 9, 21, 175, 211, 227, 232
  realism 9, 23, 106, 214–17, 218, 223,
    225, 227, 237, 238, 240, 243,
    250
  romance 9, 173, 221, 227
  working-class 3, 5, 21, 212–14, 216,
    222–3, 242
Llewellyn, Richard 214, 242
  How Green Was My Valley 177,
    213–14, 227, 234
Llewellyn, T. Lister 36, 102
Lloyd, Ellis
  Scarlet Nest 167
Lukács, Georg 216
lung diseases 79, 81–3, 84, 85, 93, 239,
    254
  asthma and 'miners' asthma' 37, 43,
    47, 119
  dust 24–5, 37–8, 52, 60, 73, 81–2,
    124, 214, 217, 219, 230–1,
    242
  'miners' consumption' 82
  'miners' lung' 4, 37
  pneumoconiosis 4, 28, 37–8, 51–2,
    60, 81–3, 87, 101, 122, 144, 145,
    148, 158, 161–2, 164, 171, 199,
    230–1, 252
  silicosis 24–5, 37, 43, 50, 74, 81–2,
    101, 107, 122, 124, 162, 186,
    224–5
  see also tuberculosis

MacDonald, Alexander 196
McLeod, Robert 'Bob' 222
  'Takkin a Rest' 222
malingering 1–2, 71, 111–12, 113,
    119–20, 124, 132, 158, 222
marches and processions 157, 161, 193,
    227, 228–39, 247
  allegorical 231–2
  and health 229, 247
  Jarrow March (1936) 229
  National League of the Blind 228–9

marriage 40, 153, 154, 173, 218
Marx, Karl 217, 240
masculinity 141–2, 146–7, 148, 150–2, 154, 157, 215, 218, 238–9
Means Test 21, 233
medical aid societies 70–1, 76–7
   Ebbw Vale Workmen's Medical Society 74, 76
   Tredegar Workmen's Medical Aid Society 70, 76, 77, 93, 96
mental health 94
mental impairment 217
Merthyr Tydfil 50, 122, 203
Middlesbrough 79
Miners' Welfare Fund 32, 88, 89, 90, 102, 163, 201
mining communities 4, 5, 66, 81, 107, 109, 115, 132, 141, 142, 145, 146, 159, 161, 163, 165, 169, 170, 199, 213, 241, 249–50, 253, 254
Mitchell, David T. 10, 215, 216, 235, 239–40, 247, 248
monstrosity 211, 217
mothers 30, 32–3, 38–40, 108, 144, 145, 149, 153, 165, 195, 200–1, 218, 219, 226, 238, 241, 253
   see also women
mutualism 77–8, 93, 108, 109, 110–12, 151, 217, 228, 231, 237, 240, 250
   'lifts' 107, 164–5, 237, 248

National Coal Board 52–3, 93, 201, 251
National Health Service 12, 69, 70, 92, 93, 213
National League of the Blind of Great Britain and Ireland 109, 228–9, 246, 254
National Unemployed Workers Movement 203, 229, 242
Newcastle-upon-Tyne 79, 80, 167, 176
normalcy 5, 42, 65, 78, 98, 217–21, 250
normate 218, 221

occupational health 5, 37, 81, 93, 197, 209
oral history 4, 155, 169
orthopaedics 12, 35, 74, 76, 81, 86, 87–92
Orwell, George 67

pain 39, 40, 58, 66, 85, 147, 156, 211, 215, 227–8
paralysis 58, 116, 119, 144, 145, 146, 148, 154, 158, 167, 171, 173, 175, 211, 237
paternalism 51, 78, 106, 109, 116, 163, 183, 205, 236
permanent relief funds 112–15
   contracting out 122
   Monmouthshire and South Wales Permanent Provident Society 113
   Northumberland and Durham Permanent Relief Fund 112, 113, 114, 122
Phillips, Marion 182
pit poetry 9
   see also miners as writers
pitmatic 9, 242
Poor Law 105, 110, 115–21, 125, 131, 132, 148–9, 155, 252
   medical services 119
   Scotland 149
prosthetics 75–8, 167, 237, 244, 250
publishing 21, 156, 166, 213–14, 240

Quayson, Ato 10, 11, 212, 224

Raine, Allen 82
   A Welsh Witch 59
rehabilitation 12, 87–92
   Berry Hill Hall Miners' Rehabilitation Centre 88, 90
   and convalescent homes 87–92
   Durham Miners' Rehabilitation Centre 90

rehabilitation (cont.)
  Inter-Departmental Committee on the Rehabilitation of Persons Injured by Accidents 89
  and orthopaedics 87
  Talygarn Rehabilitation Centre 88, 89
  Uddingston Rehabilitation Centre 88, 92
religion
  alter Christus 227
  Catholicism 166, 176
  and disability 167
  Eucharist 167, 226, 227
  nonconformity 75, 96, 147, 156, 161, 166–8, 193, 227–8, 237
    Calvinist 55, 166
    Congregationalist 166
    Presbyterian 166, 167
    Primitive Methodists 55, 116, 166, 176
  resurrection 226
  and socialism 167–8, 227
  stigmata 226, 227
  see also coalminers as Christ
rheumatism 4, 40, 118, 119, 120, 153, 199
Rhondda 1–3, 32, 33, 38, 43, 50, 52, 109, 142, 163, 178, 186, 190, 193, 194, 200, 209, 223, 232, 234
Rhys, Ernest 85, 244
  Black Horse Pit 85, 94
Rice, Margery Spring 39
Roberts, Judge Bryn 1–2
Royal Commissions
  Coal Industry Commission (Sankey Commission) (1919) 33, 34, 95, 130, 200, 201
  on the Coal Industry (1925) 24
  on the Housing of the Industrial Population of Scotland (1917) 57
  on Labour (1892) 27
  on Workmen's Compensation (1945) 122

Saunderson, Irene
  A Welsh Heroine 99, 247
Siebers, Toibin 9, 215, 234, 243, 247
Skipsey, Joseph 9, 16, 55
smart money 113, 125
Snyder, Sharon L. 10, 215, 216, 235, 239–40, 247, 248
Soviet Union 214
Stanton, Charles Butt 2
strain injuries 4, 33, 34, 37, 42, 84, 217, 220
Swan, John 26–7, 179, 195, 203, 213
  The Mad Miner 26–7

'temporarily able-bodied' 221
Thomas, Gwyn 8, 128, 168, 213, 222–3, 227, 287, 233–6
  'Oscar' 139
  Sorrow for Thy Sons 168, 233–6
Tonypandy 1
  'Riots' 211
trade unions 130, 180–1, 183–5, 186–95, 250, 252, 253
  Durham Miners' Association 71, 75, 123, 127, 186, 188, 189, 195, 245
  Fife and Kinross Miners' Association 191, 192
  membership 180–1
  Mid and East Lothian Miners' Association 75
  Miners' Federation of Great Britain 47–8, 181, 184, 188, 196–8, 199, 200
  National Union of Miners 52–3, 82–3, 230–1
  South Wales Miners' Federation 1, 51, 109, 151, 180, 184, 187, 190, 193, 194–5, 199, 250
  Trades Union Congress 184, 196–8

tuberculosis 124, 143, 235, 238
Turner, David 5, 7, 116

undisciplined body 233, 235
unemployment 20, 21–2, 48–51, 52, 53, 77, 116, 150, 168, 172, 179, 195, 217, 218, 232–4, 235, 238, 243

van Hove, Geert 221

wages and earnings 26–8, 31, 33, 41, 42, 44, 68, 109, 125–6, 131, 148, 150, 168, 183, 188, 189, 190, 194, 195, 198, 203, 217, 223, 250, 253, 254
   piece rates 26–8, 251
   sliding scale 180–1, 203
Watts Morgan, Dai 1, 178–9, 193
welfare 105–32, 159, 199–201
   mixed economy of 12, 106, 120, 125
Welsh, James C. 31, 117, 179, 213
   The King and the Miner 31
   The Morlocks 67, 99, 219
   The Underworld 59, 67, 107, 219, 237
Welsh language 4, 9, 16, 55, 67, 107, 132–3, 156–7, 166, 216, 235, 243
Wilkinson, Ellen 229
Williams, Emlyn 213
   The Corn is Green 219
Williams, Enid M. 38, 162
Williams, Raymond 212–13, 214–15, 244
Wilson, Arnold Talbot 129

women
   campaigns 30, 32–3, 144, 182–3, 199–201, 210, 238, 253
   as dependents 149
   and disability 32–3, 38–9, 58, 71, 76, 141, 141–2, 154–5, 218, 219–21
   and domestic work 6–7, 12, 30–4, 57, 108, 132, 141, 143–6, 148, 154–5, 163, 169, 243
   healers 156
   and leisure 163–4, 168–9
   maternity 38–40, 183, 199–201, 210, 253
   paid employment 23, 46, 149–50
   as storytellers and writers 17, 213, 226, 241
   Women's Co-operative Guild 182–3, 199–200
   Women's Labour League 182, 199, 200
   see also care and carers; childbirth; gender; mothers
workhouse 65, 110, 115–16, 118, 119, 155, 229, 251
working hours 27–30, 33, 68
   absenteeism 27–8, 74, 145
   shifts 28–9, 30, 33–4, 99, 107, 145
World War I 4, 17, 18, 19–20, 21, 26, 28, 42, 46–8, 77, 85, 87, 88, 108, 180, 190, 196, 199
World War II 12, 28, 51, 84, 201

Young, Edward (Eos Wyn) 156–7, 174

Zweig, Ferdynand 67, 159, 162, 169

EU authorised representative for GPSR:
Easy Access System Europe, Mustamäe tee 50,
10621 Tallinn, Estonia
gpsr.requests@easproject.com